WHAT TO EXPECT WHEN YOU'RE EXPECTING

WHAT TO EXPECT WHEN YOU'RE EXPECTING

Arlene Eisenberg
Heidi Eisenberg Murkoff
Sandee Eisenberg Hathaway, R.N.

Foreword by Caroline Flint S.R.N., S.C.M.
And a word from Dr. Richard Aubry,
Director of Obstetrics, Upstate Medical Centre,
Syracuse, New York

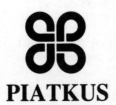

PIATKUS

To Emma, who inspired this book while still in the womb, who did her best to keep us from writing it once she was out, and who, we trust, will put it to good use one day.

To Howard, Erik, and Tim, without whom this book would not have been possible – in more ways than one.

First published in Great Britain 1986 by
Judy Piatkus (Publishers) Ltd., London

British Library Cataloguing in Publication Data

Eisenberg, Arlene
What to expect when you're expecting.
1. Pregnancy   2. Childbirth
I. Title   II. Murkoff, Heidi Eisenberg
III. Hathaway, Sandee Eisenberg
618.2'00240431   RG525

ISBN 0–86188–541–4
ISBN 0–86188–546–5 Pbk

Book Design: Sue Ryall
Text anglicized by Sue Stone

Printed and bound in Great Britain by Mackays of Chatham, Ltd
Typeset by Phoenix Photosetting, Chatham, Kent

Acknowledgements

Books and babies have a lot in common. Both take plenty of time, hard work, dedication, and care (not to mention a healthy dose of worry) to turn out the best possible product. Both also require the cooperation of a team of concerned people. We've been lucky to have a fine team involved in the creation of our book, all of whom we gratefully thank:

Elise and Arnold Goodman, our agents, for their confidence, advice, support, and friendship.

Suzanne Rafer, our editor at Workman, for her perceptive suggestions, her patience, her sense of humour (she needed it), and her endless capacity for what sometimes seemed endless work.

Ann Appelbaum (who read our chapters-in-progress during her pregnancy-in-progress and insists that credit for her beautiful end product, Abby, goes at least partially to the Best-Odds Diet), for her practical and thoughtful suggestions, particularly on the caesarean section material. Beth Falk, another encouraging reader whose nine months paralleled ours. And the hundreds of expectant parents who shared their concerns with us.

Richard Aubry, M. D., Professor of Obstetrics and Gynaecology and Director of the Division of Obstetrics: Maternal-Foetal Medicine at The Upstate Medical Center (Syracuse, NY), and Henry Eisenberg, M.D., Assistant Clinical Professor at Upstate, who reviewed the book, for their invaluable critiques, suggestions, and fact-checking. We feel privileged to have worked with two such remarkable physicians.

Howard Eisenberg, husband and father, who understood the importance of the father in pregnancy and childrearing long before it was the vogue, who taught all of us all we know about writing, and who gave us unfailing support and counsel every step of the way.

Erik Murkoff, whose worries during Heidi's pregnancy served as an inspiration to the project.

Tim Hathaway, who, though only father-come-lately to the project, has contributed much, and who spent many lonely days in Boston while his wife helped complete the book in New York.

The women who allowed us to 'shoot' their bellies, so our artist could have photographs of real pregnant woman to work from; and Peggy Levine of Great Shapes, in Manhattan, who permitted us to attend exercise classes to photograph her students.

CONTENTS

11 The Seventh Month

12 The Eighth Month

Part 3

LAST BUT NOT LEAST:
Postpartum, Fathers, and the Next Baby

Foreword

by Caroline Flint

Any total life change is frightening, any new venture into the unknown is daunting, and childbirth is the most dramatic and important experience in most women's lives, a time when a woman's whole life changes, when society's perception of her changes, and her perception of herself. It is a dynamic, life changing event and like all new experiences it is a time when people feel vulnerable and alone and insecure – and very ambivalent: now day dreaming of walking down leafy glades cooing at a beautiful smiling baby; then filled with fear at what is to come, a labour which may hurt, a baby whom the couple may not like, a burden on their lives which they may regret – a stranger who may come between them. The new parents are full of doubts and fears.

This book is a book for women written by women, it faces head on the fears and doubts every woman experiences, it provides answers and explanations, and a sense of not being alone. It answers all those questions you meant to ask your midwife or doctor but forgot when you were at the clinic – like having a midwife in your pocket to tackle every question or gnawing doubt as it arises. It deals with aspects of pregnancy that most other pregnancy books seem to leave out, facing squarely the exhaustion of the first few months: the spider naevus on the legs, the fear of harming the baby when having an aspirin, the vivid dreams, the doubts, the dread of making a fool of yourself during labour, the feelings of inadequacy when faced with the overwhelming job of parenting this child through the most formative time in his or her existence.

What to Expect when You're Expecting was originally written for an American audience and proved so popular that it was adapted for parents going through the British system of birth. It will be eagerly read by mothers- and fathers-to-be, and used as a supplement to professional advice and childbirth classes. The system of having a baby is different in the USA where midwives are very rare and most of a woman's care in childbirth is carried out by doctors and nurses. In England most women see a midwife throughout their pregnancy either on her own or with a doctor. Seventy-six per cent of women have a midwife delivering their baby – midwives are the practitioners of normal childbirth. A doctor only becomes involved if any complications develop, so half the women in English hospitals never see a doctor through their labour. Yet on both sides of the Atlantic the feelings of pregnant women are absolutely universal and just as the authors describe.

A man and woman are preparing themselves for parenthood from the time of their own births – children watch their parents with love and admiration, and learn what 'perfect' parents do. All children look upon their parent as the epitome of perfect parenthood when they are small, it is only when they reach the age of enlightenment during puberty that they suddenly discover that their parents actually know nothing and that it is up to them – the teenage children – to teach their parents how to live their lives!

We have all had parents, we have all watched parents, but at this time most couples expecting their first baby live away from their own parents – the modern couple are expected, and indeed expect themselves to be self sufficient, living apart from their family. Many families now contain only one or two children, so those children don't have the opportunity to be involved with the rearing of younger siblings. They have usually never bathed a baby brother, never seen a baby suckling at the breast, never experienced the time-consuming nature of a small baby.

Most women have never seen another woman in labour, never been the helper at their own mother's births, never been near to the emotional upheaval a new baby brings. Thus our need for sensitive and down-to-earth advice from books is greater than at any other time in history.

In our society a woman has her best friend with her during labour, and usually that 'best friend' is the father of her baby. For men, the whole experience of pregnancy, labour and birth, and afterwards can be an overwhelming and stressful experience, a time when he feels that he must be strong and supportive, but also a time when he needs support and cherishing himself.

I always notice the difference in the atmosphere when I am with a woman in labour who has women with her, compared with when she has her male partner. When the woman is surrounded by experienced women who have themselves given birth, the atmosphere is confident, humorous, full of cheery words and jokes, heavy with reminiscences and remembered feelings and experiences. I always think that this is how it must be in more primitive cultures and how it has always been, stretching back through time – women supporting and cherishing each other through a known experience. How much more difficult and stressful it is for a man who has never experienced this situation before. His fears are as great as those of his partner and he also has the burden of wondering if he will 'let her down', the fear of seeing the woman he loves in pain, the fear that most people have of hospitals – the smell of them, the atmosphere of them.

In this book are suggestions for that man: how he can become more involved; what he can do to help. Midwives are used to men being with their partners during both antenatal visits and labour, in fact most of us find it hard if he isn't there to help us. The man will be given many jobs to do, not difficult but very comforting, 'John can you go with Mary when she goes to the loo please?', 'John can you mop her face with a cool flannel because she looks really hot', 'John can you help me move this monitor over to the other side of the room please', 'John can you pour the tea for us all please?'

For Mary, all John needs to do is to be there as her partner, lover, best friend – the person who is there JUST for her, the person who cares about her more than anyone else in the world. A woman needs desperately to be cared for and loved during labour. He is the most appropriate person to do that, and his caring makes an enormous difference to the labouring woman. It means that she can relax and surrender to the enormous sensations of labour without having to worry about what is happening around her, safe in the knowledge that John is there, caring about her, and that he will alert her to anything she needs to know about. He can say soothing words, he can repeat what the midwives have said if he thinks she has missed anything, he can ensure a

peaceful atmosphere by asking her if any chatting is aggravating her. Just the familiar smell of him will be a help and comfort, the touch of his familiar hands, the brush of his familiar kiss, the sound of his familiar voice whispering encouraging words.

Childbirth is one of life's enormous moments – never before have you been present at such a miracle, never before seen the human body working at its glorious best, the cervix dilating, the baby descending through the stretched vagina, the body working in a preordained way that is amazing. If someone were to design childbirth they could never think of anything so clever. For those of us who are privileged to be present at the birth of another human being, to see that small damp head emerging, to see those enquiring eyes open and look around in fascination, to see those first breaths taken – so naturally, with such ease, as if it were an everyday thing to breathe, to see the personality of that other human being beginning to assert itself within minutes of birth, it is indeed an amazing and life-changing experience. It is an experience which is different for every couple, and from each birth that the midwife attends she learns more and more and she gains more and more respect for the design of the human body and for the uniqueness of each human personality.

Caroline Flint is a Midwifery Sister at St George's Hospital, Tooting, and Associate Midwifery Editor of Nursing Times.

A Word From the Doctor

The 1980s are the best years in history to be expecting a baby. In recent decades, there has been a remarkable improvement in the outcome of human pregnancy – for mothers as well as for infants. Women enter pregnancy healthier; they get better, more complete prenatal care; and the hospital maternity wing has replaced the kitchen table and the four-poster as the place to have a baby.

Yet more can be done. To those of us in academic medicine it is becoming increasingly clear that superior doctors and superior equipment aren't enough. Further reductions in pregnancy and childbirth risks will require actively participating expectant couples as well. In order to participate more, couples will have to be more completely and accurately informed, not just about the climactic birth experience, but about the all-important nine months that precede it, not just about the risks that pregnancy presents, but about the steps parents can take to minimize and eliminate risks; not just about the medical aspects of pregnancy, but about psychosocial and lifestyle factors as well.

How can parents become so informed? Schools and colleges have no time or place in their curricula for Babymaking. Professionals who provide obstetrical care have a time problem, too. And they are sometimes overly scientific in their explanations and insufficiently sensitive to the psychological and emotional needs of expectant parents.

Consumer advocates have vaulted into the void with books, magazine articles, and classroom instruction. They are often tremendously helpful, but almost as often they're medically inaccurate, unnecessarily alarming, and/or disproportionately focused on the inadequacies of the health care profession, driving a wedge of suspicion and doubt between parents and their obstetrical caregivers.

The need for a book that provides

accurate, up-to-date, and medically sound information with proper emphasis on nutrition, lifestyle, and the emotional aspects of pregnancy has long been apparent. Now, I believe, that need has been met in a highly readable and eminently practical month-by-month format.

The three authors – each an experienced 'consumer' of maternity care – have given us that essential consumer perspective. They have wisely concentrated on giving expectant parents the information that will allow them to intelligently play their central role in the entire process, without threatening the doctors and nurse-midwives with whom they must work closely and congenially.

What to Expect When You're Expecting is lively in style, accurate, current, and well-balanced overall. But four aspects of its structure and content deserve special comment:

☆ The book's thoughtful family-centred approach to child-bearing – with involvement of the partner throughout the pregnancy process and with a chapter responding to his special needs and problems – is excellent and important.

☆ It has a practical chronological arrangement – sensibly answering all the big and little, trying and troubling questions that come up month after month – makes for timely reassurance and easy bedside-table reference.

☆ The book's emphasis on pre-pregnancy and pregnancy nutrition and lifestyle and its common-sense approaches to lactation and the psychosocial dimensions of motherhood, make it particularly valuable and unique.

☆ Its accurate and up-to-the-minute medical detail – particularly the clarity of its sections on genetics, teratology, preterm labour, delivery, caesarean section, and again, lactation – is outstanding.

All in all, I believe that this excellent book should be *required reading* not only for expectant parents, but for doctors, midwives and nurses who are training to provide obstetrical care and for professionals already providing it. That is, I know, a long way out on a limb for a generally cautious medical school professor to go. But I say it out of strong conviction: the belief that only with properly informed and responsible consumers and providers working together can we draw near our common goal – healthy babies, mothers, and families. And, ultimately, society.

Richard Aubry, M.D., F.A.C.O.G.
Director of Obstetrics – Maternal-Foetal Medicine, SUNY, Upstate Medical Centre, Syracuse, NY

How This Book Was Born

I was pregnant, which about one day out of three made me the happiest woman in the world. And for the remaining two, the most worried.

Worried about the wine I'd sipped nightly with dinner, and the gin and tonics I'd downed more than a few times before dinner in my first six weeks of pregnancy – after two gynaecologists and a blood test convinced me that I wasn't pregnant.

Worried about the seven doses of Provera one of the doctors had prescribed to bring on what she was certain was just a tardy period, but which proved two weeks later to be a nearly two-month gestation.

Worried about the coffee I'd drunk, and the milk I *hadn't;* the sugar I'd eaten, and the protein I hadn't.

Worried about the cramps in my third month, and the four days in my fifth month when I felt not even a flicker of foetal movement.

Worried about the time I fainted while touring the hospital I was to deliver in (I never did get to see the nursery), my middle-of-the-street belly-flop in the eighth month, and a bloody vaginal discharge in the ninth.

Worried, even about feeling *good* ('But I'm not constipated. . . . I don't have morning sickness. . . . I'm not urinating more frequently – something must be wrong!').

Worried that I wouldn't be able to tolerate the pain during labour, or stand the sight of blood at delivery. And worried that because I couldn't squeeze out a drop of the colostrum all my books told me should fill my breasts by the ninth month, I wouldn't be able to breastfeed.

Where could I turn to find reassurance that all would be well? Not to the ever-growing stack of pregnancy books piled high on my bedside table. As common and normal as a few days of no foetal activity is in the fifth month, I couldn't find a single reference to it. As often as pregnant women take a tumble – almost always without harming their babies – I could find no mention of accidental falls.

When my symptoms, problems, or fears *were* discussed, it was usually in an alarming way which only compounded my concern. *Never* take Provera unless you would 'absolutely abort,' warned one volume – without adding that a woman who has taken the drug has so slight an increased risk of birth defects in her baby that an unwanted abortion need never be considered. 'There is evidence that a single drinking 'binge' during pregnancy may affect some babies, depending on the stage of development they have reached,' cautioned another book ominously – disregarding studies which show that a few drinking sprees in early pregnancy, when many women indulge unknowingly, appear to have no effect on a developing embryo.

I certainly couldn't find relief for my worries by opening a newspaper, flipping on the radio or television, or browsing through magazines. According to the media, threats to the pregnant lurked everywhere: in the air we breathed, in the food we ate, in the water we drank, at the dentist's office, even at home.

My doctor offered some solace, of course, but only when I was able to summon up the courage to phone. (I was either afraid my worries would sound silly, or afraid of what I would hear. Besides, how could I spend two days out of three on the phone badgering her?)

Was I (and my husband, Erik – who worried about everything I worried about, and more) alone in my fears?

Far from it. Worry, according to one study, is one of the most common complaints of pregnancy, affecting more expectant women than morning sickness and food cravings combined. Ninety-four out of every hundred women worry about whether their babies will be normal, and 93% worry about whether they and their babies will come through delivery safely. More women worry about their figures (91%) than their health (81%) during pregnancy. And most worry that they worry too much.

But though a little worry is normal for pregnant women and their mates, a lot of worry is an unnecessary waste of what should be a blissfully happy time. Despite all that we hear, read, and worry about, never before in the history of reproduction has it been safer to have a baby – as Erik and I discovered some seven and a half months of worrying later, when I gave birth to a healthier and more beautiful baby girl than I'd dared to dream possible.

Thus, out of our concerns, *What to Expect When You're Expecting* was born. It is dedicated to expectant couples everywhere (especially to my co-author and sister, Sandee, and her husband, Tim, whose first baby will be in a tight race with this book for publication), and written with the hope that it will help fathers- and mothers-to-be worry less and enjoy their pregnancies more.

Heidi Eisenberg Murkoff
New York City

Part I

IN THE BEGINNING

1
Are You Pregnant?

A m I really pregnant? This is the first preoccupation of the hopeful expectant parent, and it occurs the first moment one or another of the signs of pregnancy appears. Happily, it's one question that can very soon be answered, via the combination of a pregnancy test and a medical examination.

Some signs suggest the possibility you are pregnant, others the probability. *No* early signs are positive indications of pregnancy.

WHAT YOU MAY BE CONCERNED ABOUT

Signs of Pregnancy

'I only have some of the signs of pregnancy – can I still be pregnant?'

You can have all of the signs and symptoms of early pregnancy and not be pregnant. Or you can have only a few of them and be very definitely pregnant. The various signs and symptoms of pregnancy are only clues – important to pay attention to, but not to be relied upon for absolute confirmation. In fact the first sign that is proof positive of your pregnancy is your baby's heartbeat, which is audible at about 10, or more often 12, weeks with the sensitive ultrasound Doppler device, or with an ordinary stethoscope at 18 to 20 weeks.[1] Earlier signs only indicate the possibility or probability that you're carrying a child. Combined with a reliable pregnancy test and your doctor's examination, they can help provide an accurate diagnosis.

Pregnancy Tests

'My doctor said the exam and pregnancy test indicated I wasn't pregnant, but I really feel I am.'

As remarkable as modern medical science is, when it comes to pregnancy

---

1 Verification of a pregnancy can be made earlier through ultrasound, but these are not routine procedures.

diagnosis, it still sometimes takes a backseat to a woman's intuition. The accuracy of the different pregnancy tests varies, and none are accurate as early as some women begin to 'feel' that they are pregnant – sometimes within a few days of conception. There are basically three kinds of pregnancy tests available today – and a rabbit needn't give its life for any of them.

The Home Pregnancy Test. This is the most private of pregnancy tests. Very much like the urine test done in the lab, it diagnoses pregnancy by detecting the presence of the hormone HCG (Human Chorionic Gonadotropin) in the urine. It can tell you if you're pregnant as early as nine days after a missed menstrual period, or about three and a half weeks after conception. If it's done correctly –

Possible Signs Of Pregnancy

SIGN	WHEN IT APPEARS	OTHER POSSIBLE CAUSES
Amenorrhoea (absence of menstruation)	Usually entire pregnancy	Travel, fatigue, stress, fear of pregnancy, hormonal problems or illness, extreme weight gain or loss
Morning sickness (any time of day)	2–7 weeks after conception	Food poisoning, tension, infection, and a variety of diseases
Frequent urination	Usually 6–12 weeks after conception	Urinary tract infection, diuretics, tension
Tingling, tender, swollen breasts	As early as a few days after conception	Birth control pills, menstruation
Changes in colour of vaginal and cervical tissue as blood flow increases to area*	First trimester	Menstruation
Darkening of areola around nipple and elevation of tiny glands around nipple	First trimester	Hormonal imbalance
Blue and pink lines under skin on breasts and later on abdomen	First trimester	Hormonal imbalance
Food cravings	First trimester	Poor diet, imagination
Darkening of line from navel to pubis	4th or 5th month	Hormonal imbalance

* Signs of pregnancy looked for in medical examination.

and that's an important 'if' – the at-home test is about as accurate (95%) as a urine test done in a doctor's surgery or laboratory, with a positive result more likely correct than a negative one. But there are drawbacks to this test. You're less likely to feel confident in the results and more likely to want another test. The major risk is that if your test is negative (and incorrect), you may postpone a visit to the doctor and not begin taking proper care of yourself and your baby until weeks later. If you do decide on a home test, buy it the day before you plan to use it (it requires a first-of-the-morning urine sample) and follow the instructions carefully.

The Lab Urine Test. Like the home test, this test can detect HCG in the urine with an accuracy of about 95% – and as early as 20 days after conception. Unlike the home test, it's performed by a professional, who is more likely to do it correctly. (Of course, labs have been known to make mistakes, too.) You will take a urine sample to your doctor's surgery, and they will send it to the lab. You will usually be asked to phone the surgery within a few days to be given the result.

No matter which test you choose, the chances of your pregnancy being correctly diagnosed are enhanced when the test is followed up by a medical examination. The physical signs of pregnancy – an enlarging and softening of the uterus, and a change in the texture of the cervix – may be apparent to a doctor by the sixth week of pregnancy. False-negatives are more common than false-positives: The doctor is more likely to know for sure that you are pregnant than that you're not.

If you are experiencing the symptoms of early pregnancy (absent periods, full and tender breasts, morning sickness, frequent urination, fatigue) and feel, test or no test, exam or no exam, that you are pregnant, act as though you are until you find out definitely otherwise. Neither tests nor doctors are infallible. You know your own body – at least externally – better than your doctor does. Ask for a retest and another exam a week later;

Probable Signs of Pregnancy

SIGN	WHEN IT APPEARS	OTHER POSSIBLE CAUSES
Softening of uterus and cervix*	2–8 weeks after conception	A delayed menstrual period
Enlarging uterus* and abdomen	8–12 weeks	Tumour
Intermittent painless contractions	Early in pregnancy, increasing in frequency	Bowel contractions
Foetal movements	First noted 14–20 weeks of pregnancy	Wind, bowel contractions

Positive Signs of Pregnancy

SIGN	WHEN IT APPEARS	OTHER POSSIBLE CAUSES
Visualization of foetus through ultrasound*	4–6 weeks after conception	None
Foetal heartbeat*	At 10–28 weeks**	None
Foetal movements felt through abdomen*	After 16 weeks	None

* Signs of pregnancy looked for in medical examination.
** Depending on device used.

it may just be too early for a correct diagnosis.

It is possible, of course, that you can experience all of the signs and symptoms of early pregnancy and not be pregnant. None of them alone are proof positive of pregnancy. After two pregnancy tests and a second exam determine that you are not pregnant, you must consider that the 'pregnancy' may be psychological – possibly because you very strongly do, or don't, want to be pregnant. Or the symptoms may have some other biological cause, which should be investigated by your doctor. (See Signs of Pregnancy, page 24.)

Due Date

'My periods are irregular. How can I know if my due date is correct?'

Life would be a lot simpler if you knew from the onset of pregnancy the exact day you were going to give birth. But life isn't that simple very often. According to some studies only four women in a hundred give birth exactly on their due date. Most others, because a normal full-term pregnancy can last anywhere from 38 to 42 weeks, deliver within two weeks either way of that date.

That's why the medical term for 'due date' is EDC, or the *estimated* date of confinement (or delivery). The date your doctor gives you is only an educated estimate, calculated this way: Note the date of the first day of your last normal menstrual period (LMP), and add to it seven days. From that date, count back three months and you have your due date – one year later. (LMP + 7 days − 3 months + 1 year = EDC.) If your periods come every 28 days, you are more likely than most to deliver close to your estimated due date. If your cycles are longer than 28 days, you are more likely to deliver after the EDC, and if they are shorter, before it.

But if your cycle is irregular, this system may not work for you at all. Say you haven't had your period in three months and suddenly you are pregnant. When did you conceive? The only clue the doctor or midwife has to work with early in pregnancy, unless you can pinpoint the time of conception, is the size of your uterus. Later on there are other milestones that together can more accurately gauge just how pregnant you are: the first time the foetal heartbeat is heard (at about 10 to 12 weeks with a Doppler device, or at about 28 weeks with a stethoscope), the first flutter of life (at about 20 weeks with a first baby, or 16 to 18 with subsequent ones); the height of the fundus (the top of the uterus) at each visit (for example, it will reach the navel at the 20th week). If all of these indications seem to correspond to the due date you and your doctor or midwife have calculated, you can be pretty sure that it is close to accurate – that is, that you are fairly likely to deliver within two weeks of that date. But if they don't correspond, the doctor or midwife may decide to do an ultrasound scan, which can more closely pinpoint the gestational age of your foetus. (See page 54.)

As delivery nears, there will be other clues to the date of the big event: painless contractions will become more frequent (and possibly even uncomfortable), the foetus will move down into the pelvis (engagement), your cervix will begin to thin (effacement), and last of all, your cervix will begin to dilate. These clues will be helpful, but not definitive – only your baby knows for sure what his or her birthday will be. (For more information, see Lightening and Engagement, page 232); When You Will Deliver, page 234.)

WHAT IT'S IMPORTANT TO KNOW: YOUR CHOICES IN MEDICAL CARE

While it takes two to conceive a baby, it takes a minimum of three – mother, father and at least one health care professional – to make that transition from fertilized egg to delivered infant a safe and sound one. Assuming you and your partner have already taken care of conception, the next challenge you face is selecting that third member of your pregnancy team. And making sure that it's a selection you can live with – and labour with.

The pattern of care during pregnancy and childbirth was very different thirty years ago. During the 1950s many more babies were born at home, or in small maternity homes and cottage hospitals. In the 1980s, the trend is to bring the majority of women into large, centralised obstetric hospital units for the birth of their babies, and to transfer them to small local maternity homes for postnatal care before they return home. This policy means that it is very important for you to be aware of the choices that are available to you.

What Kind of Person Are You?

Your first step in deciding what choice you want to make about the way in which you would like to be cared for during your pregnancy and the birth of your child is to give some thought to the kind of person you are.

Do you believe that 'doctor knows

best' (after all, he or she's the one who went to medical school)? Would you prefer your doctor to make all the decisions without consulting you, and do you feel safest when all the latest medical technology is being used in your care? Then you will probably feel most comfortable with a doctor who has a traditional practice, a god-like aura and an unswerving dedication to his or her own obstetrical philosophy.

Or do you believe that your body and your health are your business and no one else's? Do you have definite ideas about pregnancy and childbirth and feel you'd like to run the show, from conception to delivery, with minimal interference from your health professional. Then look for a doctor or midwife who is willing to give up the starring role and serve as your consultant on the production of your baby. Someone who will step aside, though not entirely out of the picture, while you make as many of the childbirth decisions as is medically practical; who is dogmatic only when it comes to giving you a controlling vote. Don't assume however, that a doctor who leans towards more radical obstetrics is going to be any less doctrinaire in his or her beliefs than a traditional doctor.

Or perhaps you'd prefer a practitioner who'll put you in the position of partner; that is, who will make decisions based on his or her experience and knowledge, but include you in the process. Who will keep as the number one priority, your health and the health of your baby, not some inflexible medical gospel. Then the doctor for you is probably one who sees his or her role in your pregnancy

as somewhere in between. A doctor who is neither inflexible nor putty in your hands; who feels that either a natural delivery or a caesarian can be the best way, depending on the situation; who doesn't routinely withold or order pain medication. He or she should see nothing incongruous in using a foetal monitor and a birthing room at the same time – if that's what's best for mother and child. The doctor or midwife sees his or her relationship with you as an equal but definitely separate partnership in which each party contributes what he or she does best.

Whatever your preferred style, if you believe that the father-to-be should have equal billing in the pregnancy–childbirth drama, you'll also need to make sure that the caregiver you select agrees with you. His or her first attitude will be clearly apparent on the first visit. Is the father invited to participate in both the examination and consultation? Are his questions given full consideration? Is the discussion addressed to both expectant parents, not just to the mother? Is it clear that the father will be permitted to share in both labour and delivery?

Bearing these considerations in mind, it is a good idea to find out about the choices that are available to you in your area before you make your first appointment with your GP to discuss your pregnancy.

As a pregnant woman you will be asked to sign a form (EC24) which is a contract between you and your doctor for maternity care only. If your GP is not on the 'obstetric' list (available from your post office, Community Health Council, or Family Practitioner Committee) or you do not want her or him to care for you during your pregnancy, you are legally entitled to register with another GP for obstetric care only, returning to your regular GP after the baby is born.

Three main decisions need to be made: Where shall I have my baby? Who will be involved in the delivery? Who will look after me during my pregnancy?

Where to Give Birth

Depending on the facilities in your area, your own health and the progress of your pregnancy, you can choose to have your baby in one of a number of different places, and the people involved in the delivery will vary according to your choice.

Firstly, you could choose to have your baby at home. In this case, the community midwife and GP will care for you during pregnancy, the birth of your baby, and the postnatal period.

Alternatively, if you choose the DOMINO scheme (Domiciliary In or Out), you will again be cared for by your midwife and GP, but will go into hospital, with them, for the actual birth of your baby, returning home as soon after the birth as possible.

Another alternative is to book into a GP Unit. In this case a hospital midwife, rather than your community midwife will deliver your baby, together with your GP.

If you have a maternity home or small local hospital in your area, you can be booked in there. Your baby will then be delivered by a hospital midwife and doctor.

The final choice available to you is that of a consultant maternity unit. Here you will be cared for by the hospital midwives and the consultant's medical team, who will be involved in the birth of your baby.

The choice that you make will ultimately depend on a number of independent factors. These include the range of facilities available in your area, the advice of your midwife and GP, based on their knowledge of these facilities, and your own medical history and the progress of your pregnancy.

Although a home birth or domino delivery can be an ideal choice for a healthy woman who is enjoying a straightforward pregnancy, obviously if complications arise during that pregnancy, a transfer to a consultant unit may be considered necessary.

The key to making the right choice for you and your baby is to be aware of the range of possibilities available to you, and to discuss your views with your midwife and GP. Why not visit the local maternity homes and hospitals before you make your final decision? Most of them will be only too pleased to show you round and discuss their policies with you. Although it is usual to make your decision early in pregnancy, it is not essential. If you are not sure, wait a while before you make your choice. That is often much easier than transferring from one option to another once a booking has been made.

Care During Pregnancy and the Postnatal Period

The medical care you will receive during your pregnancy, and postnatally will vary according to the choice that you've made about where to have the baby.

In the case of a home birth, the community midwife and GP will care for you during the antenatal period. After the birth your midwife will visit you at home daily for at least 10 days. The GP will also make regular visits during this time, following up with a postnatal check-up at the surgery at 6–8 weeks after the birth.

For a Domino delivery the care is exactly the same as for a home birth, except that your community midwife and GP transfer you to hospital for 6–24 hours for the birth and immediate postnatal period but will continue to be responsible for your care during this time.

If you have chosen a hospital-based birth, either in a GP Unit, a maternity home, a small local hospital, or a consultant unit, you could be offered 'shared care' between the community midwife and the GP at your local surgery, as well as visits to the hospital or maternity home antenatal clinics where you will see hospital midwives, doctors and consultants. In this case it is usual to have a booking clinic at the local hospital early on in pregnancy, returning to your local surgery for the intervening months unless a complication arises, and then back to the hospital for the final weeks of pregnancy and the birth. After returning home, your community midwife will visit you at least until the 10th day postnatally, and you may have the option to have your postnatal check-up 6–8 weeks after the birth at either your GP's surgery or the hospital.

The final variation which is available to you is to be cared for throughout your pregnancy, for the birth and immediate postnatal period by the hospital midwives, doctors and consultants. If you have your baby in a large centralised consultant unit, you may be given the option to transfer to a smaller local maternity home after your postnatal stay in hospital, before returning home. After you return home, the community midwife will visit you at least until the 10th day after the birth. You will return to the hospital for your postnatal check-up 6–8 weeks after the birth.

In all cases, a health visitor will also visit you at home, probably antenatally, and then some time after the 10th day postnatally. He or she will keep in touch with you and your family until your child is five years old.

Making the Choice

In order to make an informed choice about the birth of your baby it is helpful to know more about the alternatives that are available. Here is an outline of some of the points that you should consider when making your choice. If you require more information at any point or about facilities in your area, contact the addresses listed on page 32 or your local Community Health Council or Family Practitioner Committee.

Home Birth

If you would like to have your baby at home, talk to your GP about it. If there are no medical contraindications but your doctor is not prepared to deliver your baby at home, it is possible to change your GP for obstetric care only. There are usually some GP's in most areas who would welcome you.

In order to have a safe home birth you need a willing GP and community midwife, and also an 'obstetric flying squad' (or obstetric emergency service) in case of an emergency. There should be emergency consultant teams who are on call 24 hours a day with equipment to deal with any emergency that may arise at a home delivery. Not all areas of the country offer an adequate obstetric flying squad service, so it is necessary to check the facilities in your area before you make the choice about a home birth.

If you are unable to find a willing GP, you can obtain the services of a community midwife by writing to your Area Nursing Officer and Area Medical Officer in your Area Health Authority (address in the local telephone book), stating your intention to remain at home and your desire to be attended by a midwife. A midwife is a medically-qualified practitioner in her own right, and may attend a birth on her own without GP backing, but usually would not consider doing this. If help is refused, ask for written refusal of service. Your Community Health Council or Family Practitioner Committee may be able to help and give advice. It is your legal right to have your baby at home, even your first one. If you do choose to have your baby at home, practical help and support are particularly important. Your midwife will visit you at home at least up to the 10th postnatal day. It is also worth enquiring from your local Social Services Department (address in your telephone book) about the provision of a home help. These are often also provided if you are expecting twins!

Useful addresses:

AIMS (Association for Improvements in Maternity Services),
c/o Elizabeth Key,
Goose Green Barn, Much Hoole,
Preston,
Lancashire
PR4 4TD

ARM (Association of Radical Midwives),
c/o 8A The Drive,
Wimbledon,
London SW20 8TG

The Birth Centre,
c/o Roz Claxton,
16 Simpson Street,
London SW11

National Childbirth Trust,
9 Queensborough Terrace,
London W2

Society to Support Home Confinements,
c/o Margaret Whyte,
17 Laburnum Avenue,
Durham
(0385) 61325
(Phone after 6 p.m. Send s.a.e. if writing.)

Domino Scheme

This scheme enables you to be cared for antenatally by your community midwife, in conjunction with your GP. When you go into labour your midwife or another midwife on call at the time will go with you to hospital, and deliver your baby there. She will go home with you and your baby 6–48 hours later, providing you are both in a satisfactory condition. She will then continue to visit you at home, at least up until the 10th postnatal day.

Usually the hospital used will be a GP unit, maternity home or small local or cottage hospital. However, it is also possible to have a domino delivery in a consultant unit, your community midwife working with the consultant team, so do enquire in your local area.

Not all areas of the country offer a domino service, but if yours does, it is possible to transfer to a GP who is involved in the scheme, for obstetric care only, if your usual GP is not. Information is available from the Community Heath Council or Family Practitioner Committee.

The advantage of this scheme is that it ensures continuity of care during your pregnancy, for the birth and postnatally.

GP Unit

These exist in some areas of the country, and will enable you to receive antenatal and postnatal care from your community midwife and GP, and delivery of your baby by your GP or midwifery staff in the unit. You can be booked for a short (48 hour) or long (up to 8–10 day) stay postnatally, and when you return home your community midwife will visit you at least up to the 10th day postnatally.

Some GP units are attached to a consultant unit at a hospital, and others are some distance from medical facilities. It is important to find out what sort of emergency provision and services are available at your local GP unit – see section on Home Birth (page 32) for details of emergency back-up necessary to ensure a safe delivery.

Maternity Homes and Small, Local Cottage Hospitals

Together with GP units, these homes and hospitals are being phased out in favour of centralised obstetric units in large towns. Where they do exist they all provide midwife-based care for women whom it is anticipated will have a normal healthy pregnancy and birth, i.e. in the 'low risk' category. However, in many areas they are being used primarily for antenatal and postnatal care, with most deliveries taking place in the consultant maternity units.

Your antenatal care will be shared between your GP and community midwife, and the maternity home clinic. Some clinics have regular visits from consultant obstetricians. The delivery will take place in the maternity home, and you can be booked for a short (48-hour) or long (up to 8–10 day) stay postnatally. When you return home your community midwife will visit you at least up to the 10th postnatal day.

Hospital Birth

Consultant maternity units within hospitals provide obstetrician-based care and a wide range of technology and emergency services. These facilities are provided to cater for the 'high risk' women, i.e. women whom it is anticipated may have complications during pregnancy, labour and birth.

It is possible to have your antenatal care shared between your GP and community midwife, and the maternity unit. Inevitably, more staff will be involved in this care than in a smaller hospital. However, in many hospitals nowadays some effort is made to minimise any sense of anonymity that such large institutions may generate. Take full advantage of antenatal and parentcraft classes and open evenings for you and your partner to learn more about the place where your baby is to be born.

You can be booked in for a short (48-hour) or long (up to 8–10 day) stay postnatally. When you return home your local community midwife will visit you at least up to the 10th postnatal day.

Make the Most of the Patient–Doctor/ Midwife Relationship

By thinking about the options that are open to you, it is possible for you both to make an informed choice about the birth of your child. Having made that choice, it is then important to nurture a good working partnership with your doctor or midwife.

☆ When something you think worth mentioning crops up between visits, put it on a list that you take with you to your next appointment. (It helps to keep a few lists in convenient places – the refrigerator door, your handbag, your desk at work, your bedside table – so that you'll always be within jotting distance of one.) That's the only way you can be sure that you won't forget to ask all your questions and report all your symptoms. And you won't be wasting your time, or your doctor's, while you try to recall what it was you wanted to ask.

☆ Along with your questions list, bring a pen and pad to each visit, so you can make a note of your doctor's directions. Most people are too nervous in the presence of a physician to remember directions accurately. If your doctor doesn't volunteer information, make inquiries before you leave, so there's no confusion once you get home. Ask about such things as side effects of treatments, how long to take a medication if one is prescribed, when to check back about a problem situation.

☆ Though you don't want to call your doctor at every pelvic twinge, you shouldn't hesitate to call about worries that you can't resolve by checking in a book such as this one, and that you feel can't wait until the next visit. Don't be afraid that your concerns will sound silly. Unless your doctor has just graduated from medical school, he or she's heard it all before. If you are having pain or bleeding, be very specific about location, duration, quantity (of bleeding), and quality (of pain), as well as about what makes it worse or better. Also report accompanying symptoms (such as fever, nausea, vomiting, chills, or diarrhoea). (See When to Call the Doctor or Midwife, page 110.)

☆ When you read about something new in obstetrics, don't brandish the clipping in front of the doctor saying, 'I must have this.' Instead, bring it in at your next visit, and ask your doctor if he or she feels there is any value in this new procedure. Often the media report medical advances prematurely, before they are proven safe and effective through controlled studies. If indeed it is a worthwhile advance, your doctor may already be aware of it. If not, he or she may want to find out more.

☆ When you hear something which doesn't correspond with what your doctor has told you, ask for his or her opinion on what you've heard.

Not in a challenging way, just in order to get more information.

☆ If you suspect that the doctor may be wrong about something (for example, okaying intercourse when you have a history of miscarriage), say so. Don't challenge, just open your suspicion to discussion. A doctor has many patients and may sometimes forget critical information about your particular obstetrical situation.

☆ If you have a gripe, tell your doctor about it. Letting it fester jeopardizes your relationship.

☆ If your relationship with your doctor breaks down irreparably, think about changing doctors. He or she probably doesn't enjoy the bad feelings any more than you do. Don't, however, expect to get good obstetrical care if you regularly switch from doctor to doctor trying to find one who will follow *your* orders. Consider, instead, that the problem with the care you've been receiving may originate with you.

2
Now That You Are Pregnant

WHAT YOU MAY BE CONCERNED ABOUT

Now that you no longer have to worry about whether or not the pregnancy test will be positive, you're sure to come up with a whole new set of concerns: What effect will my age or my husband's age have on my pregnancy and on our baby? How will chronic medical problems or family genetic problems affect him or her? Will our past lifestyles make a difference? Will my previous obstetrical history repeat? What can I do to lower any risks my history may present?

Your Gynaecological History

'Several years ago I had fibroids removed. I've also had a couple of D and Cs. What effect could this have on my pregnancy?'

Your past gynaecological history is important to your practitioner because it will provide clues to the cause of any problem that might come up. For the most part, however, you shouldn't expect surgery for the removal of small uterine fibroid tumours, or one or two dilatation and curettages (D and Cs) for spontaneous or therapeutic abortions, to affect your pregnancy – though unusually large fibroids that haven't been removed can keep a woman from conceiving or can cause miscarriage or preterm labour, and scarring from D and Cs can interfere with implantation.

It is possible that *deep* surgery for large fibroids could weaken the uterus enough so that it could not tolerate labour. If, on reviewing your surgical records, your doctor decides this may be true of your uterus, he or she will plan a caesarean section for you. It is also possible (though evidence is contradictory) that *repeated* D and Cs could result in a weakening of the cervix (the opening of the uterus), which could lead to a midtrimester miscarriage or preterm labour. Should an incompetent cervix be suspected, or should your cervix begin to open prematurely, suturing (stitching) the cervix closed will probably allow the pregnancy to continue until the foetus is mature, when the stitches can be safely removed.

Your Obstetrical History Repeating Itself

'I had an easy first pregnancy. Can I expect this one to go well, too?'

In general, your first pregnancy is a pretty good predictor of future pregnancies, all things being equal. If it was uneventful, subsequent pregnancies probably will be, too. If, on the other hand, you had any kind of problem the first time around, it's a good idea to ask your doctor about the possibility of a repeat and to see what can be done to prevent it. For example, if you delivered prematurely there are a great many steps that can be taken to help you go to term (see page 195). Or if you developed gestational diabetes, you can take preventive measures before sugar shows up in your urine (see page 138). On the other hand, if your problem was caused by a one-time event (such as an infection or an accident), or by something you did during your first pregnancy that you aren't doing

in the second (such as smoking), then it isn't likely to recur.

Some problems may repeat no matter what you do. For example, if a first baby was in a breech position due to an irregularly shaped uterus, subsequent babies may be, too. Or if a baby was in an occiput posterior position (back of the head toward the mother's back) because of the shape of the mother's pelvis, any future brothers and sisters may be as well – which can mean uncomfortable back labour for mum. If, however, a specific reason for the foetus being in an unusual position was not identified, then the odds of the problem repeating are probably not much greater than average.

Repeat Caesareans

'I can't have a vaginal delivery because my pelvis is abnormally shaped. I want to have six kids just like my mother did, but I understand three caesareans is the limit.'

Tell that to Ethel Kennedy, the indomitable wife of Robert F. Kennedy, who is reported to have had 11 caesareans in an era when the procedure was neither as safe nor as easy as it is today. Of course, sometimes having numerous caesareans isn't possible. Much will depend upon the kind of incision that was made and the kind of scar that formed. Talk to your obstetrician about your concern, because only someone fully familiar with your case can tell you whether or not you can do an 'Ethel Kennedy' (or even half an 'Ethel Kennedy'). You may be pleasantly surprised.

Because of your scars, however,

you should be alert for the signs of labour (contractions, bloody show, ruptured membranes; see page 239) in the final months of pregnancy. Should they occur, notify your doctor and go to the hospital immediately. You should also notify him or her at *any* time in your pregnancy if you have unexplained, persistent abdominal pain, or bleeding.

'I had my last baby by emergency caesarean. I'm pregnant again and have heard "once a caesarean, always a caesarean."'

'Once a caesarean always a caesarean' was, until very recently, an obstetrical edict engraved in stone, or rather in the uteruses of women who'd had at least one baby born through a classic vertical incision. This type of incision is very rare now. Today, though many women who've had one caesarean delivery go on to have others, many other women, usually those who have had the most commonly used low-transverse incision are able to go through a normal labour and a vaginal delivery.

Whether or not you can deliver vaginally will depend upon the reason for your first caesarean. If the reason was a one-time problem (foetal distress, premature separation of the placenta, faulty placement of the placenta, infection, breech, toxaemia), it's very possible you can have a vaginal delivery this time. If it was a chronic disease (diabetes, high blood pressure, heart disease) or a permanent problem (an oddly shaped pelvis), you will certainly have a repeat caesarean. Don't rely on your recollection of the reason – check, or

have your doctor check the medical records of the delivery. You will also probably have a repeat if the original incision was a vertical one, which is more likely to rupture than the low-transverse variety.

If you feel strongly about having a vaginal delivery with your next baby, then discuss the possibility with your doctor now. Some doctors still cling to the old adage and will not permit a woman with a caesarean-scarred uterus to labour, fearing a rupture (which, however, is very rare with low-transverse incisions). In addition to finding an amenable consultant who is willing to be with you from the very beginning of labour through delivery, you must plan to be delivered in a fully equipped hospital with round-the-clock operating facilities in case problems develop.

Your role is as important as the doctor's in assuring a safe vaginal delivery. You should:

☆ Take childbirth education classes, and take them seriously, so that you will be able to labour as efficiently as possible.

☆ Notify your doctor or midwife the moment signs of labour, such as contractions, bloody show, ruptured membranes, occur.

☆ Expect to use little or no medication (which might mask signs of impending problems).

☆ If you notice any unusual pain or tenderness *between* contractions, tell your doctor immediately.

Though your chances of a normal vaginal delivery are good, even the woman who has never had a caesarean has a 10% to 20% chance of needing one. So don't be disappointed if you end up needing a repeat. The safest possible birth of that wonderful baby of yours is what this is all about, after all.

Pregnancies Too Close Together

'I became pregnant with a second child just 10 weeks after I delivered my first. I'm worried about what effect this might have on my health and on the baby I'm carrying.'

Conceiving again before you've fully recovered from a recent pregnancy and delivery puts enough strain on your body without adding the debilitating effects of worry. So first of all, *relax*. Though conception in the first three postpartum months is rare (almost a miracle if the new baby is exclusively breastfed), it's taken other women by surprise, too. And most have delivered normal, healthy infants, little the worse for wear themselves.

However, it's essential to be aware of the toll two quickly consecutive pregnancies can take, and to do everything possible to compensate. Conception within three months of delivery puts the new pregnancy in a high-risk category, which, in this case, isn't as ominous as it sounds, particularly with the proper care and precautions, including:

☆ The best prenatal care, starting as soon as you think you're pregnant. As with any high-risk pregnancy, you're probably best off with an obstetrician, or a nurse midwife who practices with one. You should be scrupulous about following doctor's orders and not missing office visits.

☆ The Best-Odds Diet (see page 82), adhered to, if not religiously, at least faithfully. Your body may still be at a nutritional disadvantage, and you may need to overcompensate – particularly with protein (at least 100 grams a day), iron (you should take a supplement), and possibly calories (insufficient weight gain will be a clue that you need more food).

☆ Adequate weight gain. Your new foetus doesn't care whether or not you've yet shed the extra pounds his or her sibling put on you. The two of you need the same 20-to-30-pound gain this pregnancy. So don't even think about losing weight, not even early on. A carefully monitored gradual weight gain will be relatively easy to take off afterward – especially with two infants keeping you on the go.

☆ Weaning your older baby immediately, if you're nursing. He or she's already reaped many of the benefits of breastfeeding, and weaning at this age should be neither difficult nor traumatic. Some women do continue nursing, but trying to rally the nutritional forces for both nursing and pregnancy can be a losing battle for all concerned.

☆ Rest – more than is humanly (and new-motherly) possible. This will require not only your own determination, but help from your partner and possibly others as well. Let chores or other work go undone, and force yourself to lie down when your baby is napping. Have daddy take over as many nighttime feedings as he can rise for, as well as much of the cooking, housework, and baby care (particularly tasks which involve a lot of baby-lifting).

☆ Exercise – just enough to keep you in shape, but not enough to overtax you. Ask your doctor for guidelines.

☆ Eliminate or minimize all other risk factors, such as smoking and drinking. Your body doesn't need any additional strains. (See page 57.)

Tempting Fate the Second Time Around

'I had a perfect first baby. Now that I'm pregnant again, I can't get rid of the fear that I won't be so lucky this time.'

A million-dollar lottery winner isn't likely to hit the jackpot twice, though his or her odds remain as good as any other player's. A mother who has had a 'perfect' baby, however, is not only likely to win again, her odds are better than they were before – because she has now proven she can successfully complete a pregnancy. In addition, with each pregnancy she has the chance to improve her odds a little – by eliminating the negative (smoking, drinking, using drugs) and accentuating the positive (eating better, exercising, getting good medical care).

Having a Baby After 35

'I'm 38 and pregnant with my first – and probably last – baby. It's so important that it be healthy, but I've read so much about the risks of pregnancy after 35.'

Becoming pregnant after 35 puts you in good (and growing) company. While the pregnancy rate has been dropping among women in their 20s, it has been zooming among women over 35. These women are a new breed of mothers – better educated (more than half have gone to college), career oriented, and more settled. Some believe they make better parents because of their maturity and because they've already had their flings and don't resent being tied down by a baby. On the other hand, some find motherhood a strain because they are more set in their ways, have less physical stamina, and are separated by a wide generation gap from their children. Yet few regret having had their children.

If you've lived for more than 35 years, you know that nothing one does in life is completely free of risk. Pregnancy, at any age, certainly isn't. And the risks do increase somewhat as age advances. Most older mothers, however, feel that the benefits of starting a family at the time that is right for them far outweigh any risks. And they are buoyed by the fact that new medical discoveries are reducing these risks almost daily.

The most notorious risk faced by older mothers is that of having a child with Down's syndrome. The risk increases with each passing year: 1 in 10,000 for 20-year-old mothers, about 3 in 1,000 for 35-year-old mothers, and 1 in 100 for 40-year-old mothers. It's speculated that this and other chromosomal abnormalities, though still relatively rare, are more common in older women because their ova (every woman is born with a lifetime supply) are older, too, and have had more exposure to x-rays, drugs, infections, and so on. (It is now known, however, that the egg is not always responsible for such chromosomal abnormalities. An estimated minimum of 25% of Down's syndrome cases have been linked to a defect in the father's sperm. See page 42.)

While Down's syndrome (characterised by mental retardation, a flat face, and slanting eyes) isn't preventable at this time, it can, like many other genetic disorders, be diagnosed in utero, through amniocentesis (page 53). Such diagnostic testing is now offered routinely to mothers over 35 and others in high-risk categories. Often, so is an ultrasound scan (page 54). Should Down's syndrome or another abnormality show up, the parents then have the option of terminating the pregnancy and trying again. Or, if abortion is unacceptable, they can choose to continue the pregnancy, with the knowledge that children with Down's syndrome generally have the potential for living fulfilling, if somewhat sub-optimal lives. Not only are they very loving and lovable, they can often, with early training, learn to take care of themselves, even to read and write.

In addition to chromosomal aberrations like Down's syndrome, 35-plus mothers are also slightly more subject to high blood pressure and diabetes (which are more common in older groups in general), and to miscarriage, often because of a blighted embryo (one that is too defective to develop normally). Delivery may be more difficult because of a decrease in muscle tone and joint flexibility – though at least one study showed older mothers with an average rate of caesareans, a high percentage of unmedicated births, and a much lower need for forceps delivery than mothers of all ages.

In spite of the risks – which are actually far less threatening than the media make them seem – older mothers have a lot going for them. Medical science, for example. Screening for birth defects can be done in utero through amniocentesis, ultrasound, and newer procedures – foetoscopy and chorionic villi sampling (see About Prenatal Diagnosis, page 52). Drugs can forestall a preterm labour, a somewhat more common complication among both younger (under 17) and older (over 35) mothers. Electronic foetal monitoring during labour can warn of foetal distress, allowing speedy measures to be taken to protect the foetus from further trauma.

As successful as these advances have been in reducing the risks of pregnancy after 35, they pale next to the strides older mothers have taken – and can take – to improve the odds for themselves and their babies, through exercise, diet, and quality prenatal care. Advanced reproductive age alone does not necessarily put a mother in a high-risk category. But an accumulation of many individual risks can. When the older mother makes a concerted effort to eliminate or minimize as many risk factors as possible, she can take years off her pregnancy profile – making her chances of delivering a healthy baby virtually as good as those of a younger mother. (See Reducing Risk in Any Pregnancy, page 57.)

The Father's Age

'I'm only 31, but my husband is over 50. Does advanced paternal age pose risks to a baby?'

Throughout most of history, it was believed that a father's responsibility in the reproductive process was limited to fertilization. Only during this century (too late to help those queens who'd lost their heads for failing to produce a male heir) was it discovered that a father's sperm held the deciding genetic vote in determining his child's sex. And only in the last few years has it begun to be postulated that an older father's sperm might contribute to birth defects such as Down's syndrome. Like the older mother's ova, the older father's primary oocytes (undeveloped sperm) have had longer exposure to environmental hazards and might conceivably contain altered or damaged genes or chromosomes. And from the isolated studies that have been done, there is some evidence that in about 25% or 30% of Down's syndrome cases the faulty chromosome can be traced to the father. It also appears that there is an increase in the risk of Down's syndrome when the father is over 50 (or 55, depending on the study), though the association is weaker than in the case of maternal age.

But the evidence remains inconclusive – mostly because of the inadequacy of the existing research. Setting up the kind of large-scale studies required for conclusive results has been difficult so far, for two reasons. First of all, Down's syndrome is relatively rare (about 1 or 2 in 1,000 live births). Second, in the majority of cases, an older father is married to an older mother, making it tricky to clarify the independent role of paternal age.

So the question of whether or not advanced paternal age is linked to Down's syndrome and other birth defects remains largely unanswered. Experts believe that there probably is some connection (although it's not clear at what age it begins), but that the risk is almost certainly very small. At this time, genetic counsellors do not recommend amniocentesis on the basis of paternal age alone. If, however, you're going to spend the rest of your pregnancy worrying about the possible – though unlikely – effects of your husband's age on your baby, you might discuss your fears with your doctor to see if amniocentesis is warranted.

Chronic Health Problems: Diabetes

'I'm a diabetic, and I'm concerned about the effect of my condition on my baby.'

Until recently, getting pregnant was a risky business for the diabetic woman, and an even riskier business for her unborn baby. Today, if she receives continuous expert medical care, the diabetic woman has just about as good a chance of having a successful pregnancy and a healthy baby as any other pregnant woman does. In fact, diabetic women in one study took such excellent care of themselves throughout their pregnancies that they and their babies had even *fewer* problems than their non-diabetic counterparts.

Making your diabetic pregnancy a success won't be effortless. It will be more stressful than a non-diabetic pregnancy (blood sugar must be continuously monitored and insulin doses adjusted accordingly), more costly (weekly trips to your doctor and obstetrician may be necessary), and will require more self-discipline (diet must be scrupulously adhered to). But the reward for those extra efforts – a healthy baby – can make them well worthwhile.

Research has proved that the key to successfully managing a diabetic pregnancy is maintaining euglycaemia (normal blood glucose levels, usually under 100 milligrams per decilitre). The availability in the past few years of home monitoring, split dose administration of insulin, and insulin pumps has made this increasingly possible. A variety of other factors also contribute to a safe diabetic pregnancy.

Following Doctor's Orders. You'll have many more orders from your doctor than most pregnant women. And you'll have to be far more scrupulous in following them, too.

Good Diet. A diet geared to your personal needs should be carefully planned with your doctor, a nutritionist, or a nurse-practitioner who specializes in diabetes education. It will probably be high in fibre, which recent studies show may reduce insulin requirements in pregnant diabetics. This is not a time to be lax about your diet, although (especially late in pregnancy) exhaustion may tempt you to be. It is, rather, an ideal time to get your dietary act together – for you and your baby. Perfecting dietary control is so important that many specialists recommend in-hospital training for diabetic mothers-to-be prior to conception, or early in pregnancy.

If morning sickness is a problem at any time during pregnancy, don't let it interfere with nourishing your baby and keeping your blood glucose level stable. Don't fast or skip meals. Eating regularly is essential. If you have trouble getting down three large meals, take six to eight small ones, regularly spaced and carefully planned. (See page 101 for some general tips on dealing with morning sickness.)

Sensible Weight Gain. The ideal approach is to attain desirable weight before conception – something to remember before your next pregnancy. Even if it's too late for that, weight gain should be kept within strict guidelines set by your doctor. If you start your pregnancy overweight, don't use the gestational period for slimming down. Getting sufficient calories is vital to your baby's well-being.

Exercise. Your exercise programme, too, should be planned with medical assistance and in conjunction with your medication schedule and diet plan. Exercise will give you more energy, aid in stabilizing your blood sugar, and help get you in shape for delivery.

Rest. Especially in the third trimester, adequate rest is very important. avoid overtaxing your energies and try to take some time off during the middle of the day for relaxation or a nap. If you're working, your doctor may recommend beginning your maternity leave early.

Medication Regulation. Certain pregnancy hormones are antagonistic to (work against) insulin. That's the reason why your insulin dose may have to be adjusted upward during the second trimester, when the secretion of these placental hormones substantially increases. If you are taking oral hypoglycaemic (blood-sugar-lowering) drugs, which cross the placenta readily, you may be switched to injected insulin during your pregnancy, which is less likely to affect your foetus.

Reduction of Other Risk Factors. Since risk in pregnancy is cumulative – the more risk factors the higher the risk – you should endeavour to eliminate or minimize as many as possible. (See Reducing Risk in Any Pregnancy, page 57.)

Careful Monitoring. Don't be alarmed if your doctor orders a great many tests for you (in and out of the hospital), especially during the final trimester, or even suggests hospitalization for the final weeks of pregnancy. This doesn't mean something is wrong, only that he or she wants to be sure that everything stays right. The tests will primarily be directed toward continual evaluation of your condition and that of your baby, in order to determine the optimal time for delivery. Your retinas and kidney function will be checked regularly. (Retinal and kidney problems tend to worsen during pregnancy, but usually return to pre-pregnancy states after delivery.) Dropping levels of oestriol, an oestrogenic hormone (often measured several times a week), and a positive stress or non-stress test would warn of any deterioration in the condition of the placenta or foetus. Examination of amniotic fluid (through amniocentesis) will assess the stage of maturity of the foetal lungs, and readiness for delivery. Ultrasound may be used to size up your baby so that delivery is accomplished before he or she's too big for vaginal delivery.

Don't fear complications, either, if your baby is placed in a neonatal intensive care unit immediately after delivery. This is routine procedure in most hospitals for infants of diabetic mothers. Your baby will be observed for respiratory problems (which are unlikely if his lungs were found to be mature before delivery) and for hypoglycaemia (which, though more common, responds quickly and completely to treatment).

Elective Early Delivery. Because babies of diabetics tend to be too large for full-term vaginal delivery (particularly when euglycaemia is not maintained throughout pregnancy); because their placentas tend to deteriorate early (often robbing the foetus of vital nutrients and oxygen during the last weeks); and because they are subject to acidosis (abnormal acid-base balance in the blood) and other problems, they are often delivered before term, generally at about 37 weeks. The various tests mentioned above help the doctor to choose just the right time to induce labour or perform a caesarean – late enough so that the foetal lungs are sufficiently mature, not so late that the foetus is in jeopardy. Women with very mild diabetes, gestational diabetes, and even some with very well-controlled moderate disease can often carry to term safely.

Chronic Health Problems: Asthma

'I've been an asthmatic since childhood. I'm concerned that the attacks and the drugs I take for them might harm my baby.'

While it's true that a severe asthmatic condition does put a pregnancy at higher risk, studies have shown that this risk can be almost completely eliminated. Asthmatics who are under close, experienced medical supervision (preferably by their internist and/or allergist in collaboration with their obstetrician) thoughout their pregnancies have as good a chance of having normal pregnancies and healthy babies as non-asthmatics. But though asthma, if treated, has only a minimal effect on pregnancy, pregnancy often has a considerable effect on asthma. With about one third of pregnant asthmatics, the

effect is positive – their asthma improves. In another third, their condition remains about the same. In the final third (usually those with the most severe disease) the asthma worsens, generally after the fourth month.

No matter how mild or severe your condition, it will benefit from good care:

☆ Get your asthma under control before conception or, if that wasn't done, early in pregnancy.

☆ Identify possible triggering factors. The most common offenders are pollens, animal fur, dust, and moulds. Tobacco smoke, household cleaning products, and perfumes can also provoke trouble and it's a good idea to steer clear of these irritants. (See Allergies, page 140, for tips on avoiding such allergens.) Attacks brought on by exercise can be prevented by taking the proper medicines, as prescribed by your doctor, prior to exerting yourself. If your doctor began immunotherapy (allergy shots) for your allergies before pregnancy, treatment will probably be continued. A new series, however, is not likely to be initiated during gestation.

☆ Try to avoid colds, flu, and other respiratory infections. (See page 70.)

☆ If you have an asthma attack, treat it immediately with prescribed medication, to avoid cutting off oxygen to the foetus.

☆ Take only drugs prescribed by your physician *during pregnancy*, and take them only as prescribed *for pregnancy use.* If your symptoms are mild, you may not require medication. If they are moderate to severe, there are several medications, both inhaled and ingested, that are considered to be 'probably safe' for the foetus. The risks of taking these medications, if any, are quite small compared to the benefits of preventing foetal hypoxia (too little oxygen).

☆ Reduce other pregnancy risk factors. Since pregnancy risks are cumulative, you should endeavour to eliminate or minimize as many as possible. (See Reducing Risk in Any Pregnancy, page 57.)

The normal breathlessness that afflicts a majority of women in late pregnancy (see page 210) may be alarming to the asthmatic mother-to-be, but it is not dangerous. In the last trimester, as breathing becomes more laboured because of the enlarged uterus crowding the lungs, pregnant asthmatics may notice a worsening of asthmatic flareups. Proper treatment is especially important during such attacks.

The tendency toward allergies and asthma is inherited, and so it is wise for asthmatics to breastfeed their newborns exclusively for at least six months to delay the onset of allergic sensitization in their children.

Rh Incompatibility

'My doctor said the blood tests show I am Rh negative and my partner is Rh positive. He said not to worry, but my mother lost her second child because of Rh disease.'

Every pregnant woman is tested to determine whether her blood is Rh positive (has the dominant Rh factor) or negative (lacking the factor). These blood factors are inherited, and if a woman is Rh positive (85% are), or if both she and her partner are negative, there is no cause for further concern. If, however, a woman is Rh negative and her partner is positive, then all her pregnancies must be kept under careful obstetrical surveillance.

When your mother had children, the problem of Rh incompatibility was indeed an ominous one. But thanks to several medical advances, worry is now unwarranted.

First of all, if this is your first pregnancy, there is very little threat to the baby. Trouble doesn't start brewing until the Rh factor enters the mother's circulatory system during a delivery (or abortion or miscarriage) of a child who has inherited the Rh factor from his or her father. The mother, in a protective immune reaction to the 'foreign' substance, develops antibodies. The antibodies themselves are harmless, until she becomes pregnant again. If the next baby is Rh positive, the mother's antibodies can cross the placenta into the foetal system, where they attack the foetal red blood cells. This can cause very mild to very serious anaemia in the foetus, depending on the antibody levels in the mother. Rarely, antibodies can form in first pregnancies, when foetal blood leaks through the placenta into the mother's circulatory system.

Today, prevention of the development of Rh antibodies is the key to protecting the foetus when there is Rh incompatibility. Most doctors use a two-pronged attack. At 28 weeks, an expectant Rh-negative woman who shows no antibodies in her blood is given a dose of Rh-immune globulin. Another dose is administered within 72 hours of delivery or miscarriage. If the pregnancy ends in elective abortion, this vaccine is also administered.

If tests determine that a woman has developed Rh antibodies previously, amniocentesis (see page 53) can be used to check the blood type of the foetus. If it is Rh positive, and thus incompatible with the mother's, a close watch is kept on the condition of the foetus and on the mother's antibody levels. If problems seem imminent, an exchange of blood, replacing the foetus's Rh positive and Rh negative, *may* be necessary. When the incompatibility is severe, which is rare, the foetal transfusion can take place while the foetus is still in the uterus. More often, it can wait until immediately after delivery. In mild cases, when antibody levels are low, a transfusion may not be needed. But doctors will be ready to do one at delivery if necessary.

The use of Rh vaccines has reduced the need for transfusions in Rh incompatible pregnancies to less than 1%, and in the next few years may make this lifesaving procedure a modern medical miracle of the past.

Herpes

'I was anxious for a positive pregnancy test; but now that I am definitely pregnant, I'm terrified because I have genital herpes.'

Herpes has generated more frightening headlines in the past few years than almost any other disease. This presently incurable infection may soon surpass gonorrhoea and chlamydia as the most common sexually transmitted disease. Herpes in adults can be extremely painful, but it is relatively benign. It can, however, be deadly in a newborn infant, who has contracted the disease en route through the birth canal of an infected mother. Fortunately, such infection of infants, though on the increase, is still relatively rare (about 1 in 1,000) and, with proper medical care, avoidable. Today a woman with herpes need not pass on anything but her brown hair or her green eyes.

The twin keys to protecting the baby – whether it's the mother or her partner who is affected – are strict medical supervision and good personal hygiene:

☆ See an obstetrician regularly, starting before you conceive, or as early in pregnancy as possible.

☆ Refrain from sexual intercourse if you or your partner have an active infection.

☆ Wash your hands thoroughly with mild soap and water after using the toilet or having sexual relations; bathe or shower daily.

☆ Keep any lesions clean and dry, dusted with cornflour.

☆ Wear cotton underpants; avoid garments that are constricting in the crotch area.

☆ Have a weekly viral culture (a smear of vaginal secretions is taken and tested) from the 34th or 36th week on, so that the presence or absence of an active infection can be determined before delivery.

The odds are good that you won't have an active infection at delivery, in which case there should be no problem. If, however, it turns out that your infection flares up when you're ready to deliver (your physician can determine this through examination or by recent positive cultures), you will almost certainly be delivered by caesarean section. This will assure that your baby won't become infected.

Other STDs (Sexually Transmitted Diseases)

'I've heard that herpes can be dangerous to the foetus. Is this also true of other sexually transmitted diseases?'

The bad news: Yes, there are other STDs that present a hazard to the foetus. The good news. They are easily tested for and treated. Gonorrhoea has long been known to cause conjunctivitis, blindness, and serious generalized infection in the foetus allowed to deliver through an infected birth canal. For this reason, pregnant women are routinely tested for the disease at their first antenatal visit (see page 98). If disease is found, it is treated immediately with antibiotics. As an added precaution, drops of silver nitrate are squeezed into every newborn's eyes at birth.

The bone and tooth deformities, the progressive nervous system damage, the stillbirths, and the delayed brain damage caused by syphilis have long been recognized, too. And testing for this disease is also routine at the first prenatal visit. Antibiotic treatment before the fifth month, when the infection usually begins to cross the placental barrier, will prevent damage to the foetus.

More recently recognized as a potential danger to the foetus is chlamydia, an STD that is now being reported at clinics much more frequently than gonorrhoea. Like untreated gonorrhoea, the most devastating effect of untreated chlamydia is infertility, but there is also risk of eye infection or pneumonia in a baby born to an infected mother. These newborn infections are treatable, but they can be prevented entirely if the mother is given appropriate antibiotic therapy before delivery. A woman who believes she may have been infected with chlamydia (particularly if her partner is infected) should ask to be tested for the disease promptly.

An IUD Still In Place

'I've been wearing an IUD for two years and just discovered that I'm pregnant. We want to be able to keep the baby; is it possible?'

Getting pregnant while using birth control is always a little unsettling, but it does happen. The odds of it happening with an IUD are 1 to 5 in 100, depending on the type of device used and whether or not it has been properly inserted. A woman who conceives with an IUD in place and doesn't want to terminate her pregnancy has two choices – which she should discuss as soon as possible with her doctor: leaving the IUD in place or having the IUD removed. According to the research, her chances of delivering a full-term baby are better with the second choice, particularly when the IUD is removed as soon as possible after pregnancy is confirmed. When the IUD, with its removal-string protruding from the cervix, is left in for the term of the pregnancy, there is a significant chance that the foetus will spontaneously miscarry;[1] when it's removed, the risk is only 20%. If that doesn't sound reassuring, keep in mind that the rate of miscarriage in all known pregnancies is estimated to be about 15% to 20%.

If you do continue your pregnancy with your IUD left in, you should, during the first trimester, be especially alert for such signs as bleeding, cramps, or fever, because the IUD puts you at higher risk for early pregnancy complications. (See Ectopic Pregnancy, page 105, and Miscarriage, page 106.) Notify your doctor of such symptoms promptly.

Birth Control Pills in Pregnancy

'I got pregnant while using birth control pills. I kept taking them for over a month because I had no idea I was pregnant. Now I'm worried about the effect this may have on my baby.'

Ideally, you should stop using oral contraceptives three months, or for at least two normally occurring menstrual cycles, before you want to become pregnant. But conception doesn't always wait for ideal conditions, and occasionally a woman becomes pregnant while taking the Pill. In spite of what you might have read on drug insert warnings, there's no reason for alarm. Statistically, there is a very slightly increased risk of certain types of foetal malformation when the mother has conceived while on oral contraceptives, but certainly not enough to warrant eight months of worry. A discussion of the subject with your practitioner should relieve your concern.

Spermicides

'I conceived while using a spermicide with my diaphragm, and used it several times again before I knew I was pregnant. Could the chemicals have damaged the sperm before conception, or the embryo after it?'

It is estimated that between 300,000 and 600,000 women who become pregnant each year used spermicides around the time of conception and/or in the early weeks of pregnancy before finding out that they'd conceived. So the question of what effects spermicides may have during conception and pregnancy is of great significance to a great many expectant couples – and to those choosing a method of birth control.

Fortunately, the answers so far have been reassuring. No more than a tentative link has ever been suggested between the use of spermicides and the incidence of certain birth defects, specifically Down's syndrome and

---

1. If, however, the removal-string is not protruding from the cervix, the risk of miscarriage is reduced, and it may be safer to leave the IUD in place.

limb deformities. And the most recent and most convincing studies indicate that spermicides are probably *not* teratogenic, or damaging, to the unborn child. So according to the best information available, you and the other 299,000 to 599,999 mothers-to-be can relax – there appears to be nothing to worry about.

You may however, be more comfortable with a different, and perhaps more reliable, method of birth control in the future. And because any chemical exposure of embryo or foetus is suspect, if you do continue to use a spermicide, you should plan on terminating its use before you decide to become pregnant again.

Provera

'Last month my doctor gave me Provera to bring on a late period. It turns out that I was pregnant. The package insert warns that pregnant women should never take this drug. Could my baby be malformed? Should I consider an abortion?'

Having taken the progesterone drug Provera during pregnancy, though it isn't recommended, is no reason to consider an abortion – as your obstetrician will probably tell you. It's not even a reason to worry. The drug company's warnings are not only for your protection, but for theirs: to protect themselves in case of a lawsuit. It's true that some studies show a 1 in 1,000 risk of certain birth defects when an embryo or foetus has been exposed to Provera, but that is only minimally higher than the same defects occurring in any pregnancy.

Whether Provera actually does cause birth defects or not isn't even certain. Some doctors who use Provera to prevent miscarriage believe that it only *seems* to cause defects – by occasionally helping a woman to sustain a blighted pregnancy that would have otherwise miscarried. It will probably take years more study on hundreds of thousands of pregnant women to determine definitely the effects – if any – of progesterone drugs on the foetus. But from what is presently known, it is believed that if Provera is actually a teratogen, it is a very weak one (see Playing Baby Roulette, page 78). Cross this one off your worry list.

DES

'My mother took DES when she was pregnant with me. Can this affect my pregnancy or my baby in any way?'

Before the dangers of using the synthetic oestrogen drug diethylstilbestrol (DES) to prevent miscarriage were known, more than a million pregnant women took it. Now that their daughters, many of whom were born with structural abnormalities of the reproductive tract (the majority so slight that they are of no gynaecological or obstetrical significance), are of childbearing age, they are concerned about the effects DES exposure will have on their own pregnancies. Happily, these effects appear to be minimal – it is estimated that at least 80% of DES-exposed women have been able to have children. However, when the abnormalities are serious, there appears to be an increased risk of ectopic pregnancy, miscarriage (particularly midtrimester), and premature delivery. Ectopic pregnancy is uncommon, even among DES-exposed women. But because it could be life threatening, it is important to be aware of the symptoms and to get emergency medical attention immediately if they occur.

Though nothing can be done to save an ectopic pregnancy, it is possible to head off a late miscarriage or premature birth. These complications are generally related to an incompetent, or weakened, cervix. (See page 36 for treatment). Threatened premature labour can also often be successfully postponed with bed rest and the use of labour-halting drugs. To be sure that your cervix will be carefully monitored throughout your pregnancy (weekly or bi-weekly pelvic examinations may be necessary), let your obstetrician[2] know of your DES exposure at your first visit.

Genetic Problems

'I keep worrying that I might have a genetic problem and not know it. Should I get genetic counselling?'

Probably all of us carry one or more deleterious genes for mild or serious genetic disorders. But fortunately, because most disorders (for example, Tay-Sachs or cystic fibrosis) require a matching one-from-mum, one-from-dad pair of genes – an unlikely possibility – they rarely manifest themselves in our children. One or

2. Because of the slightly increased risk of complications. DES-exposed women are probably better off with an obstetrician overseeing their pregnancy care.

both parents can be tested for some of these disorders before or during pregnancy. But testing only makes sense if there is a better-than-average possibility that both parents are carriers of a particular disorder. The clue is often ethnic or geographic origin. Jewish couples, for example, whose families came originally from eastern Europe should be tested for Tay Sachs. (In most cases, a practitioner will recommend a test for one parent; the second test is necessary only if the first is positive.) Black couples can be tested for the sickle cell anaemia trait.

The diseases that can be passed on by one carrier parent (haemophilia), or by one affected parent (Huntington's chorea), have usually turned up in the family before and should be common knowledge. That's why it's important to keep records of family health histories.

Most expectant parents, happily, are at low risk for having genetic problems and need never see a genetic counsellor. In many cases, an obstetrician will talk to a couple about the most common issues, referring to a genetic counsellor those with a need for more expertise:

☆ Couples whose blood tests show them both to be carriers of a genetic disorder.

☆ Parents who have already borne one or more children with genetic birth defects.

☆ Couples who know of hereditary defects on any branch of either of their family trees.

☆ Closely related couples, because the risk of inherited disease in offspring is greatest when parents are related (for example, 1 in 8 for first cousins).

☆ Women over 35.

A genetic counsellor is a sort of heredity bookmaker, trained to give such couples the odds of bearing a healthy child and to guide them in deciding whether or not to have children. If they are already pregnant, the counsellor can suggest appropriate prenatal testing.

Genetic counselling has saved hundreds of thousands of high-risk couples from the heartbreak of bearing children with genetic or other serious problems. The best time to see a genetic counsellor is before getting pregnant, or in the case of close relatives, before getting married. But it's not too late after pregnancy is confirmed. Consult your GP if you would like to have such counselling.

If testing uncovers a serious defect in a foetus, the expectant parents are faced with the decision of whether or not to continue with the pregnancy. Though the decision is theirs, a genetic counsellor can provide important input.

WHAT IT'S IMPORTANT TO KNOW: ABOUT PRENATAL DIAGNOSIS

Is it a boy – or a girl? Will it have blond hair like grandma, green eyes like grandpa? Daddy's voice and Mummy's flair for figures or – heaven forbid! – the other way around? The questions of pregnancy far outnumber the answers, providing lively material for nine months of dinner table debate, neighbourhood speculation, and office pools.

But there's one question that isn't a topic for casual wagering. It's one most parents hesitate to talk about at all: 'Is my baby okay?'

Until recently, that question, like that of the colour of a baby's hair and eyes, could be answered only at birth. Today some (no doubt in the future it will be all) such questions are being answered as early as six weeks after conception, through prenatal diagnosis.

Because of inherent risks, small as they are, prenatal diagnosis isn't for everyone. Most parents will continue to play the waiting game, with the happy assurance that the odds are overwhelming that their babies are indeed 'okay.' But for those whose concerns represent more than normal prenatal jitters – whose age, health status, or family history makes their chances of having a baby who isn't okay greater than average – the benefits of prenatal diagnosis can far outweigh its risks.

In more than 95% of cases, prenatal diagnosis turns up no apparent abnormalities. In the remainder, the expectant couple's discovery that something is wrong with their baby isn't comforting. But, teamed with professional advice, the information can be used to make vital decisions about this and future pregnancies. Options include:

A Therapeutic Abortion. If testing

suggests a defect that is fatal or very disabling, and interpretation and/or retesting by a genetic counsellor confirms the diagnosis, many parents opt for terminating the pregnancy. Most after consulting with genetic counsellors, try again, with hopes that test results – and thus pregnancy outcome – will turn out favourable the next time around.

Continuing the Pregnancy. For some parents, an abortion just isn't an option – no matter how seriously handicapped their baby may be. Assuming the third option (see below) isn't available in their case, prenatal diagnosis gives them the advantage of being able to prepare themselves emotionally and practically for the birth of a child with special needs.

Prenatal Treatment of the Foetus. This option is available in only a few instances, though in the future it can be expected to become more and more common. Treatment may consist of blood transfusion (as in Rh disease), surgery (to drain an obstructed bladder, for instance), or administration of enzymes or medication (such as steroids to accelerate lung development in the foetus who must be delivered.)

The most commonly used methods of prenatal diagnosis follow.

Amniocentesis

The cells shed by the growing foetus into the amniotic fluid make this solution a reliable indicator of the foetal condition in the uterus. Thus, being able to extract some of the fluid

through amniocentesis so that foetal cells can be cultured (grown) and examined for genetic defects is one of the most important advances in prenatal diagnosis. It is recommended when:

☆ The mother is over age 35. Between 80% and 90% of all amniocentesis is performed solely on the basis of advanced maternal age, primarily to determine if the foetus has Down's syndrome, which is most prevalent among children of older mothers.

☆ The couple has already had a child with a chromosomal abnormality, such as Down's syndrome, or with a metabolic disorder, such as Hunter's syndrome.

☆ The couple has already had a child or has a relative with a neural tube defect. (A test to determine alphafoetoprotein, or AFP, levels in the mother's blood will probably be performed first.)

☆ The mother is a carrier of an x-linked genetic disorder, such as haemophilia, which she has a 50-50 chance of passing on to any son she bears. Amniocentesis can identify the sex of the foetus, although not whether the baby is affected. Foetoscopy (see page 56) can, however, detect some of these disorders.

☆ Both parents are carriers of autosomal recessive inherited disorders, such as Tay-Sachs disease or sickle cell anaemia, and thus have a 1 in 4 chance of bearing an affected child.

☆ It is necessary to assess the maturity of the foetal lungs (among the last organs ready to function on their own) when an early delivery is contemplated to protect the well-being of mother of child.

When Is It Done? Diagnostic second-trimester amniocentesis is usually performed between the 16th and 18th weeks of pregnancy, though occasionally as early as the 14th or as late as the 20th week. Earlier than this there would be insufficient amniotic fluid; later might prove too late for an abortion should a defect be detected. Most tests, because cells must be cultured in the laboratory, take from 24 to 35 days to be completed, though a few, such as for Tay-Sachs disease, Hunter's syndrome, and neural tube defects, can be performed immediately.

Amniocentesis can also be performed in the last trimester to assess the maturity of foetal lungs.

How Is It Done? After changing into a hospital gown and emptying her bladder, the expectant mother is positioned on the examining table on her back, her body draped so that only her abdomen is exposed. The foetus and placenta are then located via ultrasound, so that the doctor will be able to steer clear of them during the procedure. The abdomen is shaved, swabbed with antiseptic solution, and numbed with an injection (the only painful part of the procedure) of a local anaesthetic, similar to the novocaine used by dentists. Then a long, hollow needle (the only scary part of the procedure) is inserted through the abdominal wall into the uterus, and a small amount of amniotic fluid is with-

drawn. The mother's vital signs and the foetal heart tones are checked before and after the procedure, which, from start to finish, shouldn't take more than an hour.

Unless it is a necessary part of the diagnosis, parents have the option not to be told their baby's sex when the report comes back, but to find out the old-fashioned way, in the delivery room. (Keep in mind that mix-ups, though rare, do happen.)

How Safe Is It? Most women experience no more than a few hours of cramping after the procedure; rarely there is slight vaginal bleeding or amniotic fluid leak. Although fewer than 1 in 200 women experience infection or other complications that lead to miscarriage, amniocentesis, like most other prenatal diagnostic tests, should be performed only when the benefits outweigh the risks.

Ultrasound

The advent of ultrasound has made obstetrics a much more precise science and pregnancy much less worrisome for many expectant parents. Through the use of sound waves which bounce off internal structures, it allows visualization of the foetus without the hazards of x-ray. If the apparatus used has a TV-like viewing screen, it provides a unique opportunity to 'see' your baby – and maybe even get a photo to show to friends and family – though it may take an expert to make heads or buttocks out of the blurry image.

Ultrasound may be recommended when the mother has a poor obstetrical history; for example, when she's had an ectopic (tubal) pregnancy, a hydatidiform mole (the placenta developed into a grape-like bunch of cysts which couldn't support an embryo), delivered a baby with birth defects or genetic disease, or had a caesarean section. It may also be used to:

☆ Rule out pregnancy by the seventh week if there's been a suspected false-positive test result.

☆ Determine causes for bleeding or spotting in early pregnancy, such as a tubal pregnancy or a blighted ovum (an embryo that has stopped developing and is no longer viable).

☆ Locate an IUD that was in place at the time of conception.

☆ Verify a due date by checking to see if it correlates with the baby's size.

☆ Locate the foetus prior to amniocentesis and during chorionic villi biopsy (see page 58).

☆ Determine the baby's condition if no heartbeat has been detected by the 14th week with a Doppler device, or no foetal movement by the 22nd week.

☆ Diagnose the existence of multiple foetuses, especially when the mother has taken fertility drugs and/or the uterus is larger than expected.

☆ Determine if rapid uterine growth is due to an excess of amniotic fluid.

☆ Determine the condition of the placenta. A deteriorating placenta, which does not nourish the foetus adequately, might be responsible for retarded foetal growth or foetal distress. Early delivery may be necessary.

☆ Determine if bleeding late in pregnancy is due to placenta praevia, in which the placenta implants near or over the cervix.

☆ Evaluate the maturity of a foetus when early delivery, either induced or by caesarean, is being contemplated; or to evaluate the condition of a foetus that is believed to be postmature.

☆ Verify breech presentation or other uncommon foetal position prior to delivery.

When Is It Done? Depending on the indication, ultrasound is performed any time from the fifth week of gestation until delivery.

How Is It Done? The procedure itself is painless (except for the discomfort of a full bladder), and quick (5 to 10 minutes).

During the exam, the expectant mother lies on her back and her bare abdomen is spread with a film of oil or gel that improves conduction of sound. A transducer is then moved slowly over the abdomen, recording echoes as the sound waves bounce off parts of the baby. It may be possible, with the doctor's help, to see the beating of the heart, the curve of the spine, the head and arms and legs – depending on the position of the foetus. Sometimes even the genital organs are visible and the sex can be surmised. (If you don't want to know your baby's sex yet, inform the doctor in advance.)

How Safe Is It? In 25 years of clinical use and study, no known risks and a great many benefits have been associated with the use of ultrasound photography. Still, because risks may yet show up in the future, it is the position of a panel of experts who examined the use of ultrasound in pregnancy for the National Institutes of Health that the procedure should be used only when valid indications exist.

Foetoscopy

Foetoscopy is science fiction turning fast into medical fact. In a voyage as fantastic as any penned by Isaac Asimov, a miniaturized, telescope-like instrument, complete with lights and lenses, is inserted through a tiny incision in the abdomen into the amniotic sac, where it can view and photograph the foetus. At the same time, foetoscopy allows the diagnosis, through tissue and blood sampling, of several diseases which amniocentesis can't detect. Still a relatively new procedure, its usefulness in certain high-risk pregnancies is speeding its acceptance in the obstetrical community. It is most commonly recommended when there is a family history of a blood disease, particularly when one or both parents are carriers, or of certain skin disorders.

When Is It Done? Usually after the 16th week.

How Is It Done? After the abdo-men is swabbed with antiseptic and numbed with a local anaesthetic, a tiny incision is made in the abdomen. With ultrasound monitoring to guide the instrument, a fibreoptic endo-scope is passed through the incision into the uterus. With this miniature periscope, the foetus, placenta, and amniotic fluid can be observed, blood samples can be taken from the junction of the umbilical cord and the placenta, and/or a tiny bit of foetal or placental tissue removed for examination (a biopsy).

How Safe Is It? Foetoscopy is, at this point, still a relatively risky procedure, carrying between a 3% and 5% chance of foetal loss. Though this risk is greater than with other diagnostic tests, it is outweighed for the occasional woman who needs it by the benefit of discovering, and possibly treating, a defect in her foetus.

Alpha-Foetoprotein Screening

Elevated levels in the mother's blood of alpha-foetoprotein (AFP), a substance produced by the foetus, can indicate a neural tube defect, such as spina bifida (a deformity of the spinal column) or anencephaly (an absence of all or part of the brain). But since AFP levels may also be abnormally high because of a multiple pregnancy or a miscalculation of due date (levels increase later in pregnancy), the test yields many false-positives, which can prompt pregnant women to unnecessarily abort a normal foetus or foetuses.

When Is It Done? Between the 16th and 18th weeks.

How Is It Done? The first screening step is a simple maternal blood test. If AFP levels are found to be high, a second test is run. If levels are still high, then a series of follow-up procedures – including amniocentesis to obtain AFP levels in the amniotic

---

Reducing Risk in Any Pregnancy

Good Medical Care. Even a low-risk pregnancy is put at high risk if prenatal care is absent or poor. Seeing a qualified practitioner regularly, beginning as soon as pregnancy is suspected, is vital for all expectant mothers. Choose an obstetrician experienced with your particular condition if you are in a high-risk category. But just as important as having a good doctor is being a good patient. Be an active participant in your medical care – ask questions, report symptoms – but don't try to be your own doctor. (See Your Choices In Medical Care, page 28.)

Good Diet. The Best-Odds Diet (see page 82) gives every pregnant woman the best odds of having a successful pregnancy and a healthy baby. It may also help to prevent gestational diabetes, hypertension, and preeclampsia.

Fitness. It's best to begin pregnancy with a well-toned, exercised body, but it's never too late to start deriving the benefits of fitness. Regular exercise prevents constipation and improves respiration, circulation, muscle tone, and skin elasticity, all of which contribute to a more comfortable pregnancy and an easier, safer delivery. (see page 166.)

Sensible Weight Gain. A gradual, steady, and moderate weight gain may help prevent a variety of complications, including diabetes, hypertension, varicose veins, haemorrhoids, low birth weight, or difficult delivery due to an overly large foetus. (See page 132.)

No Smoking. Quitting as early in pregnancy as possible reduces the many risks to mother and baby, including prematurity and low birth weight. (See page 63.)

Abstinence From Alcohol. Drinking very rarely or not at all will reduce the risk of birth defects, particularly of foetal alcohol syndrome, the result of high alcohol intake. (See page 62.)

Avoidance of Drugs. So little is known about the effects of drugs on foetal development that it is best to avoid taking any during pregnancy that are not absolutely essential and prescribed by your doctor.

Prevention of and Prompt Treatment for Infection. All infections – from common flu to urinary tract and vaginal infections to the increasingly common venereal diseases – should be prevented whenever possible. When contracted, however, infection should be treated promptly by a doctor who knows you are pregnant.

Being Wary of the Superwoman Syndrome. Often well established in their careers and highly motivated in everything they do, today's mothers tend to be overachievers and overdoers. Getting enough rest during pregnancy is far more important than getting everything done, especially in high-risk pregnancies. Don't wait until your body starts pleading for relief before you slow down. If your doctor recommends that you begin your maternity leave earlier than you'd planned, take the advice. Some studies have suggested a higher incidence of premature delivery among women who work up until term, particularly if their job entails physical labour or long periods of standing.

fluid, and ultrasound to view the foetus – are performed to determine whether or not a neural tube defect actually exists. Out of 50 women with high readings on the initial blood test, only 1 or 2 will eventually be shown to have an affected foetus. In the other 48, the tests will show that there is more than one foetus, or that the pregnancy is further along than at first believed, or that the original readings were inaccurate.

How Safe Is It? The initial screening test poses no more risk to mother or baby than any other blood test. The major risk of the test is that a false positive result may lead to follow-up procedures that do present some risk – and in some cases, to therapeutic abortions of perfectly normal foetuses. To be sure that the diagnosis is accurate, all tests should be performed only by trained personnel using sophisticated equipment and results should be evaluated by an experienced doctor or competent genetic counsellor.

Chorionic Villi Sampling

Unlike amniocentesis, chorionic villi sampling (CVS) can detect foetal defects very early in pregnancy, when abortion is a less complicated and traumatic procedure. In certain cases (in the future, possibly in most), defects can be treated in utero, and healthy, normal babies delivered at term. Some experts believe CVS will become a routine screening procedure and will replace amniocentesis before the end of the decade.

Eventually, chorionic villi sampling will be able to detect virtually all of the 3,800 or so disorders for which a defective gene is responsible. At present, it is useful only in conditions where the detection technology exists. The indications for use are the same as those for amniocentesis, though CVS is not used to assess foetal lung maturity.

When Is It Done? Usually between the 8th and 12th week, sometimes as early as the 5th.

How Is It Done? This painless procedure may one day be performed routinely in a physician's office. At the moment it is done in major medical centres only. With the expectant mother on an examining table, a long thin catheter (tube) is inserted into her uterus through the vagina. Guided by a picture of the procedure on an ultrasound monitor, the doctor positions the catheter between the uterine lining and the chorion, the foetal membrane which will eventually form the foetal part of the placenta. A sampling of the chorionic villi (finger-like projections from this membrane) is then snipped or suctioned off for diagnostic study.

Since the villi, like the chorion, are of foetal origin, examining them can give a complete picture of the genetic makeup of the developing foetus. Because many cells are collected in CVS, cell study can take place immediately, and not after weeks of culturing, as is usually the case with amniocentesis.

How Safe Is It? This procedure was only recently introduced and its safety is still being evaluated. The chorionic villi, from which the cells are taken for the test, disappear as the foetus matures, so there is believed to be no danger in removing them. Some researchers have found no increased risk of foetal loss from the test; others speculate that the margin of risk will prove similar to that of amniocentesis, with about 1 in 200 women experiencing a complication leading to miscarriage. Most of the foetuses that have miscarried after chorionic biopsy were found to have serious defects, which were probably responsible for the spontaneous abortions.

3
Throughout Your Pregnancy

WHAT YOU MAY BE CONCERNED ABOUT

Pregnant women have always worried. What about, however, has changed considerably over the generations, as obstetrical medicine – and expectant parents – find out more and more about what does and does not affect the health and well-being of our unborn. Our grandmothers, vulnerable to a variety of old wives' tales, feared that seeing a monkey while pregnant would result in monkey-like offspring, or that slapping their bellies in fright would leave their babies with hand-shaped birthmarks. We, vulnerable instead to a daily deluge of modern media tales (usually as frightening, sometimes as unfounded), have other fears: Am I breathing in too much polluted air or drinking unsafe water? Is my job, or my husband's smoking, or that cup of coffee I had this morning hazardous to my baby's health?

What about that X-ray I had at the dentist's? As a basis for worry, these concerns can make pregnancy unnecessarily nervewracking. As a basis for action, they can give you a better sense of control and greatly improve the odds of your having a healthy baby.

'I have the terrible fear that my baby will be stillborn.'

That's not an unusual fear, though some women – and their partners – may be hesitant even to express it. However, it's a fear that today seldom becomes a reality. With such equipment as the foetal monitor to detect distress early on and quick rescues possible via caesarean section, it is rare for a foetus to die during delivery. The stillborn is more likely to die before birth, often because of some serious defect. Such death in utero is also rare, but it is generally easily detectable because the foetus stops moving. (See page 136 for checking foetal movement and when to report changes to your doctor.) As long as your baby keeps gently (or not so gently) jabbing you in the ribs and poking you in the pelvis, you can relax.

If the unthinkable happens and a foetus dies in utero, the couple will often be given time to grieve a bit at home before coming to the hospital to prepare themselves for labour. Depending upon the situation, labour may be induced almost immediately on the diagnosis of the foetal death or it may be allowed to begin naturally, which often happens within a few days. Delivery will progress normally.

Many midwives and doctors encourage patients to hold and greet their baby, and give him or her a name. This gives the parents a feeling of completion and makes grieving easier. But, of course, this is a decision the couple must make for themselves. They must also decide whether they want to arrange funeral services, or leave arrangements to the hospital.

The woman will receive her postnatal care either on the postnatal ward (in a side room if at all possible) or at home, according to her individual needs. She won't be anxious to see other newborns and their happy parents during this difficult time.

It is natural for the couple to be very upset about the loss of a baby and important for them to allow themselves to mourn. The woman particularly, because of her physical condition, will require a lot of support from family and friends. But her part-

ner should not be ignored. He is suffering, too.

A useful organisation to contact is:

SANDS (Stillbirth and Neo-natal Death Society),
Argyle House,
29–31 Euston Road,
London NW1 2SD

01–833 2851

'I'm worried that my baby will be handicapped.'

Far greater than a preference for a boy or a girl, for golden curls or a golden singing voice, for natural aptitude in athletics or in mathematics, is every parent-to-be's wish for a normal baby. Few expectant couples have gone through an entire pregnancy without the nagging fear that this wish won't be realized, and that their baby will be born with a handicap. Yet for the vast majority, this will never happen; and the odds are excellent that your baby, too, will be born completely healthy and normal.

If, however, your baby is born with a handicap, it's reassuring to know that with today's medical advances, many handicaps can be overcome or minimized. If your baby is born with a problem, it may be necessary for him or her to be taken to the SCBU (special care baby unit) soon after birth. If it's at all possible, the parents will be given a chance to cuddle and greet the infant in the delivery room first. If, however, immediate medical attention is necessary and the baby is moved to the SCBU before they've had this opportunity, they shouldn't fret. Bonding with a newborn can take place later (see page 292).

Both parents will be given every opportunity to visit and care for their baby in SCBU. A hospital paediatrician will be available to discuss the infant's illness and the likely course of treatment. If there is more than one option, that will be explained.

Parents will be linked up with any support groups that exist, either in their own communities or nationally, for parents of children with similar handicaps. Such contact gives them the opportunity to share their fears, their feelings, and their plans with those in like circumstances. When the couple returns home with their baby, the community midwife and health visitor will be able to advise them about further help that is available.

Alcohol

'I had a few drinks on several occasions before I knew I was pregnant. I'm afraid that alcohol may have harmed my baby.'

'Behold, thou shalt conceive, and bear a son; and now drink no wine or strong drink,' Samuel tells Hannah in the biblical book of Judges. Lucky Hannah. She was able to start ordering Perrier when Samson was just a gleam in his father's eye. But not many of us receive such advance notice of our pregnancies. And because we're often unaware that we're pregnant until we are into our second month, we're apt to have done things we wouldn't have done if only we had known. Like having a few, a few times too often. Which is why this concern is one of the most common brought to the first prenatal visit.

Fortunately, it's also one of the concerns that can most easily be put aside. There's no evidence that a few drinks on a couple of occasions early in pregnancy will prove harmful to your baby. And one recent study showed that women who had had two or three such drinking binges early in pregnancy weren't any more likely to have babies with structural defects or growth retardation than teetotalers.

Heavy daily doses of alcohol throughout pregnancy, such as those consumed by heavy drinkers or alcoholics, however, *are* connected with a wide variety of problems, including foetal alcohol syndrome (FAS) – a condition in which infants are born undersized, usually mentally deficient, with multiple deformities (particularly of the head and face, the limbs, and the central nervous system) and a high neonatal mortality rate. What 'heavy drinker' means varies from study to study, but it's generally considered to be a person who consumes five or six drinks – beer, wine, or distilled spirits – a day. The risks are certainly dose related: The more you drink, the more potential danger to your baby. And they are compounded by other drug use.

But even at lower daily intakes throughout pregnancy, alcohol appears to cause a variety of very serious problems, including increased risk of miscarriage, prematurity, complications during labour and delivery, and possible developmental lags in later infancy and childhood. Though many women manage to drink lightly during pregnancy – one glass of wine nightly, for instance – and still deliver healthy babies, there is no assurance that this is a wise practice. The safe daily alcohol dose in pregnancy, if any, is not known.

That's partly because each foetus, like each mother, has a different genetic makeup and responds differently to drugs like alcohol. And since alcohol enters the foetal bloodstream in approximately the same concentrations present in the mother's blood, each drink a pregnant woman takes is shared with her baby. This leads us to suggest that although you shouldn't worry about what you've already had to drink, it would be prudent to stop drinking for the rest of your pregnancy – except perhaps for a celebratory glass of wine on a birthday or anniversary. (Always taken *with* a meal, since food reduces the absorption of alcohol.)

That's as easily done as said for some women – those who develop a distaste for alcohol in early pregnancy which may linger through delivery. For others, particularly those who habitually 'unwind' with cocktails or take wine with dinner, abstinence may require a concerted effort, possibly including a change in lifestyle. If you drink to relax, for example, try substituting other methods of relaxation: music, warm baths, massage, exercise, reading. If drinking is part of a daily ritual that you don't want to give up, try a Virgin Mary (a Bloody Mary minus the vodka) at brunch, sparkling fruit juices or non-alcoholic malt beverages at dinner, a grapefruit or orange juice spritzer (half juice, half seltzer, with a twist) or a Mock Strawberry Daiquiri or Virgin Sangria (see page 96) at cocktail hour – served at the accustomed time, in the accustomed glasses, with the accustomed ceremony. If your husband joins you on the wagon (at least while in your company), the ride will be considerably smoother.

The sooner a heavy drinker stops drinking during pregnancy, the less risk to her baby. The heavy drinker who refuses to abstain or to seek help from Alcoholics Anonymous[1] or an alcoholism clinic is often advised to consider terminating her pregnancy.

Cigarette Smoking

'I've been smoking for 10 years. Will this hurt my baby?'

Happily, there's no clear evidence that smoking prior to pregnancy – even 10 or 20 years of it – will harm a developing foetus. But it's well documented that continuing to smoke during pregnancy – particularly beyond the fourth month – can cause a wide variety of antenatal complications, everything from miscarriage and bleeding early in the first trimester to premature separation of the placenta and premature rupture of the membranes in the last. There is also strong evidence that the expectant mother's smoking directly affects her baby's development in utero for the worse.

The most widespread risk is low birth weight, with all its concomitant dangers – especially perinatal death (just before, during, or after birth). But babies of three-pack-a-day smokers also have a quadrupled risk of low Apgar scores (the standard scale used to evaluate infants at birth), which means they just aren't as healthy as other babies. And there's evidence that, on the average, they may never catch up with the children of non-smokers, that they may have long-term physical and intellectual deficits, and may also be hyperactive. At age 14, one study showed, children of smokers tended to be more prone to respiratory disease, to be shorter than children of non-smokers, and to be less successful in school.

It was once believed that the reason for the difficulties these children display was poor prenatal nutrition: The mothers smoked rather than ate. But recent studies show this isn't the case; smoking mothers who eat as much and gain as much weight as non-smoking mothers still give birth to smaller babies. The cause seems to be carbon monoxide poisoning and a reduction of oxygen to the foetus through the placenta. Gaining a huge amount of weight – 40 pounds or more – may somewhat reduce the risk of a smoking mother having an undersized baby, but this excess weight poses other risks to the mother and child.

In effect, when you smoke, your baby is living in a smoke-filled womb. His heartbeat speeds, he coughs and sputters, and, worst of all, he can't grow and thrive as he should. Cutting down on the number of cigarettes you smoke may help just a bit: The more cigarettes you smoke, the greater the risk to your baby. But in most cases, cutting down is illusory because the smoker just compensates by taking more frequent and deeper puffs and smoking more of each cigarette, as she also does when she tries to reduce risk by using low-tar or low-nicotine cigarettes.

The news, however, isn't all bad. Some studies show that women who give up smoking early in pregnancy – no later than the fourth month – can reduce the risk of damage to the foetus to the level of the non-smoker. Sooner is better, but giving up even in the last month can help preserve oxygen flow to the baby during delivery. For some smoking women, giving up will never be easier than in early pregnancy, when they develop a sudden distaste for cigarettes – probably the warning of an intuitive body. If you're not lucky enough to have such a natural aversion, try giving up with the help of nicotine chewing gum or smoking cessation groups.[2]

You may experience withdrawal symptoms when you quit smoking; the exact symptoms vary from person to person. Some of the most common are a craving for tobacco, irritability, anxiety, restlessness, dullness, and sleep and gastrointestinal disturbances. Some people also find that concentration, judgment, and both physical and mental performance are impaired. In most cases, the symptoms won't last more than a few days, though occasionally some effects of withdrawal linger longer. The benefits, however, will last a lifetime – for you and your baby. (For more tips on habit breaking, see page 66.)

When Other People Smoke

'I gave up smoking, but my husband still goes through two packs a day. I keep worrying that somehow this may hurt our baby.'

2. Call your local Health Education Unit for information, or the National Society for Non Smokers (01–636 9103).

Smoking, it has become more and more apparent, doesn't just affect the person with the cigarette in his mouth – it affects everyone around him. Including a developing foetus whose mother happens to be nearby. So if your husband (or anyone else who lives in your home or works at the next desk) smokes, your baby's body is going to pick up nearly as much contamination from tobacco smoke by-products as if *you* were lighting up.

If your partner says he can't give up smoking, ask him to at least do all his smoking out of the house or in a different room, away from you. Giving up, of course, would be better, not just for his own health, but for the baby's long-term well-being. Studies show that parental smoking – mother's or father's – can cause respiratory problems in the infant and child after birth and impaired lung development into adulthood. (If you choose to nurse and smoke, tobacco poisons will contaminate the milk your baby drinks.)

You probably won't be able to get your co-workers to kick their habits, but you might be able to persuade them to take their cigarettes elsewhere when you're around. (In some communities and at some companies, you'll get official support in your efforts to create non-smoking spaces.)

Marijuana and Other Drug Use

'I've been a social smoker of marijuana – indulging only at parties – for about 10 years. Could this have altered my chromosomes enough to damage the baby I'm now carrying? And is smoking pot during pregnancy dangerous?'

As with cigarette smoking over 20 years ago, all the evidence on the effects of marijuana use is not yet in. Consequently, those who choose to smoke it today are guinea pigs testing a substance whose dangers may not be fully documented for some time to come. And since marijuana crosses the placenta, mothers who smoke it during pregnancy make guinea pigs out of their unborn children as well.

It is usually recommended that couples trying to conceive abstain from marijuana use, since it can interfere with conception. But if you are already pregnant, you needn't worry about your past smoking – there is no present evidence that it will harm your foetus.

Smoking *during* pregnancy, however, is a story that appears to have a less happy ending. Studies show that women who use marijuana at least once a month during pregnancy are: more than twice as likely to show meconium staining of the amniotic fluid during labour (a complication which can indicate foetal distress); more likely to suffer hyperemesis (severe and chronic vomiting, which can interfere seriously with prenatal nutrition), to gain inadequate weight, and to be anaemic; more likely to have dangerously rapid labour, prolonged or arrested labour, or to require a caesarean section; slightly more likely to have low-birth-weight babies; twice as likely to have babies needing resuscitation after delivery. Though it may not have a direct toxic effect on a

Breaking the Smoking Habit

Identify Your Motivation for Smoking. For example, do you smoke for pleasure, stimulation, or relaxation? To reduce tension or frustration, to have something in your hand or mouth, to satisfy a craving? Perhaps you smoke out of habit, lighting up without thinking about it. Once you understand your motivations, you should be able to substitute other satisfactions.

Identify Your Motivation for Giving Up. When you're pregnant, there's a clear one.

Choose Your Method of Withdrawal. Do you want to go cold turkey – or taper off? Either way, pick a 'last day' that isn't too far off. Plan a full day of activities for that date – things you don't associate with smoking.

Try to Sublimate Your Urge to Smoke. Use any and all of the following that you think will help:

☆ If you smoke mainly to keep your hands busy, try playing with a pencil, beads, a straw; knit, polish silver, create a nutritious recipe, write a letter, play the piano, learn to paint, make rag dolls, do jigsaw or crossword puzzles, challenge someone to a game of chess or Scrabble – anything that will make you forget to reach for a cigarette.

☆ If you smoke for oral gratification, try a substitute: raw vegetables, popcorn, a whole-wheat breadstick, gum made with sorbitol, a toothpick, an empty cigarette holder. Do avoid empty-calorie nibbles.

☆ If you smoke for stimulation, try to get your lift from a brisk walk, an absorbing book, good conversation. Be sure your diet contains all essential nutrients and that you eat frequently, to avoid feeling draggy because of low blood sugar.

☆ If you smoke to reduce tension and relax, try exercise instead. Or relaxation techniques. Or listening to soothing music while knitting. Or a long walk. Or a massage. Or making love.

☆ If you smoke for pleasure, seek pleasure in other pursuits, preferably in no-smoke situations. Go to a movie, visit baby boutiques, tour a favourite museum, attend a concert or a play, have dinner with a friend who is allergic to smoke. Or try something more active, like tennis doubles.

☆ If you smoke out of habit, avoid the settings in which you habitually smoke; frequent places with no-smoking rules instead. Stay away from heavy smokers.

☆ If you connect smoking with a particular beverage, food, or meal, avoid the food or beverage, eat the meal in a different locale. (Say you smoke two cigarettes with breakfast but you never smoke in bed. Have breakfast in bed for a few days.)

☆ When you feel the urge to smoke, take several deep breaths with a pause between each. Hold the last breath while you strike a match. Exhale slowly, blowing out the match. Pretend it was a cigarette and crush it out.

If You Do Slip Up and Have a Cigarette, Don't Despair. Just get right back on your programme, knowing that every cigarette you *don't* smoke is going to help your baby.

Look at Smoking as a Non-Negotiable Issue. When you were a smoker, you couldn't smoke in a theatre, or underground, or a department store, even in some restaurants. That was that. Now you have to tell yourself that you can't smoke, and that is that.

developing foetus, marijuana *does* affect placental function and the foetal endocrine system, and can interfere with the successful completion of pregnancy. Marijuana use during pregnancy may definitely be hazardous to a baby's health.

So treat marijuana as you would any other drug during pregnancy: Don't take it unless it is medically required and prescribed. If you have already smoked early in your pregnancy, don't worry. Since placental function becomes more important as pregnancy progresses, it's very unlikely any harm was done. Any pregnant woman who can't seem to break her marijuana habit should seek professional help as soon as the pregnancy is confirmed.

Pregnant women who use other 'recreational' drugs are also putting their babies in jeopardy. Not enough is known about their risks, and their benefits are hardly worth such potential danger. Using street drugs, the exact compositions of which are always unknown to the purchaser, presents added hazards. And addictive drugs, such as heroin, can 'hook' not only mother but foetus as well, with devastating results at birth.[3]

Caffeine

'I find it difficult to get through my day without my two cups of coffee. I've read, though, that caffeine can cause birth defects and low-birth-weight babies. Is this true?'

---

3. For further information and help contact Release, 1 Elgin Avenue, London W9 3PR (01–289–1123), or Turning Point, 9–12 Long Lane, London EC1A 9HA (01–606–3947).

What science doesn't know yet about caffeine might hurt your baby – or then again, it might not. The evidence is contradictory. What *is* known is that the drug (found in coffee, tea, colas, and, in a related form, in chocolate) does cross the placenta. Animal studies involving high doses of caffeine show numerous harmful effects on foetal development and an increase in foetal death. Studies on humans, however, have been far less conclusive.

Most pregnant coffee drinkers give birth to perfectly normal babies. And if you have been drinking small or moderate amounts of coffee or other caffeinated beverages during the first few months of pregnancy, there should be no need to worry.

Still, at least until more is known, there are more valid reasons to give up coffee (and tea and colas) for the rest of your pregnancy than to continue drinking it. First of all, caffeine's diuretic effect draws fluids and calcium – both vital to maternal and foetal health – from the body. Second, coffee and tea, especially when taken with cream and sugar are filling without being nutritious and can spoil your appetite for good food. Colas are not only filling but loaded with either empty sugar calories or questionable chemicals. Finally, the fact that many women lose their taste for coffee early in pregnancy suggests that mother nature considers the substance to be unsuitable for pregnant women.

How Do You Break the Caffeine Habit? The first step, finding your motivation, is easy in pregnancy: giving your baby the healthiest possible start in life. Next you need to determine why you indulge. If it's just a matter of taste or the comfort of a hot drink that turns you on to coffee or tea, then you can switch to a naturally decaffeinated beverage (but no more than two cups a day, unsweetened, or you won't have room for the good stuff). If you drink cola for taste we can't recommend substituting caffeine-free soft drinks, because no soft drink has a place in pregnancy; if it's refreshment you're thirsting for, you'll find that juices and plain or carbonated water are better thirst quenchers than colas, anyway. If it's the caffeine lift you crave, you'll get a more natural, longer-lasting boost from exercise and good food, especially protein, or from doing something that exhilarates you: dancing, jogging, making love. Though you'll doubtless sag for a few days after giving up caffeine, you'll soon feel better than ever. (Of course, you will still experience the normal fatigue of early pregnancy.)

Minimizing Caffeine Withdrawal Symptoms. But as any coffee, tea, or cola addict is well aware, it is one thing to want to give up caffeine and another thing to do it. If you're a heavy imbiber and quit cold turkey, you can expect to experience withdrawal symptoms, including headache, fatigue, and lethargy. But these uncomfortable side effects can be minimized:

☆ Keep your blood sugar, and thus your energy level, up. Eat frequently, especially when headache strikes, and concentrate on high protein and complex-carbohydrate foods. Vitamin supplements may help, too.

☆ Get some outdoor exercise every day. It will also, believe it or not, raise your energy level.

☆ Be sure to get enough sleep – which will probably be easier without caffeine.

☆ If you drink large quantities of coffee or other caffeine-containing beverages, cutting down over a period of a few days may be the best way to reduce the severity of withdrawal symptoms.

Microwave Exposure

'I've read that exposure to microwave ovens is dangerous to a developing foetus. Should I unplug ours until after the baby's born?'

A microwave oven can be a working mother-to-be's best friend, helping to make nutritious eating-on-the-run possible. But like so many of our modern miracles, there's talk it may also be a modern menace. Whether or not we ought to be exposed to microwaves is still very controversial. Much more research needs to be done before the answer is known. It is believed, however, that two types of human tissue – the developing foetus and the eye – are particularly vulnerable to the effects of microwaves because they have a poor capacity to dissipate the heat the waves generate. So rather than unplugging your microwave oven, you should take some precautions. First of all, be sure your oven doesn't leak. (Meters are available for checking leaks.) Second, don't stand near the oven when it is in operation. Finally, follow the manufacturer's directions very carefully.

Toxoplasmosis

'I love steak tartare and I've had it on a few occasions since becoming pregnant. I also have two cats at home. Should I get tested to see if I might have contracted toxoplasmosis?'

It's true that both cat faeces and raw meat of any kind can transmit the parasitic organism, Toxoplasma gondii, to humans. The disease the organism causes, toxoplasmosis, is so mild that its symptoms (a slight rash, some achiness, swollen glands, a low-grade fever) often go unnoticed by its victims. But whereas a woman infected during pregnancy will recover spontaneously and completely, her foetus may suffer lasting damage, serious illness, or may even die.

Fortunately, like most threats to the foetus, toxoplasmosis is both rare and preventable. Sixty percent of the small number of women who do contract the disease during pregnancy don't pass it on to their babies at all, and two out of three babies of those who do pass it on show no ill effects. And because harm to the foetus is most likely to occur late in pregnancy, exposure in the first trimester is not a reason for concern.

You also won't have to worry if you were infected, and thus developed immunity, before you became pregnant. The odds that you are immune are at least 1 in 4, higher if you regularly eat raw or very rare meat or have had cats at home. To determine if you are immune, ask your doctor for a blood test. If the test shows that you have an active infection, you and your doctor should discuss treatment plans. If it shows that you are immune, there's no chance of your infecting this or further offspring. If the test shows you are neither infected nor immune, you can avoid infection with the following steps:

☆ Don't touch other people's cats, and steer clear of stray cats.

☆ Don't garden in soil in which cats may have deposited faeces; if your children have a sandpit, keep it covered when they aren't playing in it. Wash produce grown in a home garden in detergent and rinse it thoroughly, and/or peel or cook it.

☆ If you have a cat, have it tested by a vet to see if it has an active infection. If it does, board it at a kennel or ask a friend to care for it for at least six weeks – the period of infection. If it doesn't, keep it infection-free by not feeding it raw meat or allowing it to roam out of doors, hunt mice or birds, or be in contact with other cats. As an extra precaution, you shouldn't handle the litter box, and the person who does should wear gloves.

☆ Don't eat meat that is raw or that hasn't been cooked to at least 140 degrees (rare) on an accurate meat thermometer. In a restaurant, order your meat well done.

X-rays

'I had an x-ray test at the dentist before I found out I was pregnant. Could this have hurt my baby?'

Don't worry. First of all, dental x-rays are directed far away from your uterus. Second, a lead apron shields your uterus and your baby effectively from any radiation.

The safety of other types of x-rays during pregnancy, however, is more controversial. No one knows exactly what a safe dose of radiation is, or what all the potential dangers are. There is believed to be some risk to the foetus from direct radiation, at least during the first trimester. Fortunately, the risk is being reduced as x-ray equipment is improved and refined, delivering lower doses of radiation and becoming more precise in focusing directly on the desired area.

Of course, it still isn't wise to take unnecessary risks, no matter how small. But necessary risks are another matter. If you need an x-ray:

☆ Never have an x-ray, even a dental x-ray, during pregnancy when the benefit does not outweigh the risk. Your doctor or dentist can help you determine that. (Read Weighing Risk vs. Benefit, page 79.)

☆ Do not have an x-ray if any safer diagnostic procedure can be used instead.

☆ Always inform the doctor ordering the x-ray and the technician performing it that you are pregnant.

☆ If an x-ray is necessary, be certain that it is taken in a licensed or regularly inspected facility. Equipment should be up-to-date, in good condition, and operated by well-trained, conscientious technicians under the supervision of a full-time radiologist. The x-ray beams should, when possible, be adjusted so that only the minimum area necessary is exposed to radiation; other areas, especially the uterus, should be shielded with a lead apron.

☆ Follow the technician's directions precisely, being especially careful not to move during the shot, so that retakes won't be needed.

☆ Most important, if you've had an x-ray, or need an x-ray, don't waste your time worrying about the possible consequences. Your baby is in more danger every time you forget to buckle your seat belt.

Becoming Ill

'I'm afraid that if I become ill my baby will suffer. And if I get a fever, there's nothing I can safely take.'

Pregnancy is one of those times when an ounce of prevention is worth a pound of cure – and is a lot safer, too. You won't have to worry about what to take for a cold if you avoid catching one, and the best ways to do that are:

☆ Keep your resistance up. Eat the best diet possible (see the Best-Odds Diet, page 82), get enough sleep, and don't wear yourself down by running yourself ragged.

☆ Avoid ill people like the plague. Stay away from those you know are ill (sit far from coughers and sneezers on the bus), and never shake hands with them (this exchanges not only greetings but germs).

☆ If your children are down with a

cold or flu, you can't avoid them entirely. But you can avoid handling their linens and soiled tissues, finishing up their lunches or drinking from their cups, and kissing them on the face. See that they wash their hands frequently and cover their mouths when they cough or sneeze. Use disinfectant on telephones and other commonly used surfaces. Ask your husband, mother, or a non-pregnant friend to play nurse-maid as much as possible. If a child comes down with a rash of any kind – unless you know you've already had, or been vaccinated for, German measles (rubella)[4] and chickenpox – stay away from them completely and contact your doctor at once.

If, despite all your efforts, you come down with a cold or the flu (most pregnant women do at some point in the nine months), you can feel reassured that mild illness, though uncomfortable for you, is very unlikely to be harmful to your baby.

It's the traditional medical treatments – antihistamines, aspirin, and antibiotics – that can cause problems. Don't take any of these, or any other medication, without your doctor's advice; he or she will know which are safe in pregnancy and which will be effective in your case. Aspirin use is not a good idea, particularly late in pregnancy when it could lead to childbirth complications and bleeding. If you've already taken aspirin, though, don't panic. There is no evi-

dence that a couple of them will be harmful, unless they are taken just prior to delivery. Less is known about the effects of acetaminophen (non-aspirin products like paracetamol), and many physicians okay them for very occasional use during pregnancy. Others do not. Nurofen also may be recommended by some physicians during the first six months of your pregnancy, but it shouldn't be used at all in the third trimester. (These pain relievers, incidentally, will not cure colds and will not relieve most cold symptoms. Over-the-counter cold medications and cough syrups may relieve symptoms, but they are generally not recommended – particularly early in pregnancy, before the foetus is well developed.)

Fortunately for you and your baby, some of the best cold and flu remedies are the safest ones, too:

☆ Nip your cold in the bud, before it blossoms into a nasty case of bronchitis or another secondary infection. With the very first sneeze, go to bed or at least plan on getting a little extra rest.

☆ When you're lying down or sleeping, keep your head slightly elevated to facilitate breathing.

☆ Don't starve your cold, fever – or baby. Stay on the Best-Odds Diet whether you have an appetite or not, forcing yourself to eat if need be. Be sure to have some citrus fruit or juice every day, but don't take extra vitamin C supplements without medical advice.

☆ Flood yourself with fluids. Your body will be losing fluids you and your baby urgently need through fever, sneezes, and runny nose.

---

4. Your doctor or midwife will have done a rubella titre as part of your first prenatal exam. Be sure to ask whether or not you are immune.

Keep a thermos of hot grapefruit or orangeade (½ cup unsweetened frozen juice concentrate to 1 quart of boiling water) next to your bed, and drink at least one cupful an hour. Also try the Jewish penicillin: chicken soup. Medical researchers have proven that it really does help.

☆ Keep your nasal passages moist with a humidifier, and by spraying the inside of your nose with an atomizer filled with salt water.

☆ If your throat is sore or scratchy, or you're coughing, gargle with salt water (1 teaspoon of salt to 8 ounces of water) at the temperature of hot tea.

☆ Bring down a fever naturally. Take cool showers or baths, or sponge with tepid water; drink cool beverages, and wear light bedclothes. If your fever reaches 102 degrees or more, call your doctor immediately. (High body temperature for extended periods isn't good for the baby.)

☆ If your cold or flu is really bad and interferes with eating or sleeping, or if you're coughing up greenish or yellowish sputum, call your doctor. He or she may want to prescribe a topical medication that won't cross the placenta, or if there is a risk of complications, an antibiotic or antihistamine that is safe during pregnancy.

Remember that you and your doctor must weigh risk against benefit when it comes to using medications. Don't put off calling the doctor, or refuse to take a prescribed medication you are assured is safe, because you've heard all drugs are harmful during pregnancy. They aren't.

Diarrhoea

'I've got an intestinal virus and my midwife took me off dairy products until the diarrhoea stops. Is that safe?'

A couple of days off your diet won't hurt your baby, but prolonged diarrhoea might. So take your practitioner's advice. Do take your vitamin-mineral supplements if you can, get plenty of fluids (diluted juices, water, decaffeinated teas) and as many calories as possible through dry toast, baked potato (no skins), boiled or steamed white rice, banana, and other permitted foods. Bedrest will also hasten your recovery. If your diarrhoea hasn't cleared up in 24 to 48 hours, medication may be prescribed.

Taking Medications

'How do I know which medicines, if any, are safe to take during pregnancy, and which aren't?'

No drug, prescription or over-the-counter, is 100% safe for 100% of the people 100% of the time. When you're pregnant, every time you take a drug there are two individuals at risk, one very small and vulnerable. On the other hand, even during pregnancy there are many situations in which medications are absolutely essential to life and/or health. Whether you will take a particular medication at a particular time during pregnancy will be something you and your physician will have to decide by weighing the risk a drug might pose against the benefit it offers (see page 79). You should take *no* medication without medical consultation, and only take medication that is absolutely necessary.

Which drug you take in a particular situation will depend on the latest information available on drug safety in pregnancy. The many lists of safe, possibly safe, possibly unsafe, and definitely unsafe drugs may provide some assistance, but most are outdated and unreliable by the time they're published. Package inserts and labels are of little use, since most warn not to use the product during pregnancy without a doctor's orders, even when the product is believed safe. Your best sources of information will be:

☆ A well-informed doctor or midwife (not all are familiar with drug safety in pregnancy).

☆ Consult your local Health Education Unit for further information.

Household Hazards

'The more I read, the more I'm convinced that the only way to protect my baby in this day and age is to spend the next nine months locked up in a sterile room. Even my home isn't safe.'

The threats you and your baby face from the increasing number of environmental hazards, including those in your own backyard, quickly pale when compared to those faced by your great-grandmothers, when modern obstetrical medicine was in its infancy. All of today's environmental perils combined (alcohol, tobacco, and other drugs excepted) are far less menacing to you and your baby than one untrained midwife with unwashed hands was to your ancestresses. So in spite of all the trumpeting about the perils around us, we repeat: pregnancy and childbirth have never been so safe.

But while you won't need to give up your home and move to that sterile room, a little caution is certainly warranted when dealing with household hazards:

Household Cleaning Products. Since many cleaning products have been in common use for the better part of the century and no correlation has ever been noted between clean homes and birth defects, it's unlikely that disinfecting your toilet bowl or polishing your dining-room table will in any way compromise the well-being of your baby. In fact, much of the opposite is probably true: The elimination of germ-carrying bacteria by chlorine, ammonia, and other cleaning agents can protect your baby by preventing infection.

No studies have proven that the occasional incidental inhalation of ordinary household cleansers has any detrimental effect on the developing foetus; on the other hand, no studies have proven frequent inhalation completely safe. If you've already been 'exposed' to cleansers, there's no reason for concern. But for the rest of your pregnancy, clean with prudence. Let your nose, and the following tips, be your guide in screening out potentially hazardous chemicals:

☆ If the product has a strong odour or fumes, don't breathe it in directly. Use it in an area with plenty of ventilation, or don't use it at all.

☆ Use pump sprays instead of aerosols.

☆ Never (even when you're not pregnant) mix ammonia with chlorine-based products; the combination produces very hazardous fumes.

☆ Try to avoid using products such as oven cleaners and dry-cleaning fluids whose labels are plastered with warnings about toxicity.

☆ Wear gloves when you're cleaning. Not only will they spare your hands a lot of wear and tear, they'll prevent the absorption through the skin of potentially toxic chemicals.

Tap Water. Water ranks second only to oxygen on the list of things essential to life. Though starvation certainly isn't medically recommended, humans can survive for at least a week without food, but only a few days without water. In other words, you've got more to worry about if you *don't* drink the water than if you do.

It's true that water once posed a serious threat to the lives it sustained, carrying deadly typhoid and other diseases. But modern treatment has eliminated such threats, at least in developed areas of the world. Though there are some who suspect that a new threat to the unborn now exists in the very chemicals that are used to purify water, there is no conclusive evidence that this is true. Any possible hazard is eliminated in cities that use filters

instead of chemicals in the water purification process.

Most drinking water in the United Kingdom is safe and drinkable. But in a few areas, chemical seepage from factories, dumping areas, and farms has led to potentially hazardous contamination. If this is the case in your home town, you're probably well aware of it. If so, or even if you're only suspicious, here's how to make sure you're drinking to your – and your baby's – health:

☆ Check with your local health department and water authority about the purity and safety of community drinking water. If there is a possibility that the quality of your water (because of pipe deterioration, because your home borders on a waste disposal area, or because of odd taste or colour) might differ from the rest of the community's, arrange for one or the other of these agencies to test it.

☆ If your tap water looks suspicious or has an 'off' taste, invest in a carbon filter for your kitchen sink. (It will last longer if it is used only for cooking and drinking water and not for the dishwasher and other purposes.) Or use bottled water for drinking and cooking.

Insecticides. Though some insects, such as gypsy moths, pose a considerable threat to trees and plants, and others, such as roaches and ants, to your aesthetic sensibilities, they rarely pose a health risk to human beings – even pregnant ones. And it's generally safer to live with them than to eliminate them through the use of chemical insecticides, some of which have been linked to birth defects.

Of course, your neighbours and/or your landlord (if they don't happen to be pregnant or have small children) may not agree. If neighbourhood spraying is currently being done, avoid being outdoors as much as possible until the chemical odours have dissipated, about two to three days. When indoors, keep the windows closed. If your landlord is spraying your flat or house for insects, ask him to skip yours. If he's already sprayed, stay out of the flat or house for a day or two if that's possible, and ventilate with open windows for as long as is feasible. The chemicals are only potentially dangerous as long as the fumes linger. Have someone scrub all of the food preparation surfaces in or near the sprayed area.

On your own property or in your flat, try to take the natural approach to pest control. Pull weeds instead of spraying them. Have someone remove gypsy moth larvae or other insect pests manually from trees and plants, or, as one doctor did in his neighbourhood, try to convince those responsible for spraying to use a soap-and-water mixture, which kills bugs by clogging up their breathing passages, instead of chemicals. The soap-and-water technique may take two sprayings, but it will work. Kill cockroaches and ants with boric acid (sprinkled in heavy-bug-traffic areas), which is harmless (unless ingested) to humans and human foetuses and is probably more effective than the insecticides most frequently used.

If you have been accidentally exposed to insecticides or herbicides, don't be alarmed. Brief, indirect exposure isn't likely to have done any harm to your baby. What does increase the risk is frequent, long-term exposure, the kind which working daily with such chemicals around (as in a factory) would entail.

Paint Fumes. In the entire animal kingdom, the period before birth (or egg laying) is passed in hectic preparation for the arrival of the new offspring. Birds feather their nests, squirrels line their tree-trunk homes with leaves and twigs, and human mothers and fathers sift madly through volumes of wallpaper and fabric samples.

And almost invariably (if a safe 'asexual' colour can be decided on) painting of the baby's room is involved. Which, in the days of arsenic- or lead-based paints, might have posed some threat to the health of the unborn. But modern latex paints are much safer. They dry quickly, give off fewer fumes, and rarely contain lead. Still, painting isn't the best avocation for an expectant mother – even for one who's trying desperately to keep busy in those last weeks of waiting. Balancing on ladder tops is precarious, to say the least, and paint odours can bring on an attack of nausea. Try, instead, to get the expectant father, or someone else, to handle this aspect of preparations.

While the painting is being done, try to be out of the house. Whether you're there or not, be sure to keep windows open for ventilation. Avoid entirely exposure to paint removers, which are highly toxic, and steer clear of removing paint (whether chemicals or sanders are used).

Air Pollution

'It seems it isn't even safe to breathe when you're pregnant. Will air pollution hurt my baby?'

Living in a bus terminal or sleeping nightly in a motorway service station might, of course, expose your foetus to excessive pollutants while depriving it of essential oxygen. Ordinary breathing in the big city, however, isn't as risky as you might think, particularly when you consider the alternative. Millions of women live and breathe in major cities across the nation and give birth to millions of healthy babies. Even in the 1960s, when pollution was at its worst levels, there was no documented damage to the unborn.

Day-to-day breathing, then, will have no detrimental effect on your baby. Even enough carbon monoxide to cause illness in the mother appears not to have deleterious effects on the foetus early in pregnancy (although carbon monoxide poisoning later in pregnancy might). It's common sense, however, to avoid extraordinarily high doses of most pollutants. here's how:

☆ Avoid smoke-filled rooms for extended, repeated periods. Keep in mind that cigars and pipes, because they aren't inhaled, release even more smoke into the air than cigarettes do. Ask family, guests in your home, and co-workers not to smoke in your presence.

☆ Have the exhaust system on your car checked to be sure there is no leakage of noxious fumes and that the exhaust pipe isn't rusting away. Never start your car in the garage with the door closed; keep the bar door on an estate car closed when the engine is running; avoid waiting in queues with other cars spewing out carbon monoxide; keep your car's air vent closed when driving in heavy traffic.

☆ Don't run, walk, or bicycle along congested highways, since you breathe in more air – and pollution – when you're active.

Occupational Hazards

'You hear a lot about dangers on the job, but how do you know if your workplace is safe?'

The hazards of the workplace, and the threats they may pose to the reproductive capabilities of both male and female workers and to the well-being of their unborn children, have only just begun to be explored and identified. Conclusive answers have been elusive, as they are whenever cause-and-effect connections between environmental factors and poor pregnancy outcomes are sought. First of all, it's hard to separate out all the various possible contributing risk factors in a woman's life, or to prove that an unfavourable outcome wasn't caused by a genetic accident. Second, though animal studies often yield interesting results, there's no way to ascertain whether the results apply to humans, since experiments on humans aren't, of course, feasible.

Therefore, effects on humans can

be determined only through epidemiological studies. These studies can be done in two ways: Large groups of women who are exposed to certain substances can be looked at to see if they show an increase in one or more types of poor pregnancy outcomes (miscarriages, birth defects, etc.). Or small groups of women who have poor outcomes can be studied to see if there is a common risk factor shared by all of them. Either way, such studies give us clues but not definitive answers.

From what we presently know, it is clear that some workplaces do present hazards for the pregnant woman (e.g., chemical factories, operating rooms, x-ray departments). Other workplace hazards so far have fallen into grey areas because not enough research has been done to establish their safety – or lack of it. What some of the research has already indicated, and will probably continue to indicate, is that there is a great deal of unwarranted concern about potential risks on the job.

The use of a video display terminal, such as that on a word processor or other computer, is one of the most common occupational preoccupations of pregnant women. Because display terminals emit radiation, pregnant women who worked with them daily and suffered miscarriages, or whose infants were stillborn or born with defects, have charged that the machines were responsible. Studies so far seem to indicate these problems were random and not related to the display terminals; the levels of radiation emitted, experts say, were far too low (less even than that of sunshine) to be causative

factors. It's been suggested, rather, that the stress under which many workers operate a VDT may be the real culprit in these tragedies. The issue is still, however, controversial, and surveys are being undertaken to try to clarify it. In the meantime, responsible manufacturers are striving, through technological refinement, to reduce any potential risks their machines may pose.

Of course, there are many occupational risks that are real and proven, and a pregnant woman should be alerted to them. There are a number of substances which pregnant women should avoid, among them: alkylating agents, anaesthetic gases, arsenic, benzene, carbon monoxide, chlorinated hydrocarbons, diethylstilbesterol, dimethyl sulphoxide, dioxin, ionizing radiation, organic mercury compounds, organophosphate pesticides, polychlorinated biphenyls.

Some workers, such as doctors and nurses who work in operating rooms, x-ray technicians, and certain lab or pharmacy workers are probably aware of the substances they're exposed to on the job. Others may not be. By law, you have the right to know, and your employer is under obligation to tell you. (Information on workplace hazards can also be obtained by contacting the Health and Safety Commission, Regina House, 259–269 Old Marylebone Road, London NW1 5RR (01–723 1261); information about the safety of machinery or other equipment that you operate on the job can often be secured by writing directly to the manufacturer's director.) If your job does expose you to hazards, either ask to be transferred temporarily to a safer post or, finances permitting, begin your maternity leave early.

Though chemicals pose the most direct occupational threats, they don't pose the only ones. Teachers and social workers who deal with young children are likely to come into contact with potentially dangerous infections, such as rubella. Laundry workers and those in the health care field may be exposed to a variety of infections; animal handlers, meat cutters and inspectors to toxoplasmosis. Fortunately, unlike exposure to chemicals, exposure to infection can usually be avoided, either through immunization or the use of gloves and masks or other precautions. (See the individual infections, such as Toxplasmosis, page 69.)

WHAT IT'S IMPORTANT TO KNOW: PLAYING BABY ROULETTE

When a gambler playing roulette puts down a bet on his lucky number, the odds are very high against the wheel coming to a stop there. It's the same when a pregnant woman plays baby roulette (intentionally or inadvertently), exposing her baby to teratogens, substances potentially harmful to the foetus. Almost all of the time the baby roulette wheel will pass innocuously by, and the baby won't be affected.

Although the gambler will call it luck, where the roulette wheel stops depends on the weight of the wheel, the friction it encounters, the force with which it is spun. And though baby roulette may also appear to be a game of chance, it, too, is dependent on a variety of factors:

How Strong Is the Teratogen?
Whereas thalidomide, a drug used in the early 1960s, caused very severe deformities in all foetuses who were exposed in utero at a particular time in their development, some sex hormones, also considered teratogens, cause defects in only about 1 in 1,000 foetuses. Fortunately, drugs as potent as thalidomide are extremely rare. In fact, a study of the effects of common drugs on 50,000 pregnancies found no drug similar to it in teratogenic effect. Other teratogens (such as x-ray, chemicals, and so on) also vary in the strength of their effect.

Is the Foetus Genetically Susceptible to the Teratogen?
Just as not every body exposed to cold or flu germs succumbs, not every foetus which is exposed to a teratogen is susceptible to its effects.

When Was the Foetus Exposed to the Teratogen?
Thalidomide, despite its horrifying potential, caused no damage when taken after the 52nd day of pregnancy. Malformations caused were specific to the part of the body that was developing at the time of ingestion and depended on the susceptibility of that part. Likewise, rubella virus causes conge-

nital damage in more than a third of foetuses exposed during the first month, but risk after the third month is probably under 1%.

How Much Exposure Was There? Most teratogenic effects are dose related. One brief diagnostic x-ray will be unlikely to cause a problem. A series of heavy-dose radiation treatments could. Smoking lightly for the first few months will not be likely to harm a foetus; heavy smoking for the entire pregnancy increases certain risks very significantly.

What Is the Mother's General Nutritional Status? Some animal experiments show defects apparently caused by a drug are actually caused by poor nutrition; the drug only reduced appetite, and thus water and food intake. Just as you will resist a cold virus more effectively if you are well nourished and not rundown, so will your foetus resist teratogens better if he or she is well nourished – through you, of course.

Are Several Factors Combining to Increase Risk? The trio of poor diet, smoking, and alcohol abuse, the duet of smoking and tranquilizers, and other 'losing combinations' can greatly increase risk.

Is Some Unknown Protective Factor in Play? Even when all factors appear identical, not all foetuses are affected in the same way. In experiments with foetal mice of identical genetic strains who were exposed to the same teratogens at identical stages in development and at identical dosages, only 1 in 9 were born malformed. No one knows exactly why, though perhaps someday medical science will come up with the solution to this mystery.

Weighing Risk vs. Benefit

Should today's pregnant woman fear for her baby's life and well-being because he or she is developing in a world filled with environmental threats? Absolutely not – and for several reasons. First of all, drugs and other environmental factors account for less than 1% of all birth defects. The general risk is extremely slight, even if you have already been exposed to a specific teratogen. Second, if you haven't, knowing what the risks are can help you to avoid them, improving your baby's odds still more. Third, in spite of the dire warnings making headlines and highlighting news programmes daily, never have the chances of having a healthy, normal baby been better.

Of course, nothing in life is totally without risk. But in dealing with risks, we learn to weigh them against benefits. This is never more important than during pregnancy, when each decision potentially affects the safety and well-being of not one but two lives. When you're faced with the decision of whether or not to smoke, to have a before-dinner cocktail, to nibble on a chocolate bar instead of an apple while watching TV, you are going to be weighing risk against benefit. Are the benefits, if any, you are going to derive from smoking, drinking, or junk-food snacking worth the risks to your baby?

Well, most of the time, your answer will probably be no. But once in a while you may decide that a little risk will be worth it. One glass of wine, for example, to toast your anniversary. The risk to your baby is practically nil. And the benefit (a more festive anniversary) is really important. Or a big chunk of cake for your birthday – a lot of empty calories, true. But just this once they won't really deprive baby of necessary nutrients, and after all, it *is* your birthday.

Some risk vs. benefit decisions are easy. For instance, regular heavy alcohol consumption throughout pregnancy can handicap your child for life (see page 62). Giving up the pleasure you derive from drinking may take considerable effort, but your choice is clear: Give it up, or don't have the baby.

Or say you have an infection and are running a fever that's high enough to pose a threat to your baby. Your doctor won't hesitate to use medication – the safest possible drug at the lowest effective dose – to wipe out the infection and bring down the fever. In this case, the benefit of drug use far outweighs its possible harm. A mild fever, on the other hand, won't hurt your baby and will help your body fight an infection. So before resorting to medication, your doctor will probably give your body a chance to cure itself, on the grounds that the possible risk of taking the drug outweighs its potential benefits.

Other decisions are not so clear cut. What if you have a terrible cold with sinus headaches which have been keeping you up at night? Should you take a cold tablet to help you get some rest? Or should you suffer through sleepless nights which won't do you or the baby any good? The best way to approach such decisions is:

☆ Determine if there are alternative no-risk ways of obtaining the benefits you seek – perhaps through non-drug approaches (see page 71). Try them. If they don't work, continue to evaluate your original option, in this case, cold tablets.

☆ Ask your doctor about risks and benefits. It's important to remember that not all drugs are known to cause birth defects, and that many have been used safely in pregnancy. New studies are turning up more information on drug safety, or lack of it, daily. Your doctor has access to this information.

☆ Do some research on your own. For the latest information on the safety of a particular drug during pregnancy, contact Foresight or The Women's Health Information Centre.[5]

☆ Determine if there are ways of increasing the benefits or decreasing the risks (taking the safest, most effective pain reliever in the smallest effective doses for the shortest possible time), and try to ensure that if you do take the risk, you will receive the benefit (take your cold tablet before you go to bed, when you are most likely to get that needed rest).

5. Foresight, The Old Vicarage, Church Lane, Witley, Surrey GU8 5PN (042879–4500). The Women's Health Information Centre, 52 Featherstone Street, London EC1 (01–251 6580).

☆ In consultation with your practitioner, review all the information you've gathered – weighing risks against benefits – and make your decision.

During pregnancy you will be challenged to make intelligent decisions in dozens of situations, weighing risk against benefit. Each decision you make will impact on your chance of having a healthy baby. But an occasional wrong decision isn't likely to be catastrophic – it will change the odds only very slightly. If you've already made a few not-so-terrific choices and there's no way to undo them, forget them. Just try to make better decisions for the rest of your pregnancy. And remember, the odds are very much in your baby's favour!

4
The Best-Odds Diet

There's a tiny new being developing inside you. The odds are already fairly good that he or she will be born healthy. But you have the chance to improve those odds significantly, to come as close as possible to guaranteeing your baby not just good health, but excellent health – with every bite of food you put in your mouth.

In the UK, a great deal of publicity has been given to the importance of preconceptional care. In particular the work of the charity Foresight (see footnote on page 80), which is concerned in taking steps to secure optimal health and nutritional status in both parents, prior to the conception of their baby. They are also involved in instigating research aimed at the identification and removal of potential health hazards to foetal development. Another group which is concerned about pregnancy and nutrition is the Templegarth Trust.[1]

1. Templegarth Trust, 82 Tinkle Street, Grimoldy, Louth, Lincolnshire, LN11 8TF.

A study done at the Harvard School of Public Health is a dramatic illustration of how closely the state of a baby's health at birth is tied to its mother's diet during pregnancy. Of the women in the study who had good-to-excellent diets, fully 95% had babies in excellent or good health. Only 5% of their babies were in fair or poor health. On the other hand, only 8% of women on really awful diets (composed largely of junk foods) had babies in excellent or good health, and 65% of their infants were in the poorest health condition – stillborn, premature, functionally immature, or with congenital defects.

Of course, most of the women in the American study (like most pregnant women) were on neither excellent diets nor extremely poor ones. Their diets were average, and so was the health of their children. Eighty-eight percent had babies in good or fair health. But only 6% had infants in really excellent health – which is, after all, what most of us want for our children.

If your eating habits aren't the most disciplined or virtuous to begin with, following the Best-Odds Diet will probably present you and your will-power with quite a challenge. But when you consider the results of your extra efforts – better odds for your baby's health – we think you'll agree it's a challenge worth taking. (And because the Best-Odds Diet nour-ishes your baby without putting excess weight on you, the odds of your quickly regaining your figure will also be improved.)

Nine Basic Principles for Nine Months of Healthy Eating

Make Every Bite Count. You've got only nine months of meals and snacks with which to give your baby the best possible start in life. Make every one of them count. Before you close your mouth on a forkful of food, consider, 'Is this the best I can give my baby?' If it will benefit your baby, chew away. If it'll benefit only your sweet tooth or appease your appetite, put your fork down.

All Calories Are Not Created Equal. For example, 150 empty chocolate-bar calories are not equal to the 150 calories in ¼ of a cup of mineral- and vitamin-packed raisins. Nor are the 100 calories in 10 high-fat potato crisps equal to the 100 in a baked potato. So choose your calories with care, selecting quality over quan-tity. (Your baby will benefit a lot more from 2,000 nutrient-rich calo-ries daily than 4,000 mostly empty ones.)

Starve Yourself, Starve Your Baby. Just as you wouldn't consider starving your baby after it's born, you shouldn't consider starving it in utero. The foetus can't live well off your flesh, no matter how ample. It needs regular nourishment at regular inter-vals. Never, never skip a meal.[2] Even if you're not hungry, the baby is. If persistent heartburn or a constant bloated feeling is spoiling your appe-tite, spread your daily requirements out over six small meals a day instead of three large ones.

Become an Efficiency Expert. Fill your daily nutritional requirements in the most efficient way possible within your caloric needs. Eating six table-spoons of peanut butter (if you can get it down) at 600 calories, or about 25% of your daily allotment, is a considera-bly less efficient way of getting 25 grams of protein than eating 3½ ounces of water-packed tuna at 125 calories. And eating a cup and a half of ice cream (about 450 calories) is a far less efficient way of getting 300 milligrams of calcium than drinking a glass of skim milk (90 calories). Fat, because it has more than twice as many calories per gram as either proteins or carbohydrates, is a parti-cularly inefficient food selection. Choose lean meats over fatty ones, low-fat milk and dairy products over full fat, broiled foods over fried; spread butter lightly; sauté in a teaspoon of fat rather than a quarter cup.

---

2. That means never fasting during pregnancy, either. An Israeli study showed a jump in deliveries just after Yom Kippur, the Day of Atonement, indicating that fasting late in preg-nancy could trigger an early delivery.

Carbohydrates Are a Complex Issue. Some women concerned about gaining too much weight during pregnancy mistakenly drop carbohydrates from their diets like so many hot potatoes. True, refined carbohydrates (like white bread, white rice, refined cereals, cakes, biscuits, sugars, syrups) are nutritionally weak – supplying little but calories. But complex carbohydrates (whole-grain breads and cereals, brown rice, vegetables, dried beans and peas, and, of course, hot potatoes – especially in their skins) and fresh fruit supply essential B vitamins, trace minerals, protein, and important fibre. Good not only for your baby, but for you. They'll help keep nausea and constipation in check, and because they are filling but not fattening, they'll help keep your weight down, too.

Sweet Nothings: Nothing But Trouble. No calorie is as empty, and therefore as wasted, as a calorie of sugar. In addition, researchers are finding that sugar may be not only void of value, but harmful – possibly implicated in diabetes, heart disease, depression, hyperactivity. That's why the Best-Odds Diet recommends eating no refined sugars (brown, white, honey, maple syrup, treacle) at all during pregnancy. Every calorie they supply could better come from foods which yield a higher return nutritionally for your baby.

Eat Foods That Can Remember Where They Came From. If your green beans haven't seen their native fields for months (having been boiled, processed, preserved, and canned since harvesting), they probably don't have much of their natural goodness left to offer your baby. Choose fresh vegetables first, or if they're not in season, the quick-frozen variety. To cook, steam or stir fry lightly, so they'll retain their vitamins and minerals. Fruits, too, should be eaten fresh and unsweetened. Avoid prepared foods that are full of chemicals, sugar, salt, and low in nutritive value. Choose a fresh chicken breast over chicken roll, fresh (preferably wholewheat) noodles and cheese over a dehydrated casserole mix, an unsweetened baked apple in place of a slice of apple pie.

Make Good Eating a Family Affair. If there are subversive elements at home, urging you to bake chocolate cake or to add potato crisps to your shopping list, it's a sure bet that the Best-Odds Diet won't stand a chance. To avoid sabotage, put the whole household on the diet with you. Bake naturally sweet Fruity Oatmeal Biscuits (page 95); bring home wholewheat bread or toasted sunflower seeds instead. In addition to a healthier baby and a relatively slimmer you, there will be the postpartum bonus of a fitter, trimmer husband and older children (if you have them) with better eating habits. Continue the Best-Odds Diet for the whole family after delivery and you will be giving each member the best odds for a longer and healthier life.

Don't Sabotage Your Diet. The best antenatal diet strategy in the world is easily undermined when the expectant mother ignores three potential dangers to her developing offspring: alcohol, cigarettes, and caffeine. Read about these under individual listings in this book, and reinforce your good dietary habits accordingly.

The Best-Odds Daily Dozen

Calories. The old adage that a pregnant woman is eating for two is true. But it's important to remember that one of the two is a tiny developing foetus whose caloric needs are significantly lower than yours – a mere 300 a day. That means that if you eat enough calories to sustain your pre-pregnancy weight, you only have to consume 300 to 500[3] additional calories daily during your pregnancy.[4] In spite of the numerous pregnancy diets you may see that seem to recommend you eat enough food to feed a family of four, ingesting more calories than this is not only unnecessary but unwise.

There are four exceptions to this basic formula. In each of these cases the expectant mother should discuss her calorie needs with her doctor: the overweight woman, who, with proper nutritional guidance, can possibly do with fewer calories; the seriously underweight woman, who certainly needs more; the adolescent, who is still growing herself and has special nutritional needs; and the woman carrying multiple foetuses, who will have to add 300 calories for each of them.

Having to eat 500 extra calories a day sounds like a food lover's dream, but sad to say, it isn't. By the time you've guzzled your four glasses of milk (total of 380 calories) and taken your required extra grams of protein, you've probably come close to exceeding your allowance.

Protein. The amino acids that compose proteins are the building blocks of human cells, and they are particularly important when you're building a new baby. Lack of protein seems to have as much to do with babies being small for their gestational ages as does lack of calories. So at minimum, the pregnant woman should have 75 grams of protein every day. We think 100 grams, the amount usually recommended for high-risk pregnancies, is safer since the larger quantity may help prevent your pregnancy from becoming high risk. The Best-Odds Diet Food Selection Groups shows you how easily and deliciously you can get your 100 grams – without exceeding your calorie limit. If you come up short on any particular day, simply eat a couple of hard-boiled egg whites (most of an egg's protein is found in the white), each of which will provide 3 grams of high-quality protein for a mere 15 calories.

---

3. Because metabolism speeds up in pregnancy, you may need the higher quantity, particularly in mid and late pregnancy. The only way you can tell if you are getting the right number of calories is to see if you are gaining the right amount of weight (see page 132). Adjust your intake according to your weekly gain – but be sure you never cut out necessary nutrients along with the calories.

---

4. To find out how many calories it takes to sustain your prepregnancy weight, multiply your prepregnancy weight by 12 if you're sedentary, 15 if you're moderately active, and up to 22 if you're very active.

Vitamin C Foods. You and baby both need vitamin C daily for growth, tissue repair, wound healing, development of strong bones and teeth, and various other metabolic processes. In addition to the small amount the prenatal supplement you take every day contains, eat at least one vitamin C-rich food daily. Vitamin C content is most available in foods that are fresh and uncooked, as exposure to heat, light, and air destroys it over time. (See Vitamin C Foods, page 89, for good food choices that are high in vitamin C.)

Calcium. Back in junior school you probably learned that growing children need plenty of calcium for strong bones and teeth. Well, so do growing foetuses on their way to becoming growing children. Calcium is also vital for muscle, heart, and nerve development, blood clotting, and enzyme activity. Be diligent about your four-glasses-of-milk-a-day, or the equivalent in high-calcium foods. One of the great things about milk is that it can be hidden in so many foods: soups, casseroles, breads, cereals, desserts – particularly by using non-fat dry milk, ⅓ of a cup of which equals a glass of fluid milk. (One terrific way to sneak 2 cups of milk into one: Double-the-Milk Shake, page 94.) For those who can't tolerate milk, the Food Selection Groups provide a variety of adequate equivalents.

Green Leafy and Yellow Fruits and Vegetables. These rabbit-favourites supply the Vitamin A that's important for healthy cell growth (your baby's cells are multiplying at a fantastic rate), for healthy skin, bones, and much more. They also provide vital doses of vitamin E, riboflavin, folic acid, B_6, numerous minerals, and constipation-fighting fibre. Even if you're not a vegetable lover, you're sure to find some of those that you can stomach in the Food Selection Groups. (If all vegetables are completely offensive early in pregnancy, short-term substitution of vegetable juice is acceptable.) Have two to three servings a day, one of which should be raw.

Other Fruits and Vegetables. In addition to the deep green and yellow and vitamin C produce, you should have at least one other fruit or vegetable daily – for added fibre, vitamins, and minerals. A variety are suggested in the Food Selection Groups.

Cereals and Grains. Whole-grain foods (made from wheat, oats, rye, barley, corn, rice, millet, triticale, soy, and so on) are packed with vitamins, particularly the B vitamins that are needed for just about every part of your developing baby's body. They are also rich in trace minerals like zinc and selenium, which have been getting so much publicity lately, and in the equally well-publicized fibre. Starchy grain foods may also help reduce early-pregnancy morning sickness. The different types of grains are pretty much interchangeable, but the more variety the better. Be adventurous. Bread your chicken with a mixture of wholewheat flour or breadcrumbs and wheatgerm. Just one caveat: use only *whole* grains. Refined flours, even when they are enriched, are lacking in trace minerals and fibre.

The Iron-Rich Foods. Since large amounts of iron are essential for the developing blood supply of the foetus, you'll need more during these nine months than at any other time in your life. Get as much as you can from natural sources (see Food Selection Groups). But because it's often difficult to fill your iron requirement through diet alone, make sure your vitamin supplement contains iron, too.

High-Fat Foods. This requirement is definitely easier to exceed than to fill exactly, since fat is so concentrated. A tablespoon of oil in your salad dressing and one of butter on your bread will do it for the day. Be aware that fat used in cooking counts, too. So if you've fried your eggs in a tablespoon of margarine, you must subtract that from your day's allotment. See the Food Selection Groups for the recommended quantities.

Salty Foods. At one time the medical establishment prescribed limiting salt (sodium chloride) during pregnancy, because it contributed to water retention and bloating. Now it is believed that some increase in body fluids is necessary and normal, and that a moderate amount of sodium is needed to maintain adequate fluid levels. Still, very large quantities of salt and very salty foods (such as, pickles, soy sauce, and potato crisps) aren't good for anyone, pregnant or not. High sodium intake is closely linked to high blood pressure, a condition which can cause a variety of potentially dangerous complications in pregnancy, labour, and delivery. To be sure that you are getting your quota of iodine, use iodized salt. As a general rule, salt your food only to taste.

Fluids. You're not only eating for two, you're drinking for two. If you've always been a non-drinker – one of those people who goes through the day with barely a sip of anything – now's the time to change your habits. As body fluids increase during pregnancy, so does your need for fluid intake. Your baby, too, needs fluids. Most of his body, like yours, is composed of water. Extra fluids also help keep your skin soft, lessen the likelihood of constipation, rid your body of toxins and waste products, and reduce the risk of urinary tract infection. Be sure to get at least eight glasses a day – more, if possible. Of course, they don't all have to come straight from the tap. You can count milk, fruit or vegetable juices, small quantities of naturally decaffeinated coffee (from which caffeine has been removed without the use of chemicals) or tea, soups, or plain soda water (seltzer, not club soda – which usually has added salt).

Supplements. Check with your doctor or midwife before taking vitamin or mineral supplements during pregnancy. But it is our view that even if you eat the very best diet when you're pregnant, you can't be sure of getting all the nutrients you and your baby need from your daily food intake. First of all, especially early in pregnancy, nausea, heartburn and indigestion, or food aversions may interfere with your eating the right foods. Second, storage, cooking, and exposure to air can rob food of vitamins. And third, the requirements for some nutrients in pregnancy are so high that it may well be impossible to get enough from your diet alone.

A good supplement formulation should contain, in addition to the usual vitamins and minerals found in multivitamin pills: calcium, iron, vitamin B_{12} (particularly important for vegetarians), folic acid, and such trace minerals as zinc and selenium.

Remember, however, the emphasis here is on *supplement*. No pill, no matter how power packed, can replace a good diet. It's very important that most of your vitamins and minerals come from foods, because that is the way nutrients can be most effectively utilized. Fresh foods (not processed) contain not only the nutrients that we know about and that can be synthesized in a pill, but a great many others that are as yet undiscovered. Thirty years ago, a pregnancy pill didn't contain zinc and the other trace minerals we now know to be necessary to good health. But wholewheat bread has always contained it. Likewise, food supplies fibre and water (fruits and vegetables are loaded with both) and important calories and protein – none of which come packaged in a pill.

And don't think that because a little is good, a lot is better. Any vitamin supplementation should be used only in medically-advised doses.

THE BEST-ODDS DIET FOOD SELECTION GROUPS[5]

Protein Foods

Every day have four of the following, or a combination of these foods equivalent to four servings. Servings contain between 18 and 25 grams of protein, and you should consume 75 to 100 grams a day.

3 8-oz glasses of skim or low-fat milk or buttermilk
¾ cup low-fat cottage cheese
2½ oz Parmesan or Edam cheese
3 oz Swiss or Cheddar cheese
2½ oz low-fat cheese
5 large egg whites

2 large whole eggs, plus 2 egg whites
3½ oz tuna
2½ oz chicken or turkey, without skin
3½ oz fish or shrimp
3 oz lean beef or pork
3 oz veal
4 oz fatty beef
3½ oz lean lamb or liver
5 or 6 oz tofu (bean curd)
Texturized vegetable proteins[6] (TVP)
1 serving of a complete protein combination (box, page 90)

High-Protein Snacks

Nuts and seeds

---

5. Many foods fill more than one nutritional requirement, so Food Selection Groups may overlap. The same 3 glasses of milk, for example, will give you 3 calcium servings and 1 protein portion.

6. Recipes vary; some have a high protein/calorie ratio, others low, so read nutrition labels, remembering you need 20 to 25 grams of protein per serving.

Wholegrain baked goods
Soy baked goods
Yogurt
Hard cheese
Hard-boiled eggs
Wheat germ

Vitamin C Foods

Have at last one of the following, or a combination equal to one, every day. Your body can't store this vitamin, so be careful not to skip a day.

½ large grapefruit
1 small grapefruit
1 cup grapefruit juice
1 large fresh orange
6 oz orange juice
3 tablespoons orange juice concentrate
¾ cup lemon juice
1 medium mango
⅔ cup cubed papaya
½ small cantaloupe melon
⅔ cup strawberries
1½ large tomatoes
1¼ cups tomato juice
1 cup vegetable juice
1½ cups shredded raw cabbage (or cole slaw)
1 small red or green pepper
⅔ cup broccoli
¾ cup raw or 1 cup cooked cauliflower
½ cup spring greens, cooked in minimal water
1 cup cooked kohlrabi
4 oz raw spinach

Calcium-Rich Foods

Take four-servings of these foods daily or any combination that is equivalent to four servings. Vegetarians who don't drink milk should also take a calcium supplement, because the calcium in some vegetarian products is not easily absorbed by the body. You need 1,280 to 1,300 milligrams daily.

8 oz skim or low-fat milk or buttermilk
½ cup evaporated skim or low-fat milk
1¾ cups low-fat cottage cheese
1½ oz Cheddar cheese
1¼ oz Swiss cheese
1 cup yogurt
⅓ cup non-fat dry milk
1 oz canned salmon with bones
3 oz canned sardines with bones
3½ oz tinned sardines or tuna
9 oz tofu (bean curd)
Soy milk and soy protein[7]
⅔ cup spring greens
1½ cups cooked fresh kale
1⅓ cups cooked fresh mustard or turnip greens
2 cups broccoli
2½ tablespoons blackstrap molasses

Calcium-Rich Snacks

Almonds
Apricots
Dried figs
Baked goods made with sesame seeds or soy flour

---

7. Soy formulas vary; check the nutrition label to determine calcium equivalence, remembering you need 1,280 to 1,300 milligrams daily.

For Vegetarians

The following combinations are good for all pregnant women, however, non-vegetarians should count only one serving a day as their protein allowance.

Vegetarian Complete Protein Combinations

Choose 1 serving (10 to 13 grams protein) from the legumes list plus 1 serving (10 to 13 grams protein) from the grains list for a complete protein combination.

Legumes

1 cup cooked beans: broad, black eyed
¾ cup soybeans or soy grits
¾ cup mung beans
1 cup chick peas
1 cup lentils

Grains

1½ cups grains[8]; brown rice, barley, millet, bulgur
1⅓ cups wild rice
2 oz (before cooking) soy pasta
2 to 4 oz (before cooking) wholewheat pasta (depending on protein content)
⅔ cup (before cooking) oats
¾ cup seeds: sesame, sunflower, pumpkin
1 oz pine nuts
½ cup Brazil nuts or peanuts
2 oz cashews, walnuts, or pistachios

Dairy Complete Protein Combinations

Choose 1 serving (about 10 grams protein) from the legumes and grains list and 1 serving (about 12 grams protein) from the dairy food list for a complete protein.

Legumes and Grains

1 portion beans, peas, lentils, grains, pasta, noodles (see above)
2 slices wholegrain bread
⅔ cup oatmeal
1½ oz ready-to-eat cereal

Dairy Foods

2 oz Cheddar, or low-fat cheese
½ cup cottage cheese
¼ cup Parmesan cheese
⅓ cup non-fat dry milk plus 2 tablespoons wheat germ
2½ tablespoons peanut butter
1 cup yogurt plus 2 tablespoons wheat germ
2 eggs plus 2 egg whites

8. These grains are low in protein, enrich with 2 tablespoons of wheat germ per serving.

Fruits and Vegetables

You need two or three a day, one of which should be raw. Try to eat one yellow and one green daily:

2 or 3 fresh or dried apricots
½ medium mango
1 cup cubed papaya
⅔ cup dried yellow peaches
⅔ cup broccoli or turnip greens
1 raw carrot, or ⅓ cup cooked
½ cup greens
3½ oz chicory
½ cup kale or spring greens
8 large leaves dark green leafy lettuce
3½ oz fresh spinach, ½ cup cooked
⅔ cup winter squash
1 small sweet potato or yam

Other Fruits and Vegetables

Have at least one of the following daily; two would be better:

1 apple or ½ cup unsweetened apple sauce
6 to 7 asparagus tips
1 small banana
1 cup bean sprouts
¾ cup green beans
⅔ cup blackberries, raspberries
⅔ cup Brussels sprouts
⅔ cup pitted fresh cherries
⅔ cup grapes
1 wedge honeydew melon (⅛ melon)
1 cup fresh mushrooms
1 medium nectarine or peach
9 pods okra
½ cup parsley
1 medium pear
1 medium slice fresh or tinned unsweetened pineapple
1 medium potato
⅔ cup courgettes

Whole Grains and Other Complex Carbohydrates

Have four or five of the following every day:

1 slice wholewheat, rye, other whole grain or soy bread
½ cup cooked brown rice
½ cup cooked wild rice
½ cup cooked wholegrain cereal (e.g. oatmeal)
1 oz wholegrain ready-to-eat cereal (Shredded Wheat, Grape Nuts, or other unsweetened cereal)
¼ cup wheat germ
½ cup cooked millet, bulgur
½ cup cooked whole grain pasta
½ cup beans or peas

Iron-Rich Foods

Small amounts of iron are found in most of the fruits, vegetables, grains, and meats you will eat every day. But try to have some of the following higher-iron-content foods daily, along with your supplement:

Dried fruit (raisins, apricots, prunes, peaches, currants)
Liver and other organ meats (use infrequently)
Beef
Sardines
Black treacle
Soy baked goods
Spinach

High-Fat Foods

Have 2 tablespoons a day unless you are gaining weight too quickly, in which case limit your fat intake to 1 tablespoon, selected from the following:

Polyunsaturated vegetable oils
Margarine high in polyunsaturates (limit 1 tablespoon per day)
Butter (limit 1 tablespoon per day)

Mayonnaise (limit 1 tablespoon per day)

One of the following can be substituted for a tablespoon of fat:
½ small avocado
3 tablespoons single cream
2 tablespoons double (whipping) cream
2 tablespoons cream cheese
4 tablespoons sour cream
20 almonds
3 tablespoons peanuts, pecans, or walnuts

BEST-ODDS RECIPES

These recipes are designed not only to pacify your sweet and snacking tooth, but also to give you party 'cocktail' suggestions and a few breakfast ideas.

Cream of Tomato Soup

Makes 3 servings

In a saucepan, melt over low heat:
1 tablespoon margarine or butter
Add and blend over very low heat for 2 minutes:
2 tablespoons wholewheat flour
Gradually blend in over low heat:
½ pt/300 ml/2 cups evaporated skim milk
Continue cooking over low heat, stirring occasionally, until thickened. Stir in until smooth:

¾ pt/450 ml/3 cups tomato or vegetable juice
4 tablespoons tomato paste
Salt and pepper to taste

Fresh or dried oregano and basil to taste (optional)
Continue cooking over low heat for 5 minutes, stirring frequently. Serve soup warm, topped with, if desired:
A scoop of low-fat cottage cheese
A sprinkling of Parmesan cheese or wheat germ
1 serving = 1 calcium-rich food serving plus 1 vitamin C food (plus 1 green leafy, if vegetable juice is used).

Power-Packed Oatmeal

Makes 1 serving

Bring to a boil in a small saucepan:
7 fl oz/ 200 ml/ 1¼ cups water
Add, stirring to mix thoroughly:
3 oz/75 g/½ cup rolled oats
2 tablespoons wheat germ (if constipation is a problem, substitute unprocessed bran for all or part of wheat germ)
Salt to taste

Lower the heat and cook 5 minutes or longer, according to desired texture, adding additional water if necessary. Remove the pan from the heat and stir in:

2 oz/50 g/¹/₃ cup instant non-fat dry milk

Serve immediately.

Sweet Variation: Add 2 tablespoons raisins and 1 tablespoon apple juice concentrate (optional) when you add the oats; ground cinnamon (optional) to taste when you add the milk.

Savoury Variation: Add pepper, grated Parmesan or Cheddar cheese (remember to count the Cheddar as part of your milk requirement) to taste when you add the milk.

1 serving = 1 grain serving plus 1 calcium-rich food serving plus 1 protein serving plus high fibre.

Bran Muffins

Makes 12 to 16 muffins.

In a small saucepan, simmer 5 minutes over low heat, stirring:

4 oz/125 g/²/₃ cup raisins
2 fl oz/50 ml/¹/₄ cup frozen apple juice concentrate, thawed, undiluted
4 tablespoons frozen orange juice concentrate, thawed, undiluted

Combine in mixing bowl and blend:

8 oz/250 g/1¹/₂ cups wholewheat flour
3 oz/75 g/¹/₂ cup wheat germ
8 oz/250 g/1¹/₂ cups unprocessed bran
1¹/₄ teaspoons baking soda
3 oz/75 g/¹/₂ cup chopped nuts
1 teaspoon ground cinnamon (optional)

Beat together in a separate bowl:

16 fl oz/450 ml/1¹/₂ cups low-fat buttermilk
6 fl oz/150 ml/³/₄ cup frozen apple juice concentrate, thawed, undiluted
2 egg whites, slightly beaten
2 oz/50 g/¹/₃ cup instant non-fat dry milk
2 tablespoons melted margarine or butter, cooled

Combine the dry and liquid ingredients, blending thoroughly in a few strokes. Fold in the raisins with their cooking juice. Fill non-stick patty pans to ²/₃ full. Bake in a preheated 350°C oven for about 20 minutes, or until a toothpick inserted in the centre of a muffin comes out clean.

1 large muffin = 1 grain serving plus high fibre.

Wholewheat Buttermilk Pancakes

Makes approximately 12 pancakes (3 servings)

Note: Allow 1 hour preparation time for batter to settle.

Purée in a blender:

1 cup low-fat buttermilk
1 teaspoon frozen apple juice concentrate, thawed, undiluted
4 oz/100 g/³/₄ cup wholewheat flour
5 tablespoons wheat germ
2oz/50 g/¹/₃ cup non-fat dry milk
Dash of salt to taste
Ground cinnamon to taste (optional)

Stir in:

2 teaspoons baking powder

In a mixing bowl, beat until stiff:

2 large egg whites

Quickly beat the buttermilk-flour mixture into the egg whites. Let the batter stand for 1 hour, then heat a non-stick skillet. When it is hot, brush on:

Margarine or butter

Stir the batter and spoon it onto the skillet to make pancakes of the desired size. When the surface of the pancakes begins to bubble and the undersides are nicely browned, turn and brown the other side. Continue making the pancakes until the batter is used up (you will need between 2 and 3 teaspoons more butter or margarine). Serve them with:

Unsweetened applesauce
Unsweetened preserves (fruit only)
  or apple butter
Plain low-fat yogurt

Variation: Add 1 oz/25 g/¼ cup raisins to the batter.

1 serving = 1 grain serving plus 1 protein serving plus ½ calcium-rich food serving plus high fibre.

Double-the-Milk Shake

Makes 1 serving

Note: Freeze the banana, peeled and wrapped in a plastic bag, 12 to 24 hours ahead of time.

Purée in a blender:

6 oz/175 g/1 cup skim or low-fat milk
2 oz/50 g/⅓ cup non-fat dry milk
1 frozen, overripe banana, cut into chunks
1 teaspoon vanilla extract
Dash of ground cinnamon, or to taste (optional)

Berry Variation: Add 3 oz/75 g/½ cup berries, fresh or unsweetened frozen (thawed), and 1 tablespoon frozen apple juice concentrate (thawed, undiluted) before blending; omit the cinnamon.

'Creamsicle' Variation: Add 2 tablespoons frozen orange juice concentrate (thawed, undiluted); omit the cinnamon.

One banana shake = 2 calcium-rich food servings plus ⅔ protein serving plus 1 fruit serving

One berry variation = 2 calcium-rich food servings plus ⅔ protein serving plus 2 fruit servings

Fig Bars

Makes about 36 bars

Cream together in a bowl:

1 tablespoon fructose
4 tablespoons (½ stick) margarine or butter

Add, and continue to cream:

4 fl oz/100 ml/½ cup plus 2 tablespoons frozen apple juice concentrate that has been heated until warm

Add, and mix to form a dough:

8 oz/250 g/1½ cups wholewheat flour
6 oz/175 g/1 cup wheat germ
1½ teaspoons vanilla extract

Divide dough in two, forming each half into a rectangular bar. Wrap them, separately, in wax paper and chill for 1 hour.

Combine in a saucepan, and cook together over low heat until soft:

1 pound dried figs, chopped

4 fl oz/100 ml/½ cup frozen apple juice concentrate, thawed, undiluted

Remove from the heat and add, stirring until smooth:

2 tablespoons ground almonds or other nuts

On a large non-stick baking sheet that has been lightly greased with oil or non-stick spray, roll out one rectangular bar of dough until it is very thin, evening out the edges as much as possible. Over this evenly spread the fig mixture. Roll out the second rectangle of dough between two sheets of wax paper to the same size as the first rectangle. Remove one sheet of wax paper, and flip the dough as neatly as possible over the fig mixture. Press down lightly, and even out the ends with a sharp knife.

Bake in a preheated 350°F oven for 15 to 30 minutes or until lightly browned. Cut into squares or diamond shapes while still hot.

2 or 3 cookies = 1 nutritious snack plus high fibre.

Fruity Oatmeal Biscuits

Makes 36 2-inch cookies

Place in a saucepan and simmer together until the fruit softens:

10 dates, pitted
6 tablespoons frozen apple juice concentrate, undiluted

Purée mixture in a blender or a food processor, then pour it into a bowl, and add:

2 tablespoons vegetable oil

8 oz/250 g/1½ cups rolled oats (or a mixture of oats and raw wheat flakes)
4 oz/100 g/1 cup raisins
2 oz/50/g ¼ cup to 3 oz/75 g/ ½ cup chopped nuts
Ground cinnamon to taste

Beat lightly in a separate bowl:

1 egg white

Fold gently into the biscuit mixture. Drop the batter in tablespoonsful onto a greased baking sheet. Bake in a preheated 350°F oven for 10 to 12 minutes.

2 or 3 biscuits = 1 nutritious snack plus high fibre

Fruited Yogurt

Makes about 1 cup/½ pt/300 ml

Purée in a blender:

8 fl oz/225 ml/¾ cup plain low-fat yogurt
½ teaspoon fresh grated orange peel
3 oz/75 g/½ cup fresh or frozen (thawed) unsweetened strawberries
1 tablespoon frozen orange juice concentrate, thawed, undiluted
5 teaspoons frozen apple juice concentrate, thawed, undiluted
½ teaspoon ground cinnamon, or to taste (optional)

1 cup = 1 fruit serving plus ½ calcium-rich food serving

Mock Strawberry Daiquiri

Makes 4 servings

Purée in blender:

2 cups washed, hulled fresh or frozen (unsweetened) strawberries (or substitute 2 very ripe bananas, cut into small pieces)

4 oz/100 g/ 1 cup ice cubes, cracked (decrease to ½ cup if using frozen berries) ·

2 fl oz/50 ml/¼ cup frozen apple juice concentrate, undiluted, or to taste

1 tablespoon lime juice

1 teaspoon rum extract

Serve cold in tall glasses

1 serving = 1 fruit serving

Virgin Sangria

Makes 5 to 6 servings

Combine in a large jug:

¾ pt/450 ml/3 cups unsweetened grape juice

12 fl oz/350 ml/¾ cup frozen apple juice concentrate, thawed, undiluted

1 tablespoon lime juice

1 tablespoon lemon juice

Stir to blend, and add:

1 small unpeeled lemon, sliced and seeded

1 small unpeeled orange, sliced and seeded

1 small unpeeled apple, cored, cut into eighths

Stir well, and chill. Add just before serving:

¼ pt/150 ml/¾ cup soda water

Serve in wine glasses over ice.

1 serving = 1 fruit serving

Carob Brownies

Makes 1 8 × 8-inch square or 32 1 × 2-inch brownies

Cook in a small saucepan over low heat for 10 minutes:

3 tablespoons butter or margarine

4 fl oz/100 ml/½ cup plus 1 tablespoon frozen apple juice concentrate, thawed, undiluted

2 oz/50 g/½ cup raisins

Remove from heat and add:

1 teaspoon vanilla extract

In a medium-size bowl, mix together:

3 oz/75 g/⅔ cup wholewheat flour

1 teaspoon baking powder

1 oz/25 g/¼ cup unsweetened carob powder

3 oz/75 g/½ cup chopped walnuts

Combine the apple juice mixture with the carob mixture, blending quickly. Pour into a non-stick 8 × 8-inch baking tin. Bake in a preheated 350°F oven for 10 minutes. Check with a toothpick to judge readiness. Let cool in the pan, then cut the brownies into squares.

2 squares = 1 higher-fibre, high-protein, high-iron snack

Part 2

NINE MONTHS AND COUNTING:

From Conception to Delivery

5
The First Month

WHAT YOU CAN EXPECT AT YOUR FIRST ANTENATAL VISIT

The first or booking clinic is the most comprehensive of all the antenatal visits.[1] A complete medical history will be taken, and certain tests and procedures will be performed only at this exam. You will be asked to visit your doctor or midwife monthly from 0–28 weeks, fortnightly from 28–36 weeks, and weekly from 36 weeks until the baby is delivered. Each doctor's routine will be slightly different. In general, the examination will include.

Validation of Your Pregnancy. Your practitioner will want to check the following: the pregnancy symptoms you are experiencing; the date of your last normal menstrual period, to determine your estimated date of confinement (EDC) or due date (see page 27); your cervix and uterus for signs and approximate duration of the pregnancy. If there's any question, a pregnancy test may be ordered if you haven't already had one.

A Complete History. Come prepared by checking home records and refreshing your memory of the following; your personal medical history (chronic illness, previous major illness or surgery, medications you are presently taking or have taken since conception, known allergies, including drug allergies); your family medical history (genetic disorders and chronic diseases); your social history (age, occupation, habits, such as; smoking, drinking, exercise, diet); your gynaecological and obstetrical history (age at first menstrual period, usual length of menstrual cycle, duration and regularity of menstrual periods; past abortions, miscarriages, and live births; course of past pregnancies, labours, and deliveries).

A Complete Physical Examination. This may include: assessment of your general health through examination of heart, lungs, breasts, abdo-

---

1. See appendix for an explanation of the procedures and tests performed.

men; measurement of your blood pressure to serve as a baseline reading for comparison at subsequent visits; measurement of your height and weight, usual and present; inspection of extremities for varicose veins and oedema (swelling from excess fluid in tissues), to serve as a baseline for comparison at subsequent visits; inspection and palpation of external genitalia; examination of your vagina and cervix with a speculum inserted internally; examination of your pelvic organs bi-manually (with one hand in the vagina and one on the abdomen.

A Battery of Tests This may include: Cervical smear for cancer detection, blood tests to determine blood type, Rh type, haemoglobin (to check for anaemia), and rubella titre; antibody screening if Rh negative; a VDRL (for syphilis); urinalysis to check for glucose (sugar), albumin (protein), white blood cells, blood and bacteria; sickle cell or Tay Sachs screening if indicated, and in some areas, routine ultrasound screening offered and booked.

An Opportunity for Discussion. Bring a list of questions, problems, and symptoms. This is also a good time to talk about fears, philosophy of childbirth, and so on. Below are some of the topics you may wish to cover:

– Dietary advice.
– Use of drugs, alcohol and smoking during pregnancy.
– Antenatal care – what are the risks and consequences of tests and procedures being offered?
– Availability of parentcraft or relaxation classes in your area and advice on the necessity for advance booking.

What You May Look Like

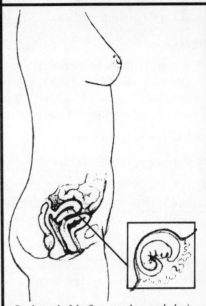

By the end of the first month, your baby is a tiny, tadpole-like embryo, smaller than a grain of rice. In the next two weeks, the neural tube (which becomes the brain and spinal cord), heart, digestive tract, sensory organs, and arm and leg buds will begin to form.

– Maternity benefits available, including free dental treatment and prescriptions, maternity grant, allowance, maternity leave and pay, referral to a social worker if needed. Details available from Maternity Alliance, 309 Kentish Town Road, London, NW5 2TJ.
– Discussion of a birth plan, to include preparation for labour, i.e. enema and shave; preferred ways of coping with contractions; pain-relieving drugs; delivery; care and feeding of the baby; and postnatal plans.

WHAT YOU MAY BE FEELING

You may feel all of these symptoms at one time or another or only one or two.

Physically:

☆ Absence of menstruation (though you may stain slightly when your period is expected or when the fertilized egg implants in the uterus[2]

☆ Fatigue and sleepiness

☆ A need to urinate frequently

☆ Nausea, with or without vomiting, and/or excessive salivation (ptyalism)

☆ Heartburn and indigestion, flatulence, and bloating

☆ Food aversions and cravings

☆ Breast changes (most pronounced in women who have breast changes prior to menstruation): fullness, heaviness, tenderness, tingling; darkening of the areola (the pigmented area around the nipple); sweat glands in the areola become prominent (Montgomery's tubercles), like large goose bumps; a network of bluish lines appear under the skin as blood supply to the breasts increases (though these lines may not appear until later)

Emotionally:

☆ Instability comparable to premenstrual syndrome, which may include irritability, mood swings, irrationality, weepiness

☆ Misgivings, fear, joy, elation – any or all of these

WHAT YOU MAY BE CONCERNED ABOUT

Fatigue

'I'm tired all the time. I'm worried that I won't be able to continue working.'

It would be surprising if you weren't tired. In some ways, your pregnant body is working harder even when you're resting than a nonpregnant body is when mountain-climbing; you just can't see its efforts. For one thing, it's manufacturing your baby's life support system, the placenta, which won't be completed until the end of the first trimester. For another, it's adjusting to the many other physical and emotional demands of pregnancy, which are considerable. Once your body is adjusted and the placenta is complete (around the fourth month), you should have more energy. Until then, you may need to work fewer hours or take a few days off if you're really dragging. But if your pregnancy continues normally,

2. It is rare, but a woman may still menstruate in the first two or three months. *Any* bleeding, of course, should be reported to your practitioner.

there is absolutely no reason why you shouldn't stay at your job. Most pregnant women are happier if they keep busy.

Since your fatigue is legitimate, don't fight it. Consider it a signal from your body that you need more rest. That, of course, is more easily suggested than done. But it is worth a try.

Baby Yourself. And your baby – as much as possible, and don't feel guilty about it. Don't try to be Super-Mum-to-Be. Getting enough rest is more important than having your house pass the white-glove-test. Keep evenings free of unessential activities. Spend them off your feet when you can, reading, watching TV, scouring baby-name books. If you have older children, play quiet games with them. If you can afford the luxury of an afternoon nap, by all means indulge. If you can't sleep, lie down with a good book. A nap at the office isn't a reasonable goal, of course, but putting your feet up at your desk or in the staff room during lunch hour is.

Let Others Baby You. Accept your mother-in-law's offer to vacuum and dust the house when she's visiting. Let your dad take the older kids to the zoo on Sunday. Enlist your partner for chores like laundry and shopping.

Get an Hour or Two More Sleep Each Night. Skip the 11 o'clock news and turn in earlier; ask your partner to fix breakfast so you can turn out later.

Be Sure That Your Diet Isn't Deficient. First-trimester fatigue is often aggravated by a deficiency in iron, protein, or just plain calories. Double check the Best-Odds Diet (page 82) to make certain you're filling all of your requirements. And no matter how tired you're feeling, don't be tempted to rev your body up with caffeine, chocolate bars, and cake. It won't be fooled for long, and after the temporary lift, your blood sugar will plummet, leaving you more fatigued than ever.

When fatigue is severe, especially when it is accompanied by fainting, pallor, breathlessness, and/or palpitations, the possibility of anaemia should be considered. (See page 139.)

Though fatigue will probably ease up by month four, you can expect it to return in the last trimester – probably as nature's way of preparing you for those long sleepless nights once the baby has arrived.

Morning Sickness

'I haven't had any morning sickness. Can I still be pregnant?'

Morning sickness, like a craving for pickles and ice cream, is one of those truisms about pregnancy that ain't necessarily so. Only one third to one half of expectant women ever experience the nausea and/or vomiting of morning sickness. If you're among those who never suffer from it, you can consider yourself not only pregnant, but lucky, too.

'My morning sickness lasts all day. I'm afraid I'm not able to keep down enough good food to nourish my baby.'

Fortunately, morning sickness (a misnamed malady, because it can strike morning, noon, or night – or even all day long) rarely interferes with proper nutrition enough to harm the developing foetus. And for most women, it doesn't last past the third month – though an occasional expectant mother won't experience it until well into the second trimester and a few, particularly those expecting twins, may enjoy its dubious pleasures for a full nine months.

What causes morning sickness? No one knows for sure, but there's no shortage of theories. It is known that the command post for nausea and vomiting is in a special area in the brain stem. A myriad of physical reasons why this area may be over-stimulated during pregnancy have been suggested, including the high level of the pregnancy hormone HCG in the blood in the first trimester and the rapid stretching of the uterine muscles. The problem is compounded by the relative relaxation of the muscle tissue in the digestive tract, which makes digestion less efficient, and excess acid in the stomach caused by not eating or eating the wrong foods.

But these physical triggers alone can't explain morning sickness, since most are common to all pregnancies and yet not all pregnant women experience nausea and vomiting. Several illuminating facts seem to support the theory that emotional factors augment the physical. For one thing, morning sickness is unknown in some more primitive societies where lifestyles are simpler, more relaxed, and less demanding (although it did exist in ancient Western civilization).

For another, many women suffering from hyperemesis, or excessive vomiting, recover without treatment as soon as they are placed in the relatively tranquil environment of a hospital, away from their families and the problems of day-to-day living. And studies also show that many of these women are highly hypnotizable, which means they are very susceptible to the power of suggestion – and our society surely suggests that morning sickness is an expected part of pregnancy. Also quite revealing is that some women suffer debilitating nausea and vomiting with unwanted, unplanned pregnancies, yet experience no morning sickness at all in pregnancies they are happy about. Physical or mental fatigue also seems to increase the possibility of nausea striking. As does carrying multiple foetuses – probably because of a multiplication of both physical and emotional stresses.

Unfortunately, medical experts are even less certain of the cure for morning sickness than they are of its cause. They do, however, agree that there are many ways of alleviating its symptoms and minimizing its effects. See which work best for you:

☆ Eat a diet high in protein and complex carbohydrates (see the Best-Odds Diet, page 82) – both of which fight nausea. So does good nutrition, so eat as well as you can under the circumstances.

☆ Take plenty of fluids – especially if you're losing them through vomiting. If they are easier to get down than solids when your stomach is upset, use them for getting your nutrients. Concentrate on any of the following you can handle: Double-the-Milk Shakes (see page 94); fruit or vegetable juices; soups, broths, and bouillons. If you find fluids make you queasier, eat solids with high water content, such as fresh fruits and vegetables – particularly lettuce, melons, and citrus fruits.

☆ Your doctor may recommend a daily ration of 50 milligrams of B_6, which seems to help relieve nausea in some women. *Do not take any medication for morning sickness*.

☆ Avoid the sight, smell, and taste of foods that make you feel queasy. Don't be a martyr and prepare sausage and onion for your husband if it makes you rush to the bathroom.

☆ Eat often – before you feel hungry. When your stomach is empty, its acids don't have anything to eat but its own lining. This can trigger nausea. So can the low blood sugar caused by long stretches between meals. Six small meals are better than three large. Carry nutritious snacks (dried fruit, whole-grain crackers) with you for convenient snacking.

☆ Eat before nausea strikes. Food will be easier to get down and, by filling your stomach, may prevent an attack.

☆ Eat in bed – for the same reasons you eat often: to keep your stomach full and your blood sugar at an even keel. Before you go to sleep at night, have a snack that is high in protein and complex carbohydrates: a glass of milk and a bran muffin, for example. Twenty minutes before you plan to get out of bed in the morning, have a high-carbohydrate snack: a few whole-wheat crackers, or rice cakes, or a handful of raisins. Keep them next to your bed so you don't have to get up for them, and in case you wake up hungry in the middle of the night.[3]

☆ Get some extra sleep and relaxation. Both emotional and physical fatigue increase morning sickness.

☆ Greet the morning in slow motion – rushing tends to aggravate nausea. Don't jump out of bed and rush out the door. Stay in bed digesting your crackers for 20 minutes, then rise slowly to a leisurely breakfast. This may seem impossible if you have other children, but try to wake up before they do to give yourself a little quiet time, or let your husband handle their early morning needs.

Frequent Urination

'I'm in the bathroom every half hour. Is it normal to be urinating this often?'

Most – though by no means all – pregnant women do make frequent detours to the toilet both in the first and last trimesters. One of the reasons for an initial increase in urinary frequency is the higher volume of body fluids and the improved efficiency of the kidneys, which helps rid the body more quickly of waste products. Another is the

---

3. If you start to associate a particular carbohydrate snack (crackers, for instance) with your nausea, switch to a different snack.

pressure of the growing uterus, which is still in the pelvis next to the bladder. The pressure is often relieved once the uterus rises into the abdominal cavity, around the fourth month. It probably won't return until the baby 'drops' in the ninth month and again presses on the bladder. But because the arrangement of internal organs varies slightly from women to woman, the degree of frequency may also vary.

'How come I'm not urinating frequently?'

No noticeable increase in the frequency of urination may be perfectly normal for you, especially if you ordinarily urinate often. You should, however, be certain you're getting enough fluids (at least eight glasses a day). Not only can insufficient fluid intake be the cause of infrequent urination, it could also lead to urinary tract infection.

Breast Changes

'I hardly recognize my breasts anymore – they're so swollen and tender. Will they stay that way, and will they sag after I give birth?'

Get used to the chest look. Although it may not be fashionable, it's one of the hallmarks of pregnancy. Your breasts are enlarging (even more than they do premenstrually) because of the increased amounts of oestrogen and progesterone your body is now producing. This, and the other changes that occur in the breasts during pregnancy, are all aimed at preparing you to feed your baby when

it arrives. The areola (the pigmented area around the nipple) darkens, spreads, and may be spotted with even darker areas. This darkening may fade but not disappear entirely after birth. The little bumps you may notice on the areola are sebaceous (sweat) glands, which become more prominent during pregnancy and return to normal afterwards. The complex road map of blue veins that traverses the breasts – often quite vivid on a fair-skinned woman – represents a mother-to-baby delivery system for nutrients and fluids. After delivery or nursing, they will disappear.

What you won't have to get used to, fortunately, is the sometimes agonizing sensitivity of your breasts. Though they will continue to grow throughout your pregnancy – possibly increasing as much as three cup sizes – they are not likely to remain tender-to-the-touch past the third or fourth month. As for whether or not they will sag after the baby is born, that is at least partly up to you. Stretching and sagging of the breast tissue result from a lack of support during pregnancy – not from pregnancy itself – though the tendency to sag may be genetic. No matter how firm your breasts are now, protect them for the future by wearing a good support bra daily. If your breasts are particularly large or have a tendency to sag, it's a good idea to wear a bra even at night.

Vitamin Supplements

'Should I be taking vitamins?'

Good supplements, formulated especially for expectant mothers, are available over-the-counter. (See page 87 for what the supplement should contain.) But never use vitamin pills to replace a good diet, only to supplement it. Any vitamins that supply more than the recommended daily allowance for pregnant women should be considered drugs and be taken only under medical supervision, when benefit outweighs risk.

Ectopic Pregnancy

'I've been having occasional cramping. Could I have an ectopic pregnancy without knowing it?'

The fear of ectopic, or tubal, pregnancy lurks somewhere in the mind of nearly every newly pregnant woman who has heard of this abnormal type of implantation. Fortunately, for the vast majority it's an unfounded fear. A fear that can be dismissed completely by the eighth week of pregnancy, by which time most tubal pregnancies have been diagnosed and terminated.

Only about 10 in 1,000 pregnancies are ectopic – that is, take place outside the uterus, usually in the fallopian tubes. A good many of these are diagnosed before a woman even realizes she is pregnant. So chances are that if your doctor has confirmed your pregnancy through a blood test and a physical exam and you've had no signs of ectopic pregnancy, then you can cross this worry off your list.

There are several factors that can make women more susceptible to ectopic pregnancies. They include:

☆ A previous ectopic pregnancy.

☆ Previous pelvic inflammatory disease.

☆ Previous abdominal or tubal surgery with postoperative scarring.

☆ Unsuccessful tubal ligation (sterilization surgery), or tubal ligation reversal.

☆ An IUD in place when conception occurs (an IUD is more likely to prevent conception in the uterus than outside it – thus the increase in the relative incidence of ectopics in IUD users).[4]

☆ Possibly, multiple induced abortions (the evidence isn't clear).

☆ Possibly, exposure to diethylstilbestrol (DES) in the womb, especially if it resulted in significant structural abnormalities of the reproductive tract.

Rare as ectopic pregnancies are, every pregnant woman – particularly those at high risk – should be familiar with the symptoms. Occasional cramping, probably the result of ligaments stretching as the uterus grows, is not one of them. But any or all of the following might be, and do require the immediate evaluation of a physician. If you can't reach your doctor, go at once to the outpatients at the hospital his or her office or service recommends.

☆ Colicky, crampy pain with tenderness, usually in the lower abdomen – on one side initially, though the pain can radiate throughout the abdomen. Pain may worsen on

---

4. But having worn an IUD previously does not appear to increase risk.

straining of bowels, coughing, or moving. If tubal rupture occurs, pain becomes very sharp and steady for a short time before diffusing throughout the pelvic region.

☆ Brown vaginal spotting or light bleeding (intermittent or persistent), which may precede pain by several days or weeks. There may be no bleeding without rupture of the tube; with rupture, heavy bleeding may begin.

☆ Nausea and vomiting in about 25% to 50% of women – though this may be difficult to distinguish from morning sickness.

☆ Dizziness or weakness, in some women. If the tube ruptures, fast weak pulse, clammy skin, and fainting are common.

☆ Shoulder pain, in some women.

☆ Feeling of rectal pressure, in some women.

Should these symptoms prove to indicate ectopic pregnancy, quick medical attention can often save the patient's fallopian tube and fertility.

The Condition of Your Baby

'I'm very nervous because I can't really feel my baby. Could it die without my knowing it?'

At this stage, with no noticeable enlargement of the abdomen or obvious foetal activity, it's hard to imagine that there's really a living, growing baby inside you. But the death of a foetus or embryo that isn't expelled from the uterus in a miscarriage is very rare. When it does happen, the woman loses all signs of pregnancy, including breast tenderness and enlargement, and may develop a brownish discharge, though no frank bleeding. Upon examination, the physician will find that the uterus, rather than growing, has diminished in size.

If at any time all of your pregnancy symptoms should disappear, call your doctor for an appointment. That's a more positive approach than sitting at home worrying.

Miscarriage

'Between what I read and what my mother tells me, I'm afraid everything I've done, am doing, and will do might cause a miscarriage.'

For many expectant women, the fear of miscarriage keeps their joy guarded in the first trimester. Some even refrain from spreading their happy news until the fourth month, when they begin to feel secure that the pregnancy will indeed continue. And for most of them – probably 90% – it will.

Though it is hard for parents to believe it at the time, when a miscarriage *does* occur it is usually a blessing. Early miscarriage is generally a natural selection process in which a defective embryo or foetus (defective because of environmental factors, such as radiation or drugs; because of poor implantation in the uterus; because of genetic abnormality, maternal infection, random accident, or unknown reasons) is discarded before it has a chance to develop.

Happily, most women who have one miscarriage do not become habitual aborters. In fact, having a miscarriage is so common that many doctors believe that virtually every woman will have at least one sometime during her reproductive life. Many of these miscarriages go unnoticed, occurring even before a woman knows she is pregnant and passing for an unusually heavy and crampy menstrual period.

There is still much to be learned about the reasons for early miscarriage, but several factors are believed *not* to cause the problem. They include:

☆ Previous trouble with an IUD. Scarring of the endometrium (the lining of the uterus) because of IUD-triggered infection could prevent a pregnancy from implanting in the uterus, but should not cause miscarriage, once implantation is well established. Nor should previous difficulty holding an IUD in position affect a pregnancy.

☆ History of multiple abortions.[5] Scarring of the endometrium from multiple abortions, as from IUD-caused infections, could prevent implantation but should not otherwise be responsible for early miscarriage.

☆ Usual and accustomed physical activity, such as hanging curtains,

moving light furniture, tennis, and so on.[6]

☆ Emotional upset – resulting from an argument, stress at work, or family problems.

☆ A fall or other minor accidental injury to the mother. But serious injury could hurt the foetus, so safety precautions – such as wearing a seat belt and not climbing on rickety chairs – should always be observed.

There are several factors, however, that *are* believed to increase the risk of spontaneous abortion. Some are one-time events and should not affect future pregnancies (for example: a severe infection such as pneumonia; a high fever; rubella, x-rays, or drugs that harm the foetus; an IUD in place when conception occurs). Other risk factors, when they are detected, can be controlled in future pregnancies (poor nutrition; smoking; Rh incompatibility; hormonal insufficiency; and certain maternal medical problems). A few miscarriage risk factors are still not easily overcome (such as a malformed uterus, though some can be surgically corrected, and certain chronic maternal illnesses).

When Not to Worry. It's important to recognize that each cramp, ache, or bit of spotting isn't necessarily warning of an impending miscarriage. Just about every normal pregnancy will include at least one of these usually

---

5. Though not a cause of early miscarriage, repeated dilatations from abortions or other procedures may result in a weakened or incompetent cervix – often a cause of late miscarriage. (See page 157.)

6. In a high-risk pregnancy, the physician may limit these activities or even prescribe strict bed rest. But you should limit activity only on direction of your doctor.

Possible Signs of Miscarriage

When to Call Your Doctor Immediately, Just in Case

☆ When you experience bleeding with cramps or pain in the centre of your lower abdomen. (Pain on one side in early pregnancy could be triggered by an ectopic pregnancy, and also warrants a call to the doctor.)

☆ When pain is severe or continues unabated for more than one day, even if it isn't accompanied by staining or bleeding.

☆ When bleeding is as heavy as a menstrual period, or staining continues lightly for more than three days.

When to Get Emergency Medical Attention

☆ When you have a history of miscarriage, and experience either bleeding or cramping or both.

☆ When bleeding is so heavy you soak several pads in an hour, or when pain is so severe you can't bear it.

☆ When you pass clots or greyish material along with the blood – which may mean a miscarriage has already begun. If you can't reach your doctor, go to the nearest emergency room or the one recommended by his or her office or source. The doctor may want you to save the material you pass (in a jar, plastic bag, or other clean container) so he or she can try to determine whether or not the miscarriage is simply threatening, is complete, or is partial and requires a D and C (dilatation and curettage) to complete it.

innocuous symptoms at one time or another:[7]

☆ Mild cramps or achiness on one or both sides of the abdomen. This is probably due to the stretching of ligaments that support the uterus. Unless cramping is severe, constant, or accompanied by bleeding, there's no need to worry.

☆ Staining a bit around the time you might have expected your period or about 7 to 10 days after conception, when the little ball of cells that is going to develop into your baby attaches itself to the uterine wall. Slight bleeding at these times is common and doesn't necessarily indicate a problem with your pregnancy – as long as it isn't accompanied by lower abdominal pain.

7. You should routinely tell your doctor about *any* pains, cramping, or bleeding. In most cases his or her response will put your worries to rest.

If You Suspect Miscarriage. If you experience any of the symptoms listed in the box above, put a call in to your doctor. If your symptoms are listed under 'get emergency medical attention' and your doctor is not available, leave a message for him or her, go straight to the nearest outpatients.

While waiting for help, lie down if you can, or rest in a chair with your feet up. This may not prevent a miscarriage if it's about to happen, but it will help you to relax. It should also help you to relax to know that most women who have episodes of bleeding in early pregnancy carry to term and have normal, healthy babies.

If, on examination, the doctor finds the cervix dilated, it will be assumed that a miscarriage has occurred or is in progress. In such a case nothing can be done to prevent the loss of the foetus. In many cases the foetus will already have died prior to the onset of miscarriage – triggering the spontaneous abortion.

On the other hand, if the foetus is shown to be alive either through ultrasound or a Doppler device and there is no dilatation, the chances are very good that the threatened miscarriage will not occur. Some physicians will suggest no particular treatment on the theory that a doomed pregnancy will abort, therapy or no, and a healthy pregnancy will hang in there (also with or without therapy). Others – particularly when a woman has a history of miscarriage, or when it is believed that implantation is imperfect – will impose bed rest and restrictions on activities, including sexual intercourse. Female hormones, once given routinely for early bleeding, are no longer used because there is doubt about their efficacy and concern that they can harm the foetus if the pregnancy continues.

Sometimes, when a miscarriage does occur, it isn't complete – only parts of the placenta, sac, and embryo are expelled. If you've had, or believe you've had, a miscarriage, and bleeding and/or pain continue, phone your doctor immediately. A D and C will probably be required to stop the bleeding. It's a simple but important procedure in which the doctor dilates the cervix and scrapes or suctions out any remaining foetal or placental tissue. Your physician will probably also want to evaluate material passed or scraped out for clues to the cause of the miscarriage.

Losing a baby, even this early, is traumatic. But don't let guilt compound your misery – *a miscarriage is not your fault*. Do allow yourself to grieve. Sharing your feelings with your spouse, your doctor, a friend, will help. In some communities, there are support groups for couples who have experienced pregnancy loss. Ask your doctor if there is one in your area[8].

Probably the best therapy is getting pregnant again soon. Before you do, discuss the possible causes of the miscarriage with your doctor and, if feasible, take steps to correct them before you conceive again.

Whatever the cause of your miscarriage, many doctors suggest waiting three to six months before starting a new pregnancy – though sexual relations can often be resumed after six weeks. Think of this waiting period positively. Take advantage of it by improving your diet and health habits. The odds are excellent that next time around you'll have a normal pregnancy and a healthy baby.

'I don't really feel pregnant. Could I have miscarried without knowing it?'

Worry that you might miscarry without realizing it, though common, is unwarranted. Once a pregnancy is established, the signs that it is aborting are not something which can be inadvertently overlooked. Simply not 'feeling pregnant' is not a reason for concern. Share your concerns with your doctor at your next visit, which will undoubtedly be reassuring.

---

8. You could also consult the Miscarriage Association, 2 West Vale, Thornhill Road, Dewsbury, West Yorkshire (0942 454510). There is a good leaflet on the subject available from the National Childbirth Trust.

When to Call the Doctor/Midwife

It's best to set up an emergency protocol with your practitioner before an emergency strikes. If you haven't, and you are experiencing a symptom that requires immediate medical attention, try the following. First call the surgery. If he or she isn't available and doesn't call back within a few minutes, call the surgery again and leave a message saying what your problem is and where you are headed. Then go directly to the nearest emergency department or call an ambulance.

When you report any of the following to your doctor, be sure to mention any other symptoms you may be experiencing, no matter how remote they may seem from the immediate problem. Also be sure to be specific, mentioning how long the symptom has existed, how frequently it recurs, what seems to relieve or exacerbate it, and how severe it is.

☆ Severe lower abdominal pain, on one or both sides, that doesn't subside: notify your practitioner the same day; if it is accompanied by bleeding, or nausea and vomiting, call immediately.

☆ Slight vaginal spotting: notify your practitioner the same day.

☆ Heavy bleeding (especially when combined with abdominal or back pain): call immediately.

☆ A gush of fluid from the vagina, which indicates the rupture of the amniotic sac: call immediately.

☆ A sudden increase in thirst, accompanied by a paucity of urination, or no urination at all for an entire day: call immediately.

☆ Swelling or puffiness of hands, face, eyes: call the same day. If very sudden and severe, or accompanied by headache or vision difficulties: call immediately.

☆ Severe headache that persists for more than two or three hours, call the same day. If accompanied by vision disturbances or sudden puffiness of eyes, face, hands: call immediately.

☆ Painful or burning urination: call the same day. If accompanied by chills and fever over 102 degrees, and/or backache: call immediately.

☆ Absence of noticeable foetal movement for more than five days through the fifth month: call the same day. From the sixth month on, absence of noticeable movement for 24 hours: call immediately.

☆ Vision disturbances (blurring, dimming, double vision) that persist for two or three hours: call immediately.

☆ Fainting or dizziness: notify the doctor or midwife the same day.

☆ Chills and fever over 100 degrees (with no cold or flu symptoms): call the same day. Fever over 102 degrees: call immediately.

☆ Severe nausea and vomiting, vomiting more often than two or three times a day in the first trimester, vomiting later in pregnancy when you haven't before: notify the doctor or midwife the same day. If vomiting is accompanied by pain and/or fever call immediately.

☆ Sudden weight gain of more than two pounds that does not seem related to excessive eating: notify the doctor the same day. If accompanied by oedema of the hands and face and/or headache or visual disturbances: call immediately.

WHAT IT'S IMPORTANT TO KNOW: GETTING REGULAR MEDICAL CARE

In the past decade, the self-care health movement has instructed us in everything from taking our own blood pressure and pulse to home-treating muscle strains and evaluating a scratchy throat or an aching ear. The impact it has had on the effectiveness of our health care has been unquestionably positive – cutting down on the number of trips we make to our doctors and making us better patients when we do go. Best of all, it's made us aware of the responsibility we each have for our own health, and it has the potential of making us a lot healthier in the years to come.

Even in pregnancy, as you can see throughout this book, there are countless steps you can take to make your own nine months safer and more comfortable, your labour and delivery easier, and your expected end product healthier. But to try to go it alone, even for a few months, is to abuse the concept of self-care – which is built on the foundation of a cooperative partnership between you and your health professional. Regular professional input in pregnancy is crucial. One major study found that women who had many antenatal visits (an average of 12.7) had bigger babies with better survival rates than those who had few prenatal visits (an average of 1.4).

A Schedule of Antenatal Visits

Ideally, your first visit to a doctor or midwife should take place while that baby is still a gleam in daddy's (and your) eye. That's an ideal many of us, especially those whose pregnancies are unplanned, can't always manage. Second best, and still very good, is a visit as soon as you suspect you have conceived. An internal exam will help confirm your pregnancy, and a physical will uncover any potential problems that may need monitoring. After that, the schedule of visits will vary depending on the practitioner you are seeing and whether or not yours is a high-risk pregnancy. In an uneventful low-risk pregnancy you can probably expect to see your doctor monthly up until the end of the 28th week. After that you may begin going every two weeks until the last month, when weekly visits are usual.

For what you can expect to happen at each antenatal visit, see the monthly chapters.

Taking Care of the Rest of You

You're understandably preoccupied with obstetrical matters during pregnancy. But though your health care should begin with your belly, it shouldn't end there. And don't just wait for problems to occur. Do pay a visit to your dentist; most dental work, particularly the preventive kind, can be done safely during pregnancy (see page 69). Your family doctor or a specialist should also be monitoring any chronic illnesses or other medical problems that don't fall under the purview of the obstetrician.

If new problems come up while you're pregnant, don't ignore them. Even if you've noticed symptoms which seem relatively innocuous, it's more important than ever to consult with your doctor or midwife promptly. Your baby needs a *wholly* healthy mother.

6
The Second Month

WHAT YOU CAN EXPECT AT THIS MONTH'S CHECKUP

If this is your first antenatal visit, see What You Can Expect at Your First Antenatal Visit (page 98). If this is your second exam, you can expect your doctor or midwife to check the following, though there may be variations depending upon your particular needs and your doctor or midwife's style of practice:[1]

☆ any unusual vaginal discharge or bleeding

☆ any urinary infection

☆ weight and blood pressure

☆ hands, feet and legs for oedema (swelling), and legs and vulva for varicose veins

☆ symptoms you have been experiencing, especially unusual ones

☆ abdominal inspection and palpation

☆ blood test for haemoglobin

☆ iron tablets usually prescribed or dispensed

☆ questions or problems you want to discuss – have a list ready

WHAT YOU MAY BE FEELING

You may feel all of these symptoms at one time or another or only one or two. Some may have continued from last month, others may be new. Don't be sur-

prised, no matter what your symptoms, if you don't feel pregnant yet.

Physically:

☆ Fatigue and sleepiness

☆ A need to urinate frequently

☆ Nausea, with or without vomiting,

---

1. See appendix for an explanation of the procedures and tests performed.

and/or excessive salivation (ptyalism)

☆ Constipation

☆ Heartburn and indigestion, flatulence, and bloating

☆ Food aversions and cravings

☆ Breast changes: fullness, heaviness, tenderness, tingling; darkening of the areola (the pigmented area around the nipple); sweat glands in the areola become prominent (Montgomery's tubercles), like large goose bumps; a network of bluish lines appear under the skin as blood supply to the breasts increases

☆ Occasional headaches, possibly due to a reaction to hormones (similar to headaches in women taking birth control pills)

☆ Occasional faintness or dizziness

☆ Clothes may begin to feel tight around waist and bust, abdomen may appear enlarged, probably due to bowel distention rather than uterine growth

Emotionally:

☆ Instability comparable to premenstrual syndrome, which may include irritability, mood swings, irrationality, weepiness

What You May Look Like

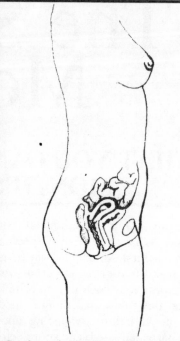

By the end of the second month, the embryo is more human-looking, about 1¼ inches long from head to buttocks (one-third of it is the head), and weighs about ½ ounce. It has a beating heart, and arms and legs with the beginnings of fingers and toes. Bone starts to replace cartilage.

☆ Misgivings, fear, joy, elation – any or all of these

WHAT YOU MAY BE CONCERNED ABOUT

Venous Changes

'Since I became pregnant I've got awful-looking spidery purplish red lines on my thighs. Are they varicose veins?'

They aren't pretty, but they aren't varicose veins. They are spider nevi, or telangiectases, which can result from the hormone changes of pregnancy. They will fade and disappear after delivery.

'I have unsightly blue lines under the skin, on my breasts and abdomen. Is that normal?'

Very normal. They are part of the network of veins that expand to carry the increased blood flow that comes with pregnancy. Not only are the veins nothing to worry about, they are a sign that your body is doing what it should. They show up earliest in very slim women. In other women the venous network may be less visible, not noticeable at all, or may not become obvious until later in pregnancy.

'My mother and grandmother both had varicose veins during pregnancy and had trouble with them ever after. Is there anything I can do to prevent the problem in my own pregnancy?'

Because varicosities often run in families, you're wise to think about prevention now. Especially since varicose veins tend to worsen with subsequent pregnancies.

Normal, healthy veins carry blood from the extremities back to the heart. Because they are working against gravity, they are designed with a series of valves that prevent back flow. In some people these valves are missing or faulty, causing blood to pool in the veins and resulting in the bulging of varicosities. Veins that are easily distended, or distensible, can further contribute to the condition. The problem is more common in people who are obese, and occurs four times more often in women than in men. In women who

are susceptible, the condition often surfaces for the first time during pregnancy. There are several reasons for this: increased pressure from the uterus on the pelvic veins; increasing pressure on leg veins; augmented blood volume; and pregnancy hormones which relax the muscle tissue in the veins, causing them to open wider.

The symptoms of varicose veins aren't difficult to recognize, but they vary a great deal in severity. The swollen veins may cause severe pain, mild achiness, a sensation of heaviness, or may even be entirely asymptomatic. A slight outline of bluish veins may be visible, or serpentine veins may bulge from ankle to upper thigh or vulva. In severe cases the skin covering the veins becomes swollen, dry, and irritated. Occasionally, thrombophlebitis (an inflammation of a vein associated with a blood clot) may develop at the site of a varicosity.

Fortunately, varicose veins during pregnancy can often be prevented, or the symptoms minimized:

☆ Avoid excessive weight gain.

☆ Avoid long periods of standing or sitting; when sitting or lying down, elevate legs above the level of the heart when possible.

☆ Wear support pantyhose or elastic stockings, putting them on before getting out of bed in the morning and removing them at night before going to sleep.

☆ Do not wear a tight girdle – especially a panty-leg girdle – or stockings or socks with elastic tops that cut off circulation.

☆ Get plenty of exercise – a brisk 20-to-30 minute walk every day.

☆ Be sure to get enough vitamin C, which some physicians believe helps to keep veins healthy and elastic.

Surgical removal of varicose veins isn't recommended during pregnancy, although it can certainly be considered afterward. Most cases, however, will clear up or improve spontaneously after delivery, usually by the time prepregnancy weight is reached.

Complexion Problems

'My skin is breaking out the way it did when I was a teenager.'

The glow of pregnancy that some women are lucky enough to exude is due not simply to happiness, but to an increased secretion of oils caused by hormonal changes. And so, alas, are the less-than-glowing breakouts of pregnancy that other women experience (particularly those whose skin ordinarily breaks out before their periods). Though such breakouts are hard to eliminate entirely, the following may help keep them to a minimum:

☆ Be faithful to the Best-Odds Diet – it's good for your skin as well as for your baby.

☆ Don't pass a tap without filling your glass – water is one of the most effective pore-purifiers around.

☆ Wash your face often with a gentle cleanser. Avoid skin-clogging greasy creams and makeups.

☆ If your practitioner approves, take a vitamin B_6 supplement (25 to 50 milligrams). This vitamin is sometimes useful in treating hormonally-induced skin problems.

For some women, dry skin, often with itching, is a pregnancy problem. Moisturizers may be helpful. So may taking plenty of fluids and keeping rooms well humidified in the heating season. Too-frequent washing or bathing, particularly with soap, tends to increase dryness, so don't overdo it.

Waistline Expansion

'Why does my waist seem to be expanding already? I thought I wouldn't 'show' until the third month at least.'

Your expanding waistline may very well be a legitimate product of pregnancy, especially if you started out slender, with little excess flesh for your growing uterus to hide under. Or it may be the result of bowel distention, very common in early pregnancy. On the other hand, it's also quite possible that your 'show' may be nothing but fat around your middle – an indication that you're gaining weight too quickly. If you've gained more than 3 pounds so far, analyze your diet – you are very likely taking in too many calories, possibly empty ones. Review the Best-Odds Diet, and read about weight gain on page 132.

Losing Your Figure

'I'm afraid I'll lose my figure forever – and so is my husband.'

This is a very understandable fear – particularly for someone who is conscious of her figure to begin with. But it is also one over which you can have complete control. Many women do look fat and flabby after childbirth because they gained too much, ate the wrong foods, or didn't get enough exercise during pregnancy – and *not* simply because they were carrying a child. The weight gain of pregnancy has just one legitimate purpose: to nurture the developing foetus. If only enough weight to serve that purpose is gained and a woman keeps physically fit, her figure should return to normal within a few months after the baby is born, especially if she is breastfeeding. See the Best-Odds Diet, and read about weight gain on page 132.

With the right prenatal care, you can look better than ever after pregnancy, because you will have learned how to take optimum care of your body. Your husband can look better after pregnancy, too, benefiting from your healthier lifestyle.

Heartburn and Indigestion

'I have indigestion and heartburn all the time. Will this affect my baby?'

While you are painfully aware of your gastrointestinal discomfort, your baby is blissfully oblivious to it and unaffected by it – as long as it isn't interfering with your eating the right foods.

Though indigestion can have the same cause (usually overindulgence) during pregnancy as when you're not pregnant, there are additional reasons why it may be plaguing you now. Early in pregnancy, your body produces large amounts of progesterone and oestrogen, which tend to relax smooth muscle tissue everywhere, including that in the gastrointestinal tract. As a result, food moves more slowly through your system, resulting in bloating. This is uncomfortable for you but good for the baby, because the slow-down allows better absorption of nutrients into your bloodstream and, subsequently, through the placenta into your baby's system.

Heartburn results when the sphincter that separates the oesophagus from the stomach becomes lax, occasionally allowing food and harsh digestive juices to back up from stomach to oesophagus. The stomach acids irritate the sensitive oesophageal lining, causing a burning sensation about where the heart is, thus: heartburn – which, of course, has nothing to do with your heart. During the last two trimesters the problem is compounded by your growing uterus, which presses up on your stomach, pushing it and its contents farther up toward the oesophagus.

It's nearly impossible to have an indigestion-free nine months; it's just one of the less pleasant facts of pregnancy. There are, however, some pretty effective ways of avoiding heartburn and indigestion most of the time, and of minimizing the discomfort when it strikes:

☆ Avoid gaining too much weight: Excess weight puts excess pressure on the stomach.

☆ Don't wear clothing that is tight around your abdomen and waist.

☆ Have small, frequent meals, and eat slowly, taking small mouthfuls and chewing thoroughly.

☆ Eliminate from your diet any food that causes discomfort. Most common offenders are: hot and highly seasoned foods; fatty foods; processed meats (hot dogs, bologna, sausage, bacon); chocolate, coffee, alcohol, carbonated beverages; spearmint and peppermint (even in the form of gum).

☆ Don't smoke.

☆ Avoid bending over at the waist; bend instead with your knees.

☆ Sleep with the head of your bed elevated about six inches.

☆ Relax.

☆ If all else fails to relieve your symptoms, ask your doctor if you can take antacids and over-the-counter medications for heartburn which have no contraindications in pregnancy. Do not take preparations containing sodium or sodium bicarbonate.

Food Aversions and Cravings

'Certain foods – particularly green vegetables – that I've always liked taste funny now. Instead, I have cravings for foods that are less nutritious.'

The pregnancy cliché of a harried husband running out in the middle of the night, raincoat over his pyjamas, for a pint of ice cream and a jar of pickles to satisfy his wife's cravings probably occurs more often in the heads of cartoonists than in real life. Not many pregnant women's cravings carry them – or their husbands – that far.

But most of us do find that our tastes in food change somewhat in early pregnancy. The long-favoured theory that these changes are signals (that our bodies are craving something they need, or warning us off something they shouldn't have) sounds reasonable. And sometimes it works. As when the black coffee that used to be the mainstay of your workday becomes totally unappealing. Or the cocktail before dinner seems too strong even when it's weak. Or you suddenly can't get enough citrus fruit. On the other hand, when you can't stand the sight of fish, or broccoli suddenly tastes bitter, or you crave ice-cream cake, you can't credit your body with sending accurate signals.

The fact is that body signals relating to food are notoriously unreliable, probably because we've departed so significantly from the food chain in nature that we can no longer interpret them correctly. Before ice-cream and sandwiches were invented, when food came from nature, a craving for carbohydrates and calcium would have steered us toward fruits or berries and milk or cheese. With the wide variety of tempting (but often unwholesome) foods available today, it's no wonder our bodies are confused.

You can't totally ignore cravings

and aversions. But you can deal with them without putting your baby's nutritional needs in jeopardy. If you crave something that's good for you and baby, by all means go ahead and eat it. If you crave something that you know isn't good, then look for a satisfactory substitute: raisins, dried apricots, or a glass of apple juice instead of a candy bar; unsalted or lightly salted whole-wheat snacks instead of the usually oversalted, nutritionally vacant variety.

If you feel a sudden aversion to coffee or alcohol or chocolate ice cream, great. It will make giving them up for the duration all the easier. If it's fish or broccoli or milk you can't tolerate, you don't have to force-feed yourself, but you do have to find compensating sources of the nutrients they supply. (See the Best-Odds Diet for substitutes.)

Most cravings and aversions disappear or weaken by the fourth month. And those that don't may be mostly triggered by emotional needs – the need for a little extra attention, for example. If both you and your husband understand this need, it should be easy to deal with. You might, instead of requesting a middle-of-the-night pint of Rocky Road, settle for some quiet cuddling or a romantic bath-for-two (or, rather, three).

Milk Aversion

'I can't tolerate milk, and drinking four cups a day would make me ill. Will my baby suffer if I don't drink milk?'

First of all, it's not the milk your baby

needs, it's the calcium. Since milk is the most convenient source of calcium in the western diet, it's the one most often recommended for filling the greatly increased requirement during pregnancy. But there are many substitutes which fill the nutritional bill just as well. Many people who are lactose-intolerant (can't digest the milk sugar, lactose) can tolerate some kinds of dairy products, such as hard cheeses, fully processed yogurts, and the new LactAid enzyme, which converts milk to a more easily digested form. If you can't tolerate these, you can still get all the calcium your baby requires by eating the non-dairy foods listed under Calcium-Rich Foods, page 89.

If your problem with milk isn't physiological, but just a matter of distaste, there are plenty of ways to get the calcium you need without offending your taste buds. You'll find them all in the Calcium-Rich Foods list.

A Meatless Diet

'I eat chicken and fish but no red meat. Can I supply my baby with all the nutrients he needs without meat?'

Your baby can be just as happy and healthy as any beef-eating mother's offspring. Fish and poultry, in fact, nourish your baby in the most efficient way possible, giving you more protein and less fat for your calories than beef, pork, lamb, and offal. And all the important nutrients found in red meats are found in plentiful supply elsewhere in a balanced diet – especially in poultry and fish, whole grains (wheat germ, whole-wheat cereals and breads, brown rice), eggs, fresh green leafy and deep yellow vegetables, dried fruits, and milk products.

A Vegetarian Diet

'I'm a vegetarian and in perfect health. But everyone – including my doctor – says that I have to eat meat and fish, eggs and milk products to have a healthy baby. Is this true?'

Vegetarians of every variety can have healthy babies without compromising their dietary principles. But they have to be even more careful in planning their diets than meat-eating mothers-to-be, particularly in being sure to get all of the following:

Adequate Protein. For the ovo-lacto vegetarian, who eats eggs and milk products, adequate protein intake can be assured by taking ample quantities of both. A vegan (a strict vegetarian who eats neither milk nor eggs) has to depend on combinations of vegetable proteins (see Vegetarian Complete Protein Combinations, page 90). Some meat analogues are good protein sources; others are low in protein and high in calories. Read the labels.

Adequate Calcium. This is no problem for the vegetarian who takes dairy products, but adroit manoeuvring is needed for those who don't. Use the Calcium-Rich Foods list, page 89, to be sure of meeting your calcium needs. Soy products are useful because they are fairly high in calcium, but don't use soy milks loaded with sucrose (sugar, corn syrup honey). Instead use a pure soybean extract. For added in surance, vegans should also take a prescribed calcium supplement.

Vitamin B_{12}. Vegetarians, particularly vegans, often don't get enough of this vitamin because it is found primarily in animal foods. So they should be certain to take a vitamin supplement that includes B_{12} as well as folic acid and iron.

Vitamin D. This vitamin is not naturally found in foods except for fish liver oils. Most milk is fortified with vitamin D, but for those who don't drink milk, this vitamin should be included in their supplement. (Be careful, however, not to take vitamin D in doses beyond pregnancy requirements, which can be toxic.)

Enough of Everything Else. Vegetarians need to have heartier-than-average appetites, because in addition to all of the above, they'll have to find room for the rest of the foods recommended for all pregnant women in the Best-Odds Diet. This doesn't mean they have to gain more weight. Since vegetarian food is generally lower in fat (and thus in calories) than meat foods, eating more of it shouldn't be more fattening.

Junk-Food Junkie

'I'm addicted to junk foods – doughnuts for breakfast; fast-food burgers, fries, and Cokes for lunch. I'm afraid that if I can't break these bad habits, my baby will be under-nourished.'

You're right to worry. Before you became pregnant, your dietary indiscretions hurt only you; now they can hurt your baby as well. Make a daily diet of doughnuts, fast-food burgers, and Cokes, and you'll be denying your baby adequate nourishment during the most important nine months of his or her life. Eat the junk food on top of a balanced diet, and baby won't be the only one growing.

Happily, any addictions can be broken. Heroin. Tobacco. Even junk food. Here are several ways to make withdrawal almost as painless as it is worthwhile:

First of All, Change the Locale of Your Meals. If you munch a pastry at your desk, have breakfast at home before you go to work. If you can't resist a burger at lunch, go to a restaurant that doesn't serve burgers, or bring a sandwich from home.

Stop Thinking of Eating as a Catch-as-Catch-Can Proposition. Start thinking of every bite as a chance to help your baby grow and thrive. Don't grab what is easiest. Plan ahead and pick what is best.

Don't Give Temptation a Tumble. Don't bring boxes of sweets, bags of chips, soft drinks, into the house (other family members will survive without it – will do better in fact). When the coffee trolley bell rings, don't answer it; keep wholesome snacks like raisins, nuts, whole-wheat breadsticks, fruit, juices, and hard-boiled eggs in your desk or purse instead. When you're about to pass your favourite cake shop, cross the street.

Don't Use Lack of Time as an Excuse for Sloppy Eating. It takes no more time to make a tuna sandwich to take to the office than to stand in a queue at Macdonalds. And in fact, it takes less time to cut a fresh peach into a container of yogurt than to bake a peach pie. If the prospect of preparing a real dinner every night seems overwhelming, cook enough for two or three dinners at once and give yourself alternate nights off. And keep it simple: fancy sauces aren't nutritious, only high in calories.

Don't Use a Tight Budget as an Excuse for Eating Junk Foods. A glass of orange juice or milk is cheaper than a can of Coke. A broiled chicken breast and baked potato cost a lot less than a Big Mac and fries.

Quit Cold Turkey. Don't tell yourself you can have just one cola today or just one doughnut. That almost never works when you're trying to break an addiction. Just make up your mind that junk food is out – at least until you deliver. You may be surprised to find, once the baby's born, that your new good eating habits will be as hard to break as your old bad ones.

Study the Best-Odds Diet. Make it part of your life.

Eating Fast Food

'I go out with friends for fast food after a movie about once a month. Do I have to skip this for the rest of my pregnancy?'

Treating yourself to an occasional

dinner at a fast-food restaurant is acceptable during pregnancy – but only if you order with care and restraint. First of all, try to pick a place that offers a salad bar. That way you will be sure to get your quota of leafy green and yellow vegetables, and possibly a serving of cheese as well. Make a main course of a single burger, a fish or chicken sandwich, a taco, or perhaps a couple of slices of pizza – preferably with whole-wheat crust. Forego the fries (you can snitch a couple from a friend), sodas, pastry pies, and shakes (they often contain little or no milk and are loaded with sugar, artificial flavours and colours, and saturated fats). Drink juice, milk, or plain water, and bring along your own fruit to munch for dessert.

Chemicals in Foods

'With additives in packaged foods, insecticides on vegetables, additives in fish and meat, and nitrates in hot dogs, is there anything I can safely eat during pregnancy?'

Reports of hazardous chemicals in just about every item in the average diet are enough to scare the appetite out of anyone – especially a pregnant woman afraid not only for her own well-being but for that of her unborn child. Thanks to the media, 'chemical' has become synonymous with 'danger,' and 'natural' with 'safe.' But neither generalization is true. Everything we eat is made up of chemicals. Some chemicals are harmless (even beneficial); some are not. And although 'natural' is often better than artificial or unnatural, it can also be deadly. A 'natural' mushroom can be poisonous; 'natural' eggs, butter, and animal fats are associated with heart disease, and 'natural' sugar and honey cause cavities.

So forget about classifying goods into natural and chemical. Think instead about foods that are safe to eat during pregnancy and those that are not. When in doubt (and for many food ingredients, safety during pregnancy is unknown), leave it out. But don't be fanatic. There are no food ingredients which in small occasional doses are known to cause birth defects. And, of course, most women eat a wide variety of foods during pregnancy – never reading a single label – and have perfectly normal babies.

Still, you will want to be as prudent as possible and avoid regularly eating foods that *might* be hazardous. Use the following as a guide in deciding what to drop into your shopping cart and what to pass up:

☆ Use the Best-Odds Diet as your basic food plan; it automatically steers you clear of most potential perils.

☆ Don't use foods sweetened with saccharine or aspartame (their effects on the foetus are not yet known).

☆ Whenever possible, cook from scratch; you'll not only avoid many questionable ingredients but you will get more nutrients from your foods.

☆ As a general rule when eating fish, ocean fish, for example tuna, sea bass, sea trout and sole are safer than river and lake varieties. Never eat raw fish or seafood, and avoid (even cooked) seafood which is sometimes contaminated, such as oysters.

☆ Generally avoid foods preserved with nitrates and nitrites: frankfurters, salami, luncheon meats, smoked fish and meats.

☆ Whenever you have the choice between products with or without artificial colourings, flavourings, preservatives, and other additives, opt for the one that's additive-free.

☆ Don't use MSG or flavour enhancers that contain it.

☆ Eat lean cuts of meat and poultry, cutting off fat and skin – they store chemicals that are fed to livestock. Don't eat offal (liver, kidneys, etc.) very often, for the same reason.

☆ Give all your fruits and vegetables a detergent bath (in the same detergent you use to hand wash dishes) and rinse thoroughly before using them, to remove chemical residues; scrub skins when possible. It is not necessary to buy organically grown produce; studies show it often has as much chemical residue as supermarket fruits and vegetables, and it is much more costly.

Reading Labels

'I'm eager to feed my baby well, but I find that it's difficult to know what I'm getting when I go to the supermarket.'

Labels aren't always designed to help you as much as to sell you. Be aware when buying and learn to read the small print, including the list of ingredients and the nutritional label.

The ingredients listing will tell you, in order of predominance, exactly what is in the product. You will know whether the first ingredient in a cereal is sugar (you'll want to pass that one by), or a whole grain (you may want that one). You will also have a rough idea of whether a product is high in salt, fats or additives.

The nutritional label appears on more than half the products on your grocer's shelves, and it is particularly valuable for a pregnant woman counting her protein and calories. A food high in a wide variety of nutrients is a good product to purchase.

While it's important to read the small print, it's just as important to ignore the large print. when a box of scones trumpets loudly 'made with wholewheat, bran, and honey,' reading the small print may show that the major (first) ingredient is *white*, not wholewheat, flour and that the muffins contain precious little honey or bran (these are near the bottom of the ingredient list).

'Enriched' and 'fortified' are also banners to be wary of. Adding a few vitamins to a poor food doesn't make it a good food. That's true of cereals that are 50% sugar (the nutritional label also gives you information on the percentage of sugar in many products) but have a few pennies' worth of vitamins added. You're much better off with a bowl of oatmeal which has acquired its vitamins naturally.

WHAT IT'S IMPORTANT TO KNOW: PLAYING IT SAFE

The home. The streets. The garden. The most significant risks faced by pregnant women are not medical but accidental.

Accidents often seem 'accidental,' that is, to happen by chance. Yet most are the direct result of carelessness – often on the part of the victim herself – and many can be avoided with a little extra caution and common sense. There are a wide variety of steps you can take to prevent injuries and accidents:

☆ Recognize that you're not as agile as you were prepregnancy. As your abdomen grows, your centre of gravity will shift, making it more difficult for you to keep your balance. You will also find it difficult to see your feet. These changes will contribute to your becoming more accident-prone.

☆ Always fasten your seat belt in cars and on aeroplanes.

☆ Never climb on a shaky chair or ladder, or better still, never climb.

☆ Don't wear high, spiky heels, sloppy slippers, or thongs that can snap, all of which encourage falls and twisted ankles. Don't walk on slippery floors in your stocking feet or in smooth-soled shoes.

☆ Be careful getting in and out of the tub; be sure your tub and shower are equipped with non-skid surfaces and sturdy grab bars.

☆ Check your house and garden for hazards: rugs without skid-proof bottoms, especially at the top of stairs; toys or junk on stairways; poorly lit stairs and hallways; wires strung across the floor; overwaxed floors; icy pavements and steps.

☆ Observe the safety rules of whatever sport you play; follow all the tips for safe exercise and activity on pages 166–174.

☆ Don't overdo. Fatigue is a major contributor to accidents.

7
The Third Month

WHAT YOU CAN EXPECT AT THIS MONTH'S CHECKUP

This month you can expect your doctor to check the following, though there may be variations depending upon your particular needs and your doctor or midwife's style of practice:[1]

☆ Weight and blood pressure

☆ Urinalysis

☆ Foetal heartbeat

☆ Size and shape of uterus, by abdominal palpation, to see how it correlates to due date or estimated date of confinement (EDC)

☆ Ultrasound scan performed now if need indicated

☆ Height of fundus (the top of the uterus)

☆ Hands and feet and legs for oedema (swelling), and legs for varicose veins

☆ Vaginal discharge, bleeding, urinary symptoms

☆ Questions or problems you want to discuss – have a list ready

WHAT YOU MAY BE FEELING

You may feel all of these symptoms at one time or another, or only a few of them. Some may have continued from last month, others may be new. You may also have additional, less common symptoms.

Physically:

☆ Fatigue and sleepiness

☆ A need to urinate frequently

1. See appendix for an explanation of the procedures and tests performed.

☆ Nausea, with or without vomiting, and/or excessive salivation (ptyalism)

☆ Constipation

☆ Heartburn and indigestion, flatulence, and bloating

☆ Food aversions and cravings

☆ Breast changes: fullness, heaviness, tenderness, tingling; darkening of the areola (the pigmented area around the nipple); sweat glands in the areola become prominent (Montgomery's tubercles), like large goose bumps; network of bluish lines under skin expands

☆ Additional veins visible as blood supply to abdomen and legs also increases

☆ Occasional headaches

☆ Occasional faintness or dizziness

☆ Clothes begin to feel tight around waist and bust, if they hadn't previously; abdomen may appear enlarged by end of month

☆ Increasing appetite

Emotionally:

☆ Instability comparable to premenstrual syndrome, which may include irritability, weepiness

---

What You May Look Like

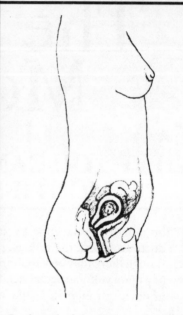

By the end of the third month, this tiny human, now a foetus, is 2½ to 3 inches long and weighs about ½ ounce. More organs are developing, circulatory and urinary systems are operating; the liver produces bile. Reproductive organs are developed, but the gender is difficult to distinguish externally.

☆ A new sense of calmness

☆ Misgivings, fear, joy, elation – any or all of these

WHAT YOU MAY BE CONCERNED ABOUT

Constipation

'All my pregnant friends seem to have problems with constipation. I don't; in fact, I've been more regular than ever. Is my system working right?'

Pregnant women are so programmed by mothers, friends, books, even doctors, to expect constipation that those who do become constipated accept it as normal and inevitable, and those who don't worry that there's something wrong.

There's a sound rationale for this programming, and for constipation being such a common complaint of pregnancy. For one thing, relaxation of the musculature of the bowel, due to the high levels of certain hormones circulating during pregnancy, makes elimination sluggish and less efficient. For another, the pressure from the growing uterus on the bowels inhibits their normal activity.

But there's no sound reason for believing constipation is inevitable with every pregnancy. Many women never experience it – probably because they are compensating for the sluggishness of their bowels with proper diet and exercise. Some of these women may also have more frequent bowel movements because of the additional food and the added fibre they are eating.[2] As long as the stools aren't loose, watery, bloody or mucusy, there's no cause for alarm.

Women who *do* suffer from constipation can overcome the problem and head off one of the common results of irregularity, haemorrhoids (see page 179). Here's how:

Enlist Fibre into Your Diet. Eat fresh fruits and vegetables (lightly cooked or raw, with skins left on when possible), whole grains (cereals and breads), and dried fruits (raisins, prunes, apricots). In general, follow the Best-Odds Diet – it also gives you the best odds against constipation. But if you usually eat little fibre, add high-fibre foods to your diet gradually or you may find your stomach upset.

2. Iron supplements may contribute to diarrhoea *or* to constipation. If your supplement seems to unsettle your system, ask your practitioner to suggest a different formula.

Drown Your Opponent. Constipation doesn't stand a chance against an ample fluid intake. Most fluids – particularly water and fruit and vegetable juices – are effective in softening stool and keeping food moving along the digestive tract. Some people find cups of hot water flavoured with lemon (but no sugar) especially useful. If constipation is severe, prune juice may do the trick.

Start an Exercise Campaign. Fit a brisk walk of at least half an hour into your daily routine; supplement it with as much as you like of any exercise you enjoy that is safe during pregnancy (see Exercise During Pregnancy, page 166).

Flatulence (Gas)

'I'm very bloated from gas and worry that the pressure, which is so uncomfortable for me, might also be hurting the baby.'

Snug in a safe uterine cocoon, protected by impact-absorbing amniotic fluid, your baby is impervious to your intestinal distress. If anything, he or she probably is soothed by the bubbling and gurgling of your gastric Muzak.

The only possible threat to your baby's well-being is if bloating – which often worsens late in the day – is preventing you from eating regularly and properly. To avoid this risk (and to minimize your own discomfort), take the following measures:

Stay Regular. Constipation is a common cause of gas and bloating.

Don't Gorge. Large meals just add to the bloated feeling. They also overload your digestive system, which isn't at its most efficient to begin with during pregnancy. Instead of three large meals a day, eat six small ones.

Don't Gulp. When you rush through meals or eat on the run, you're bound to swallow as much air as food. This captured air forms painful pockets of gas in your gut.

Keep Calm. Particularly during meals: Tension and anxiety can make you swallow air.

Steer Clear of Gas-Producers. Your stomach knows what they are – possibly onions, cabbage and cabbage-family members such as Brussels sprouts and broccoli, fried foods and sugary sweets (which you shouldn't be having now anyway), and, of course, the notorious beans.

Weight Gain

'I only gained one pound in my first trimester. My friend, who's also pregnant, gained six. What's enough, and what's too much?'

Weight gain that is just enough for one woman may be too much or too little for another. The extremely underweight woman is probably doing her baby a favour by gaining 6 pounds (as long as they're gained by eating highly nutritious foods) in the first trimester, or doing him or her an injustice by gaining only 1. The obese mother-to-be, on the other hand, is doing no one a favour by gaining weight rapidly, and can probably afford to gain only 1 pound (or even none) in the first trimester (as long as she eats adequate amounts of nutritious foods) without jeopardizing her baby's health. For the woman who is average, however, 6 pounds is probably too much and 1 not enough. Two to 4 would be just right (see page 132).

Stretch Marks

'I'm afraid I'm going to get stretch marks. Can they be prevented?'

For many women – especially those who favour bikinis – stretch marks are more to be dreaded than flabby thighs. Nevertheless, 90% of all women will develop these pink or reddish, slightly indented streaks on their breasts, hips, and/or abdomen sometime during pregnancy.

As their name implies, stretch marks are caused by stretching of the skin, generally due to a large and/or rapid increase in weight. Expectant mothers who have good, elastic skin tone (because they either inherited it or earned it through years of excellent nutrition and exercise) may slip through several pregnancies without a single telltale striation. Others may be able to minimize, if not prevent, stretch marks by keeping weight gain steady, gradual, and moderate. Promoting elasticity in your skin by nourishing it well with the Best-Odds Diet (page 82) may help, but no expensive cream, lotion, or oil will prevent or alleviate stretch marks – although they may be fun for your husband to rub on your tummy, and will prevent your skin from drying.

If you do develop stretch marks during pregnancy, you can console

THE THIRD MONTH 129

yourself with the knowledge that they will gradually fade to a silvery sheen after delivery. It may also help to think of them less as a disfigurement than as a medal of motherhood.

Aspirin, Non-Aspirin, and Headaches

'Last week I took two aspirins for a pounding headache. Now I read that aspirin can cause birth defects. Could I have hurt my baby?'

Of the millions of people who opened their medicine cabinet today and reached for a bottle of aspirin, few thought twice – or even once – about its safety. And for most people occasional aspirin use is very helpful and perfectly harmless. But during pregnancy, aspirin, like so many other ordinarily innocuous over-the-counter remedies, becomes a potential hazard.

If you've unwittingly taken one or two aspirins on one, or even a few, occasions in the first two trimesters, don't worry – they won't hurt your baby. For the rest of your pregnancy, however, be aware that like any drug, aspirin should be taken only when absolutely necessary, and then only with your doctor's approval.

Research shows that there may be a link between frequent doses of aspirin taken at any time during gestation and problems in foetal development. But during the third trimester, even one or two aspirins can be risky. Because it is an antiprostaglandin, and prostaglandins are involved in the mechan-

ism of labour, aspirin can prolong both pregnancy and labour and lead to other complications during delivery. And since it interferes with blood-clotting, if taken during the two weeks before delivery, aspirin may lead to haemorrhage during labour and bleeding problems in the newborn.

Taking an aspirin-substitute in place of aspirin isn't the logical solution in pregnancy. It *is* known that it can cause liver damage in the user, and there is speculation that it might also damage the liver of a foetus whose mother takes it in large doses during pregnancy. So take paracetamol only if absolutely necessary, and then *only* with the approval of your practitioner.

Both aspirin and paracetamol are hidden ingredients in a myriad of popular remedies, including Alka-Seltzer, cold-and-allergy-relief medicines (many of which are not recommended during pregnancy anyway), and pain relievers, such as Anadin and Panadol. Read labels carefully – a good habit not only during pregnancy but all of the time.

Headaches are extremely common during pregnancy. Often they are due to tension or other stresses on your body and to hormonal changes. Sinus headaches, too, may be more frequent because of the congestion of the mucous membranes caused by pregnancy hormones. But just because it isn't a good idea to find relief for your headaches in a pill doesn't mean you have to grin and bear them. There are many non-drug ways of overcoming (and preventing) headaches, many of which fit the cure to the cause:

Eat Regularly. Hunger often generates headaches.

Get Enough Rest. Lack of sleep, staying on the go all day without a break, can lead to headaches.

Seek Some Peace and Quiet. Stay away from loud music, noisy parties, crowded department stores.

Don't Get Stuffy. If overheated, smoke-filled, unventilated rooms trigger a headache, step outside for a stroll.

Relax. Most pregnancy headaches are – not surprisingly – of the tension variety. Ordinary relaxation (lying down in a dark, quiet room) may help. Even better are meditation, yoga, and other relaxation techniques. You can take a course or read a book on relaxation methods, or simply try this: Sit with eyes closed. Relax muscles starting with feet and working up through legs, torso, neck, and face. Breathe only through the nose. As you breathe out, repeat the v ɪrd 'one' to yourself. Continue for 1ɔ to 20 minutes.

For Relief from Sinus Headaches. Apply hot and cold compresses alternately to the aching area, 30 seconds each for 10 minutes, four times a day.

If your headache persists, returns very often, is very severe, or is accompanied by visual disturbances or puffiness of the hands and face, notify your doctor about it.

German Measles (Rubella)

'I was exposed to German measles. Should I get an abortion?'

That's a question only one out of seven pregnant women need ever confront. The other six are, happily, immune to rubella, or German measles, having contracted it at some other time in their lives (usually during childhood) or because they were vaccinated (usually in early adolescence or when they were married). You may not know whether or not you are immune, but you can find out via a rubella antibody titre – a test which measures the level of antibodies to the disease in your blood and is performed routinely at the first prenatal visit by most doctors. If a test was not performed, it should be now.

If it turns out you're not immune, you still needn't immediately consider drastic measures. Exposure alone cannot harm your baby. For the virus to do its damage, it has to infect you. And if you contract the illness after the third month, the risk is very slight.

Unfortunately, there is no way of actively preventing an exposed woman from coming down with rubella. Gamma globulin shots, which were once given routinely, have been found to be inconsistent in preventing infection. Should you contract rubella in the first trimester (this can be determined only through blood tests, since symptoms may be nonexistent), the chance of your baby developing serious congenital malformation is high – about 35% in the first month and 10% to 15% by the third.

You should discuss this risk with your doctor; but in the end, it is you and your husband who must decide whether to continue the pregnancy.

If you are not immune and do not contract the disease, avoid this dilemma entirely in subsequent pregnancies by having your doctor vaccinate you after this delivery. As a precaution, you will be instructed not to become pregnant for two or three months following vaccination. But should you conceive accidentally during this time – or if you were vaccinated early in this pregnancy, before you knew you had conceived – don't worry. There have been no cases of congenital rubella reported in babies whose mothers were inadvertently vaccinated early in pregnancy or conceived right after vaccination.

Sexual Desire

'All of my pregnant friends say that they had an increased desire for sex early in pregnancy – some had orgasms and multi-orgasms for the first time. How come I feel so unsexy?'

Pregnancy is a time of change in many aspects of your life, not the least of them sexual. Some women who have never had either orgasm or much of a taste for sex suddenly experience both for the first time when pregnant. Other women, accustomed to having a voracious appetite for sex and to being easily orgasmic, suddenly find that they are completely lacking in desire and are difficult to arouse. These changes in sexuality can be disconcerting, guilt-provoking, wonderful, or a confusing combination of all

three. And they are perfectly normal.

As you will see by reading Making Love During Pregnancy (page 145), there are many logical explanations for such changes and for the feelings that they may provoke. Some of these factors may be strongest early in pregnancy, when nausea and fatigue make you feel understandably unsexy, when being able to make love without worrying about trying to get (or trying not to get) pregnant frees you of inhibitions and makes you sexier than ever, when guilt results because you're feeling sexy and you think you should be feeling motherly instead. Other factors, such as the physical alterations that make orgasm easier to achieve, more powerful, or more elusive, continue throughout gestation.

Most important is recognizing that your sexual feelings – and your husband's as well – during pregnancy may be more erratic than erotic; you may feel sexy one day and not the next. Mutual understanding and open communication will be needed to see you through.

Oral Sex

'I've heard that oral sex is dangerous during pregnancy. Is this true?'

Cunnilingus is safe throughout pregnancy as long as your mate is careful not to blow any air into your vagina. Doing this could force air into your bloodstream and cause an embolism (an obstruction of a blood vessel), which might prove deadly to both mother and baby.

Fellatio, because it doesn't involve the female genitalia, is always safe during pregnancy and for some couples is a preferred substitute when intercourse isn't permitted.

Cramp After Orgasm

'I get an abdominal cramp after orgasm. Is this a sign that sex is hurting my baby? Will it cause a miscarriage?'

Cramping – both during and after orgasm, and sometimes accompanied by backache – is as harmless during a normal low-risk pregnancy as it is common. Its cause can be physical – a combination of the normal venous congestion in the area and the equally normal congestion of sexual arousal and orgasm. Or it can be psychological – a result of anxiety that having intercourse and orgasm may injure your baby.

The cramping is not a sign that sex is hurting the foetus. Most experts agree that sexual relations and orgasm during a normal, low-risk pregnancy are perfectly safe and are not a cause of miscarriage. If the cramps bother you, ask your husband for a gentle low back rub. It may relieve not only the cramps but any tension that might be triggering them, too.[3] (For more about sexual relations, see Making Love During Pregnancy, page 145.)

Baby's Heartbeat

'My friend's doctor picked up her baby's heartbeat at two and a half months. I'm a week ahead of her and my doctor hasn't heart my baby's yet.'

It's possible to pick up the baby's heartbeat as early as the 10th or 12th week with a highly sensitive instrument called a Doppler (a hand-held ultrasound device which magnifies the sound). But an ordinary stethoscope isn't powerful enough to detect the heartbeat until the 17th or 18th week at the earliest. Even with sophisticated instruments, the heartbeat may not be audible this early because of the baby's position or other interfering factors, such as excess layers of maternal fat. It's also possible that a slightly miscalculated due date may be causing the delay. Wait until next month. By then, the miraculous sound of your baby's heartbeat is certain to be available for you to listen to with pleasure.

WHAT IT'S IMPORTANT TO KNOW: WEIGHT GAIN DURING PREGNANCY

Put two pregnant women together anywhere – in a doctor's waiting room, on a bus, at a business meeting – and the questions are certain to start flying.

'When are you due?' 'Have you felt the baby kicking yet?' 'Have you been

3. Some women also experience crampiness in the legs after intercourse. See page 178 for tips on relieving such discomfort.

feeling sick?' And, perhaps the favourite query of all, 'How much weight have you gained?'

The comparisons are inevitable, and sometimes a little disturbing. Women who started off with a bang – enthusiastically eating their way to 10-pound first-trimester gains – wonder 'what's too much?' Others who, appetites daunted by bouts with morning sickness, ended up with net gains which barely registered on the practitioner's scale (perhaps even with a slight weight loss) wonder 'what's too little?' All wonder 'what's just right?'

Total Increase. Though it was once in medical vogue to limit a woman's pregnancy weight gain to 15 pounds, it is now recognized that this was insufficient to guarantee good infant health. Babies whose mothers gain under 20 pounds are more likely to be premature, small for gestational age, and to suffer growth retardation in the uterus.

Almost as hazardous, however, is the present vogue: eat to your heart and soul's content and gain any amount of weight. There are serious risks in gaining too much weight: assessment and measurement of the foetus become more difficult; excess weight overworks muscles and results in backaches, leg pains, increased fatigue, and varicose veins; if the diet is high in fat and carbohydrates and low in protein, toxaemia may result; the baby may become too large for a vaginal delivery; if surgery, such as caesarean section, is needed, it becomes more difficult, and postoperative complications more common;

after pregnancy the excess weight may be hard to shed.

Though a woman with an enormous weight gain may have an oversized baby, the mother's weight gain and the weight of her infant don't always correlate. It's possible to gain 40 pounds and deliver a 6-pound baby, or to gain 20 and have an 8-pounder. The quality of the food that contributes to the weight gain is more important than the quantity.

The sensible and safe weight gain for the average woman is between 20 and 30 pounds. That would allow about 6 to 8 pounds for the baby and 14 to 24 pounds for the by-products of pregnancy and for body changes in the mother (see box, page 134). It also assures a speedier return to prepregnancy weight for the woman.

Women who begin pregnancy either extremely under- or overweight, who expect twins, or who have special medical problems will probably need to have this figure adjusted by their physician or nurse-midwife.

Rate of Increase. The average-weight woman should gain approximately 3 to 4 pounds during the first trimester, and about a pound a week, 12 to 14 pounds in all, during the second trimester. Weight gain should continue at about 1 pound a week during the seventh and eighth months, and in the ninth month drop off to 1 pound or 2 – or even none at all – for a total of 8 to 10 pounds during the third trimester.

Rare is the woman who can keep her weight gain tailored precisely to the ideal formula. And it's fine to fluctuate a little – ¾ pound one week,

Breakdown of Your Weight Gain
(All weights are approximate)

Baby	7½ pounds
Placenta	1½ pounds
Amniotic fluid	1¾ pounds
Uterine enlargement	2 pounds
Maternal breast tissue	1 pound
Maternal blood volume	2¾ pounds
Fluids in maternal tissue	3 pounds
Maternal fat	7 pounds
Total average	26½-pound overall weight gain

1¼ pounds the next. But the goal of every pregnant woman should be to keep weight gain as steady as possible, without any sudden jumps or drops. If you don't gain any weight for two weeks or more during the fourth to eighth months, or if you gain more than 3 pounds in any week in the second trimester, or more than 2 pounds in any week in the third, check with your doctor.

Beware of the doctor who tells you at your first visit that you can eat all you like, and not to worry about your weight. When you then gain 30 pounds before the end of the sixth month, he or she may be the first to warn you to restrict your diet – at a time when your baby needs good nutrition most for optimal brain development. Monitor your weight carefully from the beginning, and you'll never have to put your baby on a diet to keep yourself from getting fat.

8
The Fourth Month

WHAT YOU CAN EXPECT AT THIS MONTH'S CHECKUP

This month you can expect your practitioner to check the following, though there may be variations depending upon your particular needs and upon your practitioner's style of practice:[1]

☆ Weight and blood pressure

☆ Urinalysis

☆ Foetal heartbeat

☆ Size and shape of uterus, by abdominal palpation, to see how it correlates to due date or estimated date of confinement (EDC)

☆ AFP (alpha-foetoprotein) test (16–18 weeks)

☆ Height of fundus (top of the uterus)

☆ Blood tests for haemoglobin

☆ Hands and feet for oedema (swelling), and legs for varicose veins

☆ Date of first foetal movement

☆ Symptoms you've been experiencing, especially unusual ones

☆ Vaginal discharge, bleeding or urinary symptoms

☆ Questions or problems you want to discuss – have a list ready

WHAT YOU MAY BE FEELING

You may feel all of these symptoms at one time or another or only a few of them. Some may have continued from last month, others may be new. Your may also have other, less common symptoms.

Physically:

☆ Fatigue

☆ A decrease in urinary frequency

---

1. See appendix for an explanation of the procedures and tests performed

☆ A decrease in, or end to, nausea and vomiting (in a few women, 'morning sickness' will continue; in a very few it is just beginning)

☆ Constipation

☆ Heartburn and indigestion, flatulence, and bloating

☆ Breasts continue to enlarge, but tenderness and swelling usually subside

☆ Occasional headaches

☆ Occasional faintness or dizziness, particularly with sudden change of position

☆ Nasal congestion and occasional nosebleeds; ear stuffiness

☆ Increase in appetite

☆ Mild oedema (swelling) of ankles and feet, and occasionally hands and face

☆ Varicose veins of legs and/or haemorrhoids

☆ Slight whitish vaginal discharge (leukorrhoea)

☆ Foetal movement near the end of month (but usually this early only if you are very thin or this is not your first pregnancy)

Emotionally:

☆ Instability comparable to premenstrual syndrome, which may include irritability, mood swings, irrationality, weepiness

☆ Joy and/or apprehension – if you have started to feel pregnant at last

☆ Frustration – if you don't really feel pregnant yet but are too big for your regular wardrobe and too small for maternity clothes

☆ A feeling you're not quite together. You're a scatterbrain, you forget things, drop things, have trouble concentrating

WHAT YOU MAY BE CONCERNED ABOUT

Elevated Blood Pressure and Preeclampsia

'My doctor said my blood pressure is up. Should I be concerned?'

A slight increase in blood pressure at one visit probably doesn't mean much of anything. Perhaps you were just nervous, or were late for your appointment and ran all the way, or were worrying about a report you had

to finish at work. If your pressure were taken the next day, or even later that same day, it might very well have been normal. Because it is often difficult to determine the cause of an isolated elevated reading, your practitioner may advise you to take it easy until the next visit.

If your blood pressure remains slightly elevated, however, you may be among the 1% to 2% of pregnant women who develop transient high blood pressure during pregnancy (gestational hypertension). This type

What You May Look Like

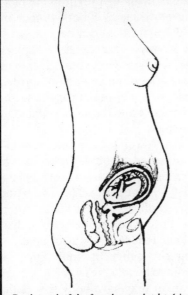

By the end of the fourth month, the 4-inch foetus, now nourished by the placenta, is developing reflexes, such as sucking and swallowing. Body growth begins to out-strip that of the head; tooth buds appear; fingers and toes are well defined. Though human-looking, it cannot survive outside the uterus.

of hypertension is perfectly harmless, as far as is known, and disappears after delivery.

What is considered normal blood pressure in pregnancy varies some-what over the course of nine months. A baseline pressure (what is normal for you) is obtained at the first prenatal visit. Generally the pressure drops a little over the next several months. But as delivery nears, somewhere about the seventh month, it usually begins to rise a bit.

During the first or second trimester, if pressure rises 30 mmHg systolic (the upper number) or 15 mmHg diastolic (the lower number) over the baseline reading (or by more than that in the third trimester) and stays up for at least two readings taken at least six hours apart, the pregnant woman's condition warrants close observation, and possibly treatment.

If increased blood pressure is accompanied by sudden weight gain (more than 3 pounds a week in the second trimester, or more than 2 pounds a week in the third), severe oedema (swelling because of water retention), particularly in hands and face, as well as ankles, and/or protein in the urine,[2] the problem may be pre-eclampsia. In women who receive regular medical care, this disorder is generally diagnosed before it pro-gresses to the more serious symp-toms, of blurred vision, headaches, irritability, and severe gastric pain.

No one knows what causes pre-eclampsia in pregnancy, or why it develops most often in first pregnan-cies. (Some research ties it to poor nutrition, particularly inadequate protein, but the evidence is not con-clusive.) It is known that it can pro-gress to the much more serious eclampsia – characterized by convul-sions and even coma – rather quickly. If preeclampsia is suspected, treatment at home may be tried first. But when a definite diagnosis of pre-eclampsia is established, partial or complete bed rest in the hospital, and medication if needed, is likely to be ordered.

If the pregnancy has not yet reached the 35th week, this conserva-

2. See appendix for explanation of protein in the urine.

tive treatment may continue until the foetus gains sufficient maturity to survive outside the uterus. But because prolonged precclampsia can lead to deteriorating environmental conditions in the uterus, permanent vascular damage to the mother, and also increases the risk of hazardous convulsions, induced delivery is desirable once the mother's condition has stabilized or improved. Thanks to modern medical treatment, the chances that both mother and baby will do well are excellent.

Woman who begin pregnancy with hypertension (high blood pressure) are classified as high risk but usually do well with increased rest, a low-sodium diet, careful monitoring, and if needed, appropriate medication and bed rest.

Sugar in the Urine

'At my last office visit the doctor said that there was sugar in my urine. She said not to worry, but I'm convinced I have diabetes.'

Take your doctor's advice – don't worry. A small amount of sugar in the urine on one occasion during pregnancy does not a diabetic make. What is probably happening is that your body is doing just what it's supposed to do: trying to make sure that your foetus, which depends on you for its fuel supply, is getting enough glucose (sugar).

Since it is insulin that regulates the level of glucose in your blood and ensures that enough is taken in by your body cells for nourishment, pregnancy triggers *anti*-insulin mechanisms to make sure enough sugar remains circulating in your bloodstream to nourish your foetus. It's a perfect idea that doesn't always work perfectly. Sometimes the anti-insulin effect is so strong that it leaves more than enough sugar in the blood to meet the needs of both mother and child – more than can be handled by the kidneys. The excess is 'spilled' into the urine. Thus your 'sugar in the urine' – a not uncommon occurrence in pregnancy, especially in the second trimester, when the anti-insulin effect increases.

In most women, the body responds to increased blood sugar levels with increased production of insulin, which will meet the challenge before the next office visit. But some, especially those who are diabetic or have diabetic tendencies, may be unable to produce sufficient quantities of insulin to handle the increase in blood sugar, or may have body tissues that are insulin-resistant. Either way, they continue to show high levels of sugar in both blood and urine. In women who were not previously diabetic, this is known as gestational diabetes.

If sugar appears in your urine at your next visit, your doctor may test your blood for sugar and may order a glucose-tolerance test, a procedure which accurately reflects the body's response to sugar in the bloodstream. Symptoms that may point to the development of diabetes in pregnancy include; excessive hunger and thirst, more frequent urination in the mid-trimester, recurrent monilial infections of the vagina, and increase in blood pressure.

About 1% to 2% of pregnant women develop gestational diabetes, and the incidence increases with maternal age (diabetes is more common as we get older). This type of diabetes usually disappears after delivery, but it sometimes recurs later in life. Women who have developed gestational diabetes in a pregnancy should be aware of this possibility so that they can take measures in the future that may prevent this, such as maintaining ideal weight, cultivating good diet and exercise habits, and having regular medical check-ups.

Though diabetic mothers-to-be and their foetuses were once at great risk, this is no longer the case. When blood sugar is closely controlled, diabetic mothers can have normal pregnancies and deliver healthy babies. (See page 42 for more on diabetes and pregnancy.)

Anaemia

'A friend of mine became anaemic during pregnancy. How can I tell if I am, and can I prevent it?'

Though nearly 20% of all pregnant women suffer from iron-deficiency anaemia, it's a condition that can be easily avoided – in most cases simply by eating a good diet and swallowing one pill, or several, each day.

A blood test for anaemia is administered at the first antenatal visit, but few women turn out to be iron-deficient at this time. Some may have come into pregnancy with the condition (common during the childbearing years because of monthly menstrual blood loss). But with conception and the cessation of menstruation, iron stores – if dietary intake is adequate – are replenished. It isn't until the 20th week (when the stores can deplete because of increased foetal requirements) that most cases of iron-

deficiency anaemia develop.

In a mild anaemia, there may be no symptoms. But when iron deficiency is more severe, a woman may be pale, tired, weak, and suffer from palpitations, breathlessness, and even fainting spells. In either case, it's the mother who falls victim to the lack of iron, as her oxygen-carrying red blood cells are depleted. Since this is one of the few instances where the nutritional needs of the foetus are met first (at the expense of its mother), it rarely suffers.

While all pregnant women are susceptible to iron-deficiency anaemia, certain groups are at particularly high risk: those who have had several babies in quick succession, those who vomit a lot or eat poorly because of morning sickness, those who are carrying more than one foetus, and those who are inadequately nourished before and/or during pregnancy.

To prevent iron-deficiency anaemia, all expectant mothers should take a daily iron supplement of 30 to 60 mgs. In addition, your diet should include a variety of iron-rich foods (see the Best-Odds Diet, page 91). This same regimen will probably be prescribed by your practitioner if you become anaemic.[3]

Nosebleeds and Nasal Stuffiness

'My nose has been congested a lot and sometimes it bleeds for no apparent reason. I'm worried because I know bleeding can be a sign of illness.'

---

3. Iron supplements can cause diarrhoea or constipation. Switching formulas may solve the problem, ask your practitioner.

Nasal congestion, often with associated nosebleeds, is a common complaint in pregnancy. It is probably because the high levels of oestrogen circulating in your body bring increased blood flow to the mucous membranes of your nose, causing them to soften and swell – much as your cervix does in preparation for childbirth.

You can expect the stuffiness to get worse before it gets better – which won't be until after delivery. You may also develop a postnasal drip, which can occasionally lead to nocturnal coughing or gagging. Don't use medication or nasal sprays to deal with the problem. But do be sure your fluid intake is adequate to compensate for any loss through sneezing or a runny nose. The congestion and bleeding are more common in winter, when heating systems force hot, dry air into the house, drying delicate nasal passages. Using a humidifier can help overcome this dryness.

Taking an extra 250 mg of vitamin C (with your practitioner's approval) along with your usual citrus fruits may help to strengthen your capillaries and reduce the chance of bleeding. (But don't take megadoses of the vitamin.) You might also try lubricating each nostril with a dab of Vaseline. Sometimes a nosebleed will follow overly energetic nose-blowing. Correct nose-blowing is an art, which you would do well to master: First, gently close one nostril with the thumb, and then carefully blow the mucus out the opposite side. Repeat with the other nostril, continuing to alternate until you can breathe through your nose.

Allergies

'My allergies seem to have worsened since my pregnancy began. My nose is runny and my eyes tear all the time.'

You may be mistaking the normal nasal stuffiness of pregnancy for allergy. Or, pregnancy – a major stress on the body – may have aggravated your allergies (though some lucky women find temporary relief from allergies during pregnancy). If your allergies worsen, you often can't rely on your usual medication. Check with your doctor to see what you can safely use to relieve severe symptoms. Some antihistamines and other medications appear to be relatively safe for use in pregnancy. But, because no tests for safety are absolutely conclusive, drugs should be used only when all else fails. If your nasal discharge is heavy or you're sneezing a lot, increase your fluid intake to compensate for any loss and to thin secretions.

In general, however, the best approach to dealing with allergies in pregnancy is preventive – avoiding the offending substance or substances, assuming you know what they are:

☆ If pollens or other outdoor allergens trouble you, stay indoors in air-conditioned and air-filtered space during your susceptible season as much as you can. Wash your hands and face if you've been out of doors, and wear big curved sunglasses to keep pollens from floating into your eyes.

☆ If dust is a culprit, try to have

someone do the dusting and sweeping for you. A vacuum cleaner, damp mop, or a damp, cloth-covered broom kicks up less dust than an ordinary broom, and an absorbent cloth will do better than a feather duster. Stay away from musty places like attics and libraries full of old books. Have someone pack away things in your home that are dust collectors, like draperies and rugs.

☆ If you're allergic to certain foods, stay away from them, even if they are good foods for pregnancy. Consult the Best-Odds Diet (page 88) for equivalent substitutes.

☆ If animals bring on allergy attacks, let friends know of the problem in advance so that they can rid the room of both pets and their dander before you visit. And, of course, don't keep a pet in your own home, unless it has a completely separate living area.

☆ Tobacco-smoke allergy is easier to control these days since fewer people smoke and more smokers oblige if they are asked to refrain. To tame your allergy, as well as for the benefit of your baby, there should be no one smoking in any area you spend time in. Don't be embarrassed to say. "Yes, I mind very much if you smoke."

Vaginal Discharge

'I've noticed a slight vaginal discharge that is thin and whitish. I'm afraid I have an infection.'

A thin, milky, mild-smelling discharge (called leukorrhoea) is normal throughout pregnancy. It's much like the discharge many women have prior to their menstrual periods and/or at the time of ovulation. Since it increases until term and may become quite heavy, some woman are more comfortable wearing sanitary pads during the last months of pregnancy.

Aside from the offence to your aesthetic sensibilities (and possibly to your husband's – who may be turned off oral sex by the unusual taste and odour), the discharge should be of no concern. It is important to keep the genital area clean and dry: cotton, or cotton-crotched, underwear may help to do this.

If you develop a vaginal discharge that is yellowish, greenish, or thick and cheesy, has a foul odour, or is accompanied by burning, itching, redness, or soreness – infection is likely. Notify your doctor or midwife so that the infection can be treated (probably with vaginal suppositories or gels, ointments, or creams inserted with an applicator). You may be able to hasten your recovery by maintaining scrupulous cleanliness, especially after going to the lavatory (always wipe from front to back), and by following the Best-Odds Diet – being especially careful to avoid refined sugars (which may help to create a breeding ground for infectious organisms). If the infection is a sexually transmittable one, avoiding intercourse until both you and your husband are infection-free is generally recommended. Unfortunately, though medication may banish the infection temporarily, it often returns. But simple vaginitis does not pose a risk to your baby.

If your vaginitis is caused by a yeast called monilia, your doctor will be careful to treat it with medication so you won't pass the infection on to your baby (in the form of thrush) during delivery.

Foetal Movement

'I haven't felt the baby moving yet; could something be wrong? Or could I just not be recognizing the kicking?'

Foetal movement may be the greatest source of joy in your pregnancy and, at the same time, the greatest cause of anxiety. More than a positive pregnancy test, an expanding belly, or even the sound of the foetal heartbeat, its presence affirms that you've got a new life growing inside you. Its absence breeds terror that the new life is not thriving.

Though the embryo begins to make spontaneous movements by the seventh week, these movements do not become apparent to the mother until they are much stronger. That first momentous sensation of life, or 'quickening,' can occur anywhere between the 14th and 26th weeks, but generally closer to the average of 18 to 20 weeks. Variations on that average are common. A woman who's been pregnant before is likely to recognise movement earlier (because she knows what to expect) than one who is expecting her first child. A very slender woman may notice very early, weak movements, while an obese woman may not be aware of movements until they've become more vigorous.

Sometimes the first perception of movement is delayed slightly because of a miscalculated due date. Or because of the foetus's position in the uterus. Or sometimes it's delayed because a woman has failed to recognize foetal movement when she felt it.

Nobody can tell a first-time mother-to-be exactly what she can expect to feel; a hundred pregnant women may describe that first quickening in a hundred different ways. Perhaps the most common descriptions are 'a fluttering in the abdomen' and 'butterflies in the stomach.' But early foetal movements have also been described as 'a bumping or nudging,' 'a twitch,' 'a growling stomach,' 'someone hitting my stomach,' 'a bubble bursting,' 'the squirmies,' 'like being turned upside down on an amusement park ride.' Often the first noticeable movements are mistaken for gas or hunger pains. And one woman recalls, 'I thought a bug was on my shirt, but when I went to brush it off, I realised it was the baby moving.'

Although it isn't unusual to be unaware of foetal movements until the 20th week or later, your practitioner may order an ultrasound scan to check on the baby's condition if you haven't felt anything – and he or she hasn't been able to elicit foetal response – by the 21st week. If the foetal heartbeat is strong, however, and everything else seems to be progressing normally, he or she may hold off even longer on testing.

'I felt little movements every day last week, but for the last few days I haven't felt a thing. Could something have gone wrong?'

Anxiety   over   when   the   first

movement will be felt is later replaced by other anxieties: that foetal movements don't seem frequent enough, or that they haven't been noted for a few days. While such anxieties are understandable, they're really unnecessary. At this stage of pregnancy, frequency of movement may vary a great deal, and there's no need to panic if the baby hasn't been heard from for three, four, even five days. Though the foetus is stirring almost continuously, only some of these movements may be strong enough for you to feel. Others may be missed because of the foetal position (facing and kicking inwards, for instance, instead of outwards). Or because of your own activity (when you're walking or moving about a lot, the baby is usually rocked to sleep; and even if he or she isn't, you may be too busy to notice the movements). It's also possible that you're sleeping right through your baby's most active period – which is, for many foetuses, the middle of the night.

From the sixth month on, foetal activity becomes stronger and more regular, so that 24 hours without movement, while not automatically cause for alarm, is a reason to call your doctor.

Appearance

'I get depressed when I look in the mirror or step on a scale – I'm so fat.'

In a society as obsessed with slenderness as ours, where those who can 'pinch an inch' despair, the weight gain of pregnancy can often become a source of depression. It shouldn't. There's an important difference between pounds added for no good reason (other than willpower gone astray) and pounds gained for the best and most beautiful of reasons: your child and its support system growing inside you.

Yet in the eyes of many, a pregnant woman isn't just beautiful inside but outside as well. Many women and their husbands consider the newly rounded pregnant reflection as the most lovely – and sensuous – of feminine shapes.

As long as you're eating right and not exceeding the recommended limits for pregnancy weight gain (see page 133), you needn't feel 'fat' – just pregnant. The added inches you're seeing are all legitimate by-products of pregnancy and will disappear rapidly once the baby appears. If you *are* exceeding the limits, self-defeating depression won't keep you from getting fatter (and may even fuel your appetite), but careful scrutiny of your eating habits might. (See the Best-Odds Diet, page 82.)

Reality of Pregnancy

'Now that my abdomen is swelling, the fact that I'm really pregnant has finally sunk in. Even though we planned this pregnancy, I suddenly feel scared, trapped by the baby – even antagonistic toward it.'

Even the most eager of expectant parents may be surprised (and guilt-ridden) to find themselves with second thoughts as their pregnancy starts to become a reality. An unseen little intruder has suddenly come between them, turning their lives upside down, depriving them of freedoms they'd always taken for granted, making more demands – both physically and emotionally – than anyone ever has before. Every aspect of the life they have become accustomed to – from how they spend their evenings, to what they eat and drink, to how often they make love – is being altered by this child even before it's born. And the knowledge that these changes will become still more imposing after delivery compounds their mixed feelings, deepens their apprehension.

Not only is a little ambivalence, a little fear, even a little antagonism, normal, it's healthy – as long as these feelings are confronted and acknowledged. And now is the best time to do that. Work out your resentments (over not being free to stay out late on Saturday nights, to pick up and go on a weekend trip when the spirit moves you, to work full time, or to spend your money any way you please) before the baby's born, and you won't find yourself venting them after he or she's arrived. Sharing your feelings with your partner is the best way to do this – and encourage him to do likewise.

It's true that your life is never going to be the same again once your 'two' is turned to 'three.' But as some parts of your world become more constricted, others will open up. You may find yourself reborn with your baby's birth. And this new life may turn out to be the best yet.

Unwanted Advice

'Now that everyone can see I'm expecting, everyone – from my mother-in-law to strangers in the street – has advice for me. It drives me crazy.'

Short of taking up a reclusive existence on a desert island, there's no way for a pregnant woman to escape the unsolicited advice of those around her. There's just something about a bulging belly that brings out the 'expert' in all of us. Take your morning jog around the park and someone is sure to chide: 'You shouldn't be running in your condition!' Lug home two bags of groceries from the supermarket and you're bound to hear: 'Do you think you ought to be carrying such heavy bundles?' Or reach up for a subway strap and you may even be warned: 'If you stretch that way the cord will wrap around your baby's neck and strangle it.'

Between such gratuitous advice and the inevitable predictions about the sex of the baby, what's an expectant mother to do? First of all, keep in mind that most of what you hear is probably nonsense. Old wives' tales that *do* have foundation in fact have been scientifically substantiated and have become part of medical practice. Those that do not, though still tightly woven into the tapestry of pregnancy mythology, can be confidently dismissed. Those recommendations that leave you with a nagging doubt – 'What if they are right?' – and are therefore impossible to dismiss are best checked with your doctor or antenatal teacher.

Whether it's possibly plausible or obviously ridiculous, however, don't let unwanted advice get your dander up. Neither you nor your baby will profit from the added tension. Instead, keeping your sense of humor handy, you can take one of two approaches. Politely inform the advice-giver that you have a trusted physician who counsels you on your pregnancy and that you can't accept suggestions from anyone else. Or, just as politely, smile, say thank you, and go on your way, letting their comments go in one ear and out the other – without making any stops in between.

But no matter how you choose to handle unwanted advice, you'd also do well to get used to it. If there's anyone who attracts a crowd of advice-givers faster than a pregnant woman, it's a woman with a new baby.

WHAT IT'S IMPORTANT TO KNOW: MAKING LOVE DURING PREGNANCY

Religious and medical miracles aside, every pregnancy begins with the sexual act. So why is it that what got you into this situation in the first place may now have become one of your biggest problems?

Whether sex suddenly becomes better than ever, virtually nonexistent, or just a little uncomfortable, almost every expectant couple finds that their sexual relationship undergoes some kind of change during the nine months of pregnancy.

Variations in sexual appetites and reactions before conception are wide to begin with. What is a satisfying sex life to one couple, 'obligatory' relations once a week, for instance, would be completely unsatisfactory for another, for whom once a day might not always be enough. After conception, these variations may be even more exaggerated. And to further complicate matters sexual, physical and emotional upheaval may leave the once-a-day couple less in the mood for love than the once-a-week couple, and vice versa.

Though intensity differs from couple to couple, there is a general down-up-down pattern of sexual interest during the three trimesters of pregnancy. It's not surprising that diminution of sexual interest is common early in pregnancy (in one survey, 54% of women reported reduced libido in the first trimester). After all, fatigue, nausea, vomiting, and painfully tender breasts do make less than ideal bedfellows. In women with comfortable first trimesters, however, sexual desire often remains more or less the same. And a sizable minority of expectant women find it increases significantly – often because the early hormones of pregnancy leave the vulva engorged and ultra-sensitive, and/or because the heightened breast sensitivity that is painful for other women is pleasurable for them. These women may experience orgasms or multi-orgasms for the first time.

Interest often – but not always – picks up during the midtrimester, when the couple is physically and psychologically better adjusted to the pregnancy. It usually wanes again as delivery nears, even more drastically than in the first trimester – for obvious reasons: first, the bulk of the abdomen is more and more difficult to 'get around'; second, the aches and discomforts of advancing pregnancy are capable of cooling even the hottest passion; and third, it's hard to concentrate on anything but that eagerly and anxiously awaited event.

Sexual pleasure, like sexual interest, seems to diminish in some – but certainly not all – couples. In one group of women, 21% received little or no pleasure from sex before conception. The percentage of these women finding sex not pleasurable rose to 41% at 12 weeks of gestation, and 59% going into the ninth month. The same study found that at 12 weeks, about 1 in 10 couples were not having sex at all; by the ninth month, more than a third were abstaining. But also the study found that more than 4 in 10 women were still enjoying sex at this point – more than half of these with *no* problems.

So you may find that sex during pregnancy is the best you've ever had. Or something you wish you could enjoy but find difficult. Or it may become an uncomfortable obligation. You may even abandon it altogether. 'Normal' in pregnancy lovemaking, as in so many other aspects of pregnancy, is what is right for you.

Understanding Sexuality During Pregnancy

Unfortunately, some practitioners are as inhibited about sexuality as the rest of us. Often they don't tell expectant couples what to expect, or not to expect, in the intimate part of their relationship. And that leaves many couples uncertain how to proceed.

Understanding why making love during pregnancy is different than it is at other times can help ease fears and worries, and make having intercourse (or not having it) more acceptable and more pleasurable.

First of all, there are many physical changes that affect both interest and actual sexual pleasure. Some can be dealt with to minimize their interference in your sex life; others you may just have to learn to live with – and love with.

Nausea and Vomiting. If your morning sickness stays with you day and night, you may just have to wait its symptoms out. (In most cases, queasiness will start letting up by the end of the first trimester.) If it strikes just at certain hours, keep your schedule flexible, and put the good times to good use. Don't pressure yourself to feel sexy when you're feeling lousy; morning sickness is often aggravated by emotional stress. (See page 101 for tips on minimizing morning sickness.)

Fatigue. This, too, should pass by the fourth month. Until then, make love while the sun shines (when the opportunity presents itself), instead of trying to force yourself to stay up late for romance. If your weekend afternoons are free, cap off a nap with a lovemaking session. (See page 100 for more on fatigue.)

The Changing Shape. Making love can be both awkward and uncomfortable when a bulging belly seems to loom as large and forbidding as a Himalayan mountain. As pregnancy progresses, the gymnastics required to scale the growing abdomen may not seem, to some couples, worth the effort. (But there are ways to get around the mountain; see page 150.) In addition, the woman's full-figured silhouette may actually turn off one or both partners. This is a socially conditioned reflex you may be able to psych yourself out of by thinking: big (in pregnancy) is beautiful.

The Engorgement of Genitals. The increased blood flow to the pelvic area can heighten sexual response in some women. But it can also make sex less satisfying (especially later in pregnancy) when a residual feeling of uncomfortable, unrelieved fullness may persist after orgasm, leaving a woman feeling as though she didn't quite make it. For males, too, the engorgement of the pregnant woman's genitalia may increase pleasure (he feels pleasantly and snugly caressed), or reduce it (he feels the fit is too tight, and he loses his erection).

Breast Tenderness. In early pregnancy, the breasts may have to be avoided during love play because they are painfully tender. (Be certain to communicate this discomfort to your partner, rather than suffering, and resenting his touch in silence.) However, as the tenderness diminishes toward the end of the first trimester, the extreme sensitivity of the breasts enhances sex for some couples. Others revel throughout in the fun of full-and-firm-for-the-first-time breasts.

Alterations in Vaginal Secretions. These secretions increase in volume and change in consistency, odour, and taste. The increased lubrication may make intercourse more enjoyable for the couple if the woman's vagina has always been dry and/or uncomfortably narrow. Or it might make the vaginal canal so wet and slippery that a man may have trouble holding an erection. The heavier scent and taste of the secretions may also make cunnilingus unpleasant to some men. Massaging scented oils into the area may help disguise the problem.

Bleeding Caused by the Sensitivity of the Cervix. The mouth of the uterus also becomes engorged during pregnancy – crisscrossed with many additional blood vessels to accommodate increased blood flow to the uterus – and much softer than before pregnancy. This means that deep penetration can occasionally cause bleeding, particularly late in pregnancy when the cervix begins to ripen for delivery. If this occurs (and possible miscarriage or any other problem is ruled out by your practitioner), simply avoid deep penetration.

Leakage of Colostrum. This occurs during sexual stimulation of the breast in some women, and it can be disconcerting in the middle of foreplay. It's nothing to worry about, of course, but if it bothers you or your partner, it can easily be avoided by refraining from breast play.

There are also a full complement of psychological hangups that can interfere with sexual enjoyment during pregnancy. These, too, can be minimized.

Fear About Hurting the Foetus or Causing a Miscarriage. In normal pregnancies sexual intercourse will do neither. The foetus is well cushioned and protected inside the amniotic sac, which is securely sealed off from the outside world with a mucous plug.

Fear That Having an Orgasm Will Stimulate Miscarriage or Early Labour. Although the uterus does contract following orgasm – and these contractions can be quite pronounced in some women, lasting as long as half an hour after intercourse – such contractions are not a sign of labour. Orgasm, particularly the more intense kind triggered by masturbation, may be prohibited in pregnancies at high risk for miscarriage or premature labour.

Fear That the Foetus is 'Watching' or 'Aware.' Though a foetus may enjoy the gentle rocking of uterine contractions during orgasm, it can neither see nor understand what is happening during intercourse, and will certainly have no memory of it.

Foetal reactions (slowed movement during intercourse, then furious kicking and squirming and speeded up heartbeat after orgasm) are based solely on hormonal and uterine activity.

Fear That the Introduction of the Penis into the Vagina Will Cause Infection. As long as the male does not have a sexually transmittable disease, there appears to be no danger of infecting either mother or foetus through intercourse during the first seven or eight months. The baby is safely sealed within the uterus in the amniotic sac, which can't be penetrated by either semen or infectious organisms. Most doctors believe this is true even during the ninth month – as long as the sac remains unbroken (the membranes haven't ruptured). But because they could rupture at any time, some suggest that a condom be worn during intercourse in the last four to eight weeks of pregnancy, as added insurance against infection.

Anxiety Over the Coming Attraction. Both the mother- and father-to-be are subject to mixed feelings over the coming event; about the responsibilities and lifestyle changes in store; about the financial and emotional cost of bringing up a baby – all of which can inhibit relaxed lovemaking. This ambivalence, which many expectant parents experience, should be confronted and talked through openly rather than being brought to bed.

The Changing Relationship Between Husband and Wife. A couple may have trouble adjusting to the idea that they will no longer be just lovers, or husband and wife, but mother and father as well. The connection between parenthood and sex may be a difficult one for either or both partners to make. (After all, many of us still avoid associating our own partners with sex, though we are living proof that such an association exists.) On the other hand, some couples may discover that a new dimension in their relationship brings a new intimacy into bed with them – and with it, a new excitement.

Subconscious Hostility. Of the expectant father toward the expectant mother, because he is jealous that she has become the centre of attention. Or of mother-to-be toward father-to-be because she feels she is doing all the suffering (particularly if the pregnancy has been a rough one) for the baby they both wanted and will both enjoy. Such feelings must be talked out, but not in bed.

Belief That Intercourse During the Last Six Weeks of Pregnancy Will Cause Labour to Begin. It *is* true that the uterine contractions triggered by orgasm become stronger as pregnancy proceeds. But unless the cervix is 'ripe,' these contractions do not appear to bring on labour – as many overdue couples who have hopefully tried obligatory nightly sex can attest. However, since no one knows exactly what initiates labour, and because some studies do show an increase in premature births among couples having intercourse in the last weeks of pregnancy, abstinence is often prescribed for women with a tendency toward preterm delivery.

Fear of 'Hitting' the Baby Once the Head Is Engaged in the Pelvis. Even couples who were relaxed about having intercourse earlier can tighten up now because the baby is too 'close' for comfort. Many doctors suggest that though you can't really hurt the baby, deep penetration won't be comfortable at this time and should be avoided.

Psychological factors can also affect sexual relations for the better:

Switching from Procreational to Recreational Sex. Some couples who worked hard at becoming pregnant may be delighted at being able to have sex just for pleasure – free from thermometers, charts, calendars, and anxiety. For them, sex becomes fun for the first time in months, or even years.

Though sexual intercourse during pregnancy may be different from what you've experienced before, it is in most cases perfectly safe. In fact, in many ways it's good for you: it keeps you and your spouse close; it helps you get in shape, preparing your pelvic muscles for delivery; and it's relaxing – which is beneficial for everyone concerned, baby included.

Since lovemaking has so much to offer the expectant couple, it would be ideal if every couple could take advantage of it throughout pregnancy. Alas, for the exceptional few this isn't possible. In high risk pregnancies, intercourse may be restricted at certain times, or even throughout the nine months. For others, intercourse may be permitted without orgasm for the wife, or petting may be allowed as long as penetration is avoided. Knowing precisely *what* is safe and *when* is essential; if your doctor instructs you to abstain, ask why and whether he or she is referring to intercourse, orgasm, or both, and whether the restrictions are temporary or meant for the entire gestation.

When Sexual Relations May Be Limited

☆ Any time unexplained bleeding occurs.

☆ During the first trimester if a woman has a history of miscarriages or threatened miscarriage, or shows signs of a threatened miscarriage during her current pregnancy.

☆ During the last 8 to 12 weeks if a woman has a history of premature or threatened premature labour, or is experiencing signs of it in this pregnancy.

☆ If foetal membranes (the bag of waters) have ruptured.

☆ When placenta praevia is known to exist (the placenta is in an abnormal position, near or over the cervix, where it could be prematurely dislodged, threatening mother and baby).

☆ In the last trimester if multiple foetuses are being carried.

Enjoying It More, Even if You're Doing it Less

Good, lasting sexual relationships – like good, lasting marriages – are rarely built in a day (or even a really terrific night). They grow with practice, patience, understanding, and love. This is true, too, of an already established sexual relationship that undergoes the emotional and physical assaults of pregnancy. Here are a few ways to 'stay on top':

☆ Remember that the quality of lovemaking is always more important than the quantity – but never more so than during pregnancy. Never allow how frequently you have or don't have intercourse to interfere with other aspects of your relationship.

☆ Keep the emphasis on love, rather than lovemaking. If one or both of you don't feel like having intercourse, or if intercourse isn't fully satisfying, find alternative routes to intimacy. The possibilities are far more numerous than positions in a sex manual. For example: old-fashioned kissing and necking, hand holding, back rubs, foot massage, sharing a milkshake in bed (see page 94 for the recipe), reading love poems, watching television while cuddling under a blanket, taking a shower together, going out (or staying in) for a romantic candlelit dinner, meeting for a quiet lunch – or whatever else makes the lovebird in you coo.

☆ Recognise the possible strains that expectant parenthood may have placed on your relationship, and acknowledge any changes in the intensity of sexual desire that either or both of you may be feeling. Discuss the problems openly; don't hide them under the bedcovers. If the problems seem too big to handle by yourselves, seek professional help.

☆ When you start worrying that making love may be harmful, think positive: It's good physical preparation for labour and delivery. (Not many athletes have this much fun in training.)

☆ Think of having to try new positions during pregnancy as an adventure. But give yourselves time to adjust to each position you try. (You might even consider a 'dry run' – trying out a new position fully clothed first, so that it'll be more familiar when you try it for real.) Usually comfortable positions include: male on top, but off to one side or supported by his arms (to keep his weight off the woman): woman on top (but avoid too-deep penetration); both partners on their side – front-to-front or front-to-back.

☆ Keep your expectations within reality's reach. Though some women achieve orgasm for the first time during pregnancy, at least one study showed that most women are less likely to achieve orgasm *regularly* during pregnancy – parti-

cularly in the last trimester, when only one out of four women reach climax consistently – than before conception. Your goal doesn't always have to be orgasm; sometimes just physical closeness can satisfy.

☆ If the doctor has ruled out sexual intercourse during any period of your pregnancy, ask if orgasm is okay – via mutual masturbation. If it isn't (if there is worry about potential miscarriage, orgasm through masturbation can cause more violent contractions than orgasm through intercourse), you might still get pleasure out of pleasuring your husband in this way.

☆ If the doctor has prohibited orgasm but not coitus, you might still want to enjoy lovemaking without your reaching climax. It's a way of feeling close to each other. Another possibility: intercourse between the thighs.

Even if the quality, or quantity, of your sexual relations isn't quite what it once was, understanding what is going on in the dynamics of a relationship during pregnancy can keep the relationship strong – even strengthen it – without spectacular or frequent coitus.

9
The Fifth Month

WHAT YOU CAN EXPECT AT THIS MONTH'S CHECKUP

This month you can expect your doctor or midwife to check the following, though there may be variations depending upon your particular needs and upon your practitioner's style of practice:[1]

☆ Weight and blood pressure

☆ Urinalysis

☆ Foetal heartbeat

☆ Size and shape of uterus, by abdominal palpation

☆ Height of fundus (top of the uterus)

☆ Feet, hands and legs for oedema (swelling), and legs for varicose veins

☆ Foetal movement

☆ Blood tests

☆ Vaginal discharge, bleeding or urinary symptoms

☆ Symptoms you've been experiencing, especially unusual ones

☆ Questions or problems you want to discuss – have a list ready

WHAT YOU MAY BE FEELING

You may feel all of these symptoms at one time or another or only a few of them. Some may have continued from last month, others may be new. Still others may hardly be noticed because you've become so used to them. You may also have other, less common symptoms.

Physically:

☆ Foetal movement

---

1. See appendix for an explanation of the procedures and tests performed

☆ Increasing whitish vaginal discharge (leukorrhoea)

☆ Lower abdominal achiness (from stretching ligaments)

☆ Constipation

☆ Heartburn and indigestion, flatulence and bloating

☆ Occasional headaches, faintness or dizziness

☆ Nasal congestion and occasional nosebleeds; ear stuffiness

☆ Hearty appetite

☆ Leg cramps

☆ Mild oedema (swelling) of ankles and feet, and occasionally hands and face

☆ Varicose veins of legs and/or haemorrhoids

☆ Increased pulse (heart rate)

☆ Easier – or more difficult – orgasm

☆ Backache

☆ Skin pigmentation changes on abdomen and/or face

Emotionally:

☆ An acceptance of the reality of pregnancy

☆ Fewer mood swings, but irritability still occasionally occurs; continued absentmindedness

What You May Look Like

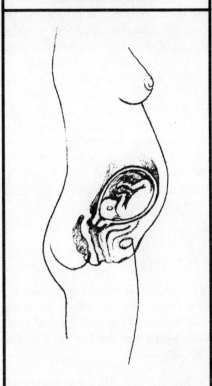

By the end of the fifth month, the activity of this 8- to 10-inch foetus is strong enough to be felt by its mother. Soft downy lanugo covers its body; hair begins to grow on its head; brows and white eyelashes appear. A protective vernix coating covers the foetus.

WHAT YOU MAY BE CONCERNED ABOUT

Fatigue

'I get tired when I am exercising or doing heavy cleaning; should I stop?'

Not only should you stop when you get tired, you should, whenever possible, stop before then. Exerting yourself to the point of exhaustion is never a good idea. During pregnancy it's a particularly bad one, since over-work takes its toll not only on you but on the baby. Pay careful attention to your body's signals. If you become breathless when you're jogging, or find the vacuum suddenly feels as though it weighs a ton, take a break.

Instead of marathon activity sessions, pace yourself. Work or exercise a bit, rest a bit. Most of the time the work, or the workout, will get done, and you won't feel drained afterward. If occasionally something doesn't get done, you're getting good training for the days when the demands of parenthood will often keep you from finishing what you start.

Faintness and Dizziness

'I feel dizzy when I get up from a sitting down or lying-down position. And yesterday I nearly fainted while I was shopping. Am I okay? Can this hurt my baby?'

On late-show movies, a fainting spell is a more reliable indicator of pregnancy than a dead rabbit. Screen-writers in the '40s were, however, misinformed. Though dizziness and fainting are fairly common in pregnancy, they are not likely to appear until the second trimester, when the mother's total blood volume increases dramatically.

The dizziness that occurs on rising from a sitting or prone position is called postural hypotension. It's a drop in blood pressure, caused by a sudden shifting of blood away from the brain. The cure is as simple as the explanation: Always get up very gradually. Jumping up quickly to answer the phone is likely to land you right back on the sofa.

You might also feel dizzy because your blood sugar has dropped. Generally this is caused by going too long without food and can be controlled by taking more frequent, smaller meals or eating snacks between your usual meal times. Carry a box of raisins, a piece of fruit, some wholewheat crackers or breadsticks in your bag for quick blood-sugar lifts.

Dizziness can strike, too, in an overheated store or bus, especially if you are overdressed. The best way to handle such dizziness is to get out in the fresh air, or to an open window. Taking off your coat and loosening your clothes – especially around the neck and waist – should help, too. If you feel lightheaded and/or think you are going to faint, you should try to increase circulation to your brain. Lie down, if possible, with your feet (not your head) elevated, or sit down and put your head between your knees until dizziness subsides. If there's no place to lie or sit, kneel on one knee and bend forward as though you were trying to tie your shoe. Actual fainting is rare, but if you do faint, there is no need for worry or concern – although the flow of blood to your brain is temporarily being reduced, this will not affect your baby.[2]

Tell your practitioner about any faintness you experience when you see him or her next. Report actual fainting promptly. Frequent fainting – occasionally a sign of severe anaemia or illness – needs to be evaluated by a doctor.

---

2. First aid for mothers-to-be who've actually fainted is the same as the preventive measures.

Sleeping Position

'I've always slept on my stomach. Now I'm afraid to. And I just can't seem to get comfortable any other way.'

Giving up your favourite sleeping position during pregnancy can be as traumatic as giving up your teddy bear was when you were six. You're bound to lose some sleep over it – but only until you get used to the new position. And the time to get used to it is now, before your expanding belly makes getting comfortable even more difficult.

Two common favourite sleeping positions – on the belly and on the back – are not recommended during pregnancy. The belly position, for obvious reasons: as your stomach grows, sleeping on it would be about as comfy as sleeping on a watermelon. The back position, though more comfortable, rests the entire weight of your pregnant uterus on your back, your intestines, and the inferior vena cava (a vein responsible for returning blood from the lower body to the heart). This can aggravate backaches and haemorrhoids, inhibit digestive function, interfere with breathing and circulation, and possibily cause hypotension, or low blood pressure.

This doesn't mean you have to sleep standing up. Curling up or stretching out on your side – preferably the left side – with one leg crossed over the other and with a pillow between them, is best for both you and the foetus. It not only allows maximum flow of blood and nutrients to the placenta, but also enhances efficient kidney function, which means

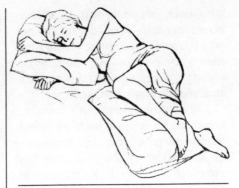

Sleep on your side.

better elimination of waste products and fluids and less oedema (swelling) of ankles, feet, and hands.

Very few people, however, manage to stay in one position through the night. Don't be alarmed if you wake up and find yourself on your back or abdomen. No harm done – just turn back to your side. And don't be concerned if you feel uncomfortable for a few nights. Your body will soon adjust to the new position.

Backache

'I'm having a lot of backaches. I'm afraid I won't be able to stand up at all by the ninth month.'

The aches and discomforts of pregnancy are not designed to make you miserable. They are the side effects of your body's preparation for that momentous moment when your baby is born. Backache is no exception. During pregnancy, the usually stable joints of the pelvis begin to loosen up to allow easier passage for the baby at delivery. This, along with your oversized abdomen, throws your body off balance. To compensate, you tend to bring your shoulders back and arch your neck. Standing with your belly thrust forward – to be sure that no one who passes fails to notice you're pregnant – compounds the problem. The result: a deeply curved lower back, strained back muscles, and pain.

Even pain with a purpose, however, hurts. And without defeating the purpose, you can conquer (or at least subdue) the pain. the best approach, as usual, is prevention. Come into pregnancy with strong abdominal muscles, good posture, and graceful body mechanics. But if it's too late for that, there's still plenty you can do. In general, your goal will be to keep your pelvis from tilting forward and the small of your back from curving inward. Your pelvis should instead tip back and cradle the baby. The following should also help:

☆ Don't gain more than the recommended amount of weight. Excess poundage will only add to the load your back is struggling under.

☆ Don't wear very high heels, or even very flat ones without proper support. Some doctors recommend wide two-inch heels to help keep the body properly aligned.

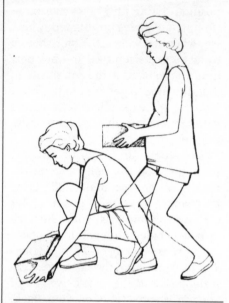

Bend at the knees.

☆ Learn the proper way to lift heavy loads (packages, children, laundry, books, etc.). Don't lift abruptly. Stabilize your body first by assuming a wide stance (feet shoulder-width apart) and tucking your buttocks in. Bend at the knees, not at the waist, and lift with the weight on your arms and legs rather than on your back. (See illustration.) If backache is a problem, try to limit the carrying you do.

☆ Don't stretch to put dishes back into the cupboard or to hang a painting. Instead, use a low, steady

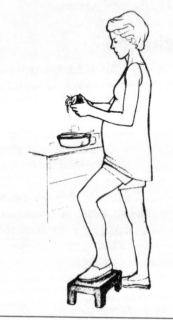

Take an anti-backache position.

footstool. Stretching puts a strain on the back muscles.

☆ Learn to walk, sit, lie, without putting stress on your back muscles. That means with buttocks tucked under and abdomen tilted inward.

☆ Do simple exercises that strengthen your abdominal muscles and tilt your pelvis the right way. (See the Pelvic Tilt, page 168.)

☆ Don't stay on your feet for long periods. If you must, keep one foot up on a stool, your knee bent. This will prevent your lower back from curving in. When standing on a hard-surfaced floor, as when cooking or washing dishes, put a small skid-proof rug underfoot as a cushion.

☆ Use a heating pad (wrapped in a towel) or warm (but not hot) baths to temporarily relieve muscle discomfort and spasm.

☆ Sleep on a firm mattress, or put a board under an oversoft one.

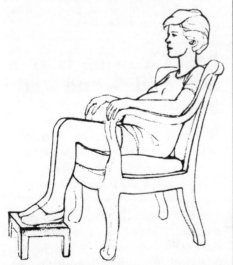

Sit comfortably.

Late Miscarriage

'I know they say that once you pass the third month, you don't have to worry about miscarriage. But I know someone who lost her baby in the fifth month.'

While it's essentially true that there's little reason to worry about miscarriage after the first trimester, it does occasionally happen that a foetus is lost between the 12th and 20th weeks. This is known as a *late* miscarriage, which accounts for fewer than 25% of all spontaneous abortions and is rare in an uneventful, low-risk pregnancy. After the 20th week, when the foetus usually weighs over 500 grams (17½ ounces) and there is the possibility that it can survive with special care, delivery is considered a premature birth and not a miscarriage.

Unlike the causes of early miscarriages, which are frequently related to the foetus, the causes of second-trimester miscarriages are usually related to either the placenta or the mother.[3] The placenta may separate prematurely from the uterus, be implanted abnormally, or fail to produce adequate hormones to maintain the pregnancy. The mother may have taken certain drugs, or undergone surgery that affects the pelvic organs. Or she may suffer from serious infection, uncontrolled chronic illness, severe malnutrition, endocrine dysfunction, untreated Rh incompatibility with the foetus, myomas (tumours of the uterus), an abnormally shaped uterus, or an incompetent cervix that

3. Many maternal causes of late miscarriage can be prevented by good medical care.

opens prematurely. Serious physical trauma, as in accidents, appears to play only a small role in miscarriage at any stage.

Early symptoms of a midtrimester miscarriage include a pink discharge for several days, or a scant brown discharge for several weeks. At this point, bed rest is often prescribed. If the spotting passes, this is an indication that it wasn't related to miscarriage, and resumption of normal activity is usually permitted. If, however, the cervix is found to have begun to dilate, a diagnosis of incompetent (or weak) cervix may be made and cerclage (the suturing closed of the cervix until a few weeks before the due date) performed. This can frequently prevent the threatened miscarriage. If, on the other hand, the spotting turns to heavier bleeding and is accompanied by cramping a miscarriage is imminent, and probably inevitable. Hospitalization may be necessary to prevent haemorrhaging; continued cramping and bleeding following such a miscarriage indicate it is incomplete, and a D and C may be required to evacuate the uterus.

If the cause of a late miscarriage can be determined, it may be possible to prevent a repeat of the tragedy. If a previously undiagnosed incompetent cervix was responsible, future miscarriages can be prevented by cerclage early in pregnancy, before the cervix begins to dilate. If hormonal insufficiency was to blame, hormone replacement may allow future pregnancies to progress normally. Chronic disease, such as diabetes or hypertension, can be better controlled, and acute infection or malnutrition avoided. Rh incompatibility can be treated in utero, if necessary. And an abnormally shaped or myomatous uterus may, in some instances, be corrected by surgery.

Abdominal Pain

'I'm very worried about the pains I've been getting on the sides of my pelvis.'

What you are probably feeling is the stretching of muscles and ligaments supporting the uterus – something most pregnant women experience. It may be crampy or sharp and stabbing, and often is most noticeable when you are getting up from a bed or chair, or when you cough. It may be brief, or last for several hours. As long as the pain is occasional and not persistent – and is not accompanied by fever, chills, bleeding, faintness, or other unusual symptoms – there's no cause for concern. Getting off your feet and resting in a comfortable position should bring some relief. You should, of course, mention the pain to your practitioner at your next visit.

Fast-Growing Hair and Nails – and Red Palms

'It seems to me that my hair and nails never looked so good. My palms, however, seem to be red all the time. Is it my imagination?'

The bounteous circulation caused by pregnancy hormones is feeding your skin cells well. Two of the happy effects of this increased nourishment are nails that grow faster than you can manicure them, and hair that grows faster than you can secure appointments with your stylist. (Some pregnant women find hair flourishing everywhere, even on once smooth abdomens.)

A not-so-happy effect is redness and itching of the palms (and the soles of the feet), which gives the appearance of dishpan hands, even if you never wash a dish. All of these effects will disappear after delivery.

Changes in Skin Pigmentation

'In addition to the dark line down the centre of my abdomen, I now have dark spots on my face. Is this discolouration normal, and will it remain after pregnancy?'

Again, it's those pregnancy hormones at work. Just as they darkened the areola around your nipples, they are now colouring the linea alba – the white line you probably never noticed, which runs down your abdomen to the top of your pubic bone. From now on, it will be called the linea nigra, or black line.

Some women, usually those with darker complexions, will also find patches of darkened skin on their foreheads, noses, and cheeks. (In black women, these may appear as white patches.) These botches , called chloasma, or the 'mask of pregnancy,' will fade after delivery. In the meantime, bleaching probably won't lighten chloasma, though cover-up makeups may disguise it. Sun can intensify the colouration, so use a sunblock containing PABA (para aminobenzoic acid) in sunny weather. Since there is some evidence that the excess pigmentation may be related to folic acid deficiency, be sure that your vitamin supplement contains folic acid and that you are eating enough green leafy vegetables, oranges, and wholewheat bread or cereal daily.

Dental Problems

'My mouth suddenly seems to have become a disaster area. My gums bleed when I brush, and I think I have a cavity. But I'm afraid to go to the dentist because of the anaesthesia.'

With so much of your attention centred on your abdomen during pregnancy, it's easy to overlook your mouth – until it begins to scream for equal time, which it frequently does because of the heavy toll a normal pregnancy can take on teeth and gums.

Gums can take the worst beating – swelling as a result of increased hormone production. (This swelling is similar to that which takes place in the nasal and vaginal mucous membranes during pregnancy.) Sensitive gums may become inflamed and bleed. And teeth, too, occasionally fall victim to the maternal condition.

You should see your dentist every 4–6 months during pregnancy, even if you don't experience any problems. If you do suspect a cavity or other incipient trouble, make an appointment right away. Sometimes there's actually more risk to the foetus in putting off necessary dental work than there is in having it done. For example, badly decayed teeth that are not taken care of can be a source of infection that spreads throughout the system, putting both mother and foetus in danger. And impacted wisdom teeth that are either infected or causing severe pain should also be attended to promptly.

However, special precautions must be taken when dental work is done during pregnancy to ensure that the supply of oxygen to the foetus is not compromised through the use of general anaesthetics, and that no anaesthetic is used that is known to cause harm to the foetus. In most cases a local anaesthetic will suffice. If a general anaesthetic is absolutely required, then it should be administered by an experienced anaesthetist. Discuss the anaesthesia with both your dentist and your doctor to ensure safety.

If after the dental work you're left with chipmunk cheeks and can't chew solids, you're going to have to make some special dietary alterations. On a fluid-only diet you can obtain adequate nutrients (temporarily) by sipping high-protein-and-vitamin milkshakes (see Double-the-Milk Shake, page 94). Supplement the shakes with citrus juices (if they don't burn your gums) and homemade 'creamed' soups made from vegetables puréed with cottage cheese, yogurt, or skim milk. Once you can manage soft foods, add puréed vegetables and meats, scrambled eggs, unsweetened yogurt, apple sauce, mashed bananas, mashed potatoes, and creamy cooked cereals enriched with non-fat dry milk.

Of course, for all dental difficulties, the best treatment is prevention. A programme of preventive dental care that is carefully followed throughout pregnancy – and preferably throughout life – will avert most dental problems.

☆ See your dentist at least once during the nine months, preferably early on (be sure to inform him or her that you're pregnant). Have your teeth cleaned. Avoid x-rays unless they are absolutely necessary, and then take the special precautions suggested on page 69. Routine repair work requiring anaesthesia should be postponed, because even a local anaesthetic can enter your bloodstream, and thus the foetus's.

☆ Follow the Best-Odds Diet, eating little or no refined sugar, particularly between meals, and plenty of foods high in vitamin C. Sugar contributes to both decay and gum disease; vitamin C strengthens gums, reducing the possibility of bleeding. Also be sure to fill your calcium requirements daily (see page 89). Calcium is needed throughout life to keep teeth and bones strong and healthy.

☆ Floss and brush regularly, according to your dentist's prescription. (If your dentist does not instruct you in such preventive measures, you are probably going to the wrong dentist.)

☆ To further reduce bacteria in the mouth, brush your tongue when you brush your teeth. This will also help keep your breath fresh.

Travel

'Is it safe for me to go ahead with the holiday my husband and I had planned for this month?'

For most women, travel during the midtrimester is not only safe, but the perfect chance to get away with their husband for a last fling (at least for a while) as a twosome. And with no nappies, no bottles, no jars of messy baby food to worry about, it'll certainly never be as easy to holiday with your baby again.

Of course, you will need your doctor's permission; if you have high blood pressure, diabetes, or other medical or obstetrical problems, you may not get the green light. (That doesn't mean you can't holiday at all. If you can't travel pick a hotel or resort within an hour's drive of your doctor's office – and enjoy!) Even in a low-risk pregnancy, travelling a great distance isn't a terrific idea in the first trimester, when the possibility of miscarriage is greatest and when your body is still making its initial adjustment to the physical and emotional strain of pregnancy. Likewise, travel is usually not recommended in the last trimester because, should labour begin early, you would be far from your doctor and hospital.

Travel to high altitudes isn't recommended at any time during pregnancy, since the adjustment to the decrease in oxygen may be too taxing for both mother and foetus. If you must make such a trip, you should plan on limiting exertion for several days after arrival, which may minimize the risk of acute mountain sickness (AMS).[4] If you are in your last trimester, your doctor may recommend you have a non-stress test on arrival, then daily for the next two days, then semi-weekly. Any signs of foetal distress will probably warrant the administration of oxygen and a move to a lower altitude.

Once you have your doctor's permission, all you'll need is a little advance planning and a few precautions to ensure a safe and bon voyage for you and your baby:

Plan a Trip That's Relaxing. A single destination is preferable to a Grand Tour which takes you to nine cities in six days. A trip on which you set the pace is a lot better than a group tour that sets it for you. A few hours of tiring sightseeing or shopping should be alternated with time spent sitting reading or napping.

Take Your Best-Odds Diet with You. You may be on vacation, but your baby is working as hard as ever at growing and developing, and has the same nutritional requirements he or she always has. Total self-sacrifice isn't required at mealtimes, but prudence is. Order carefully, and you will be able to savour the local cuisine while fulfilling your baby's requirements. (See Eating Out Best-Odds Style, page 164). Don't skip breakfast or lunch in order to save up for a lavish dinner.

Don't Drink the Water if you're travelling to a foreign country – unless

---

4. Symptoms of AMS include: lack of appetite, nausea, vomiting, gassiness, restlessness, headache, lassitude, shortness of breath, scanty urine and psychological changes.

you're certain it's safe. (But do substitute fruit juices and bottled water to get your daily fluids.) In some regions, it may not be safe to eat unpeeled fresh fruit or raw vegetables. For complete information on such restrictions, on other foreign health hazards, and on immunizations, contact the Royal College of Obstetricians and Gynaecologists, 27 Sussex Place, London NW1 4RG (01-262 5425).

Pack a Pregnancy Survival Kit. Make sure you bring enough vitamins and iron tablets to last the trip; packets of dry skimmed milk if you're afraid you won't be able to find fresh milk; a small jar of wheat germ to enrich white bread or cereal in case whole grains aren't available; medication for traveller's stomach *prescribed by your doctor*; your favourite pregnancy book for reference; comfortable shoes roomy enough to accommodate feet swelled by sightseeing; and a spray disinfectant in case you have to sanitize a communal toilet.

Have the Name of a Reliable Local Obstetrician Handy. Just in case. You doctor may be able to provide you with one. If not, contact the local medical association in the city you're travelling to for the names of English-speaking doctors throughout the world. Some major hotel chains can also provide you with this kind of information. If for any reason you find yourself in need of a doctor in a hurry and can't find one, call the nearest hospital or head for its emergency department.

Head Off Traveller's Irregularity. Changes in schedule and diet can compound constipation problems. To avoid this, make sure you get plenty of the three most effective constipation-combators: fibre, fluids, and exercise. (See Constipation, page 126.) It may also help to eat breakfast a little early, so you'll have time to use the lavatory before you set out for the day.

When You've Got to Go, Go. Don't encourage urinary tract infection by postponing trips to the bathroom. Go as soon as you feel the urge.

If You're Travelling by Car: keep a bagful of nutrious snacks and a thermos of juice or milk handy; stop at least every 2 hours and walk for 5 or 10 minutes to revive circulation; wear your seat belt at all other times.

If You're Travelling by Plane: check with the airline in advance to see if it has special regulations concerning pregnant women (many airlines do). Arrange ahead of time for a seat in the front of the plane, or if seating is not reserved, ask for pre-boarding. *Do not fly in an unpressurized cabin.* All commercial jets are pressurized; but small private or feeder airline planes may not be, and changes in pressure may rob you – and your baby – of oxygen. Drink plenty of water, milk, and fruit juice to counter the dehydration caused by air travel, and bring along healthful snacks and fresh fruit to supplement starchy airline food. (Special-order ovo-lacto vegetarian meals are usually more nutritious.) Get up and stretch your legs for at least 5 or 10 minutes every couple of hours to keep your circulation going. Wear your seat belt comfortably fastened below your abdomen. If you're travelling to a different time zone, take jet lag into account. Rest up in advance, and plan on taking it easy for a few days once you arrive.

If You're Travelling by Train: check to be sure there's a dining car with a full menu. If not, bring adequate meals and snacks along. Take a stroll every couple of hours for circulation's sake. If you're travelling overnight, arrange for a sleeper. You don't want to start your holiday exhausted.

Wearing a Seat Belt

'Is it safe to fasten my seat belt in the car or on an airplane?'

What's the major cause of death among pregnant women? Childbirth? Toxaemia? Puerperal fever? Actually, none of the above. The most common way for a pregnant woman to lose her life is in a car accident. And the best way to avoid such a fatality – as well as serious injury to you and your unborn child – is to always buckle up. Statistics prove conclusively that it is a lot safer to fasten your seat belt than not to fasten it.

For maximum safety and minimum discomfort, fasten your belt below your belly, across your pelvis. If there is a shoulder harness, use it. And don't worry that the pressure of the belt in a short stop will hurt the baby – he or she is well cushioned.

Sports

'I like to play tennis and swim. Is it safe to continue?'

In most cases, pregnancy doesn't mean giving up the sporting life – just living it with a little common sense and moderation. Most practitioners permit patients whose pregnancies are progressing normally to continue participating in sports they are proficient at for as long as is practical – but with several caveats. Among the most important: 'Never exercise to the point of fatigue.' Keeping fit is certainly recommended for anyone; for the pregnant woman there are many bonuses. (See Exercise During Pregnancy, page 166.)

Eating Out

'I try hard to stay on a proper diet, but with a business lunch nearly every day, it seems impossible.'

For most pregnant women it isn't substituting Perrier for the two martinis that poses a challenge at business lunches (or when dining out after hours); it's trying to put together a meal that's nutritionally sound from a menu of cream sauces, elegant but empty starches, and tempting sweets. But with the following cues, it is possible to take the Best-Odds Diet to lunch or dinner:

☆ Push away the bread basket, unless it's filled with whole grains. Even whole grains should be restricted to whatever remains of your daily quota. Butter or margarine, too, should not exceed your

Eating Out Best-Odds Style

☆ **Best** are seafood; American; continental; and steak-house restaurants where broiled fish, poultry, and veal are served, along with fresh vegetables, salads, and potatoes.

☆ **Next Best** are ethnic restaurants where meats, fish, and poultry are featured rather than lost in stews, sauces, or casseroles. Included in this group are Italian (if pasta is eschewed for fish, chicken, and veal dishes); French (nouvelle is preferable to classic French); Jewish (if you avoid fatty meats and gravies, superfluous starches, and salty pickles); and Middle Eastern (if you order baked or grilled fish, meats, and poultry accompanied by bulgur wheat and brown rice). Health food restaurants can fit into this category, but they don't always. The items on their menus – cheese for example – are often low in protein and high in fat; desserts that boast 'no sugar' usually contain hives-full of honey. Be discriminating.

☆ **Least Best,** restaurants to frequent infrequently during pregnancy, include: Chinese (when you do, make sure you get enough protein, request no MSG, don't order sweet-and-sour sauces or deep-fried dishes, skip the white rice, and forego adding soy sauce, which is very high in sodium); Japanese (sushi, as all uncooked fish and meat, is completely taboo, and teriyaki and sukiyaki dishes, soaked in soy sauce, should be avoided); German (steer away from empty calories in breading, dumplings, gravies, and the fat and nitrates in sausages and wursts); Mexican and Spanish (it's usually difficult to identify your protein in sauces and stews, and white rice, the starch of choice in these restaurants, is of little nutritional value.

A very occasional dining-out indiscretion won't upset the odds of your Best-Odds diet. But frequent ones will.

---

allowance; when spreading, keep in mind that there may be other fats in your meal (for example, salad with dressing and vegetables with butter).

☆ Order salad as a first course, with the dressing on the side, or dress it yourself with oil and vinegar. Stay within the Best-Odds Diet guidelines for fat intake.

☆ If you're ordering soup, opt for a clear consommé or broth, or a vegetable-, milk-, or yogurt-based soup. Generally steer clear of cream soups (unless you know they're made with milk) and onion soup laden with cheese and white bread.

☆ Select a high-protein, low-fat main course. Fish, chicken, and veal are usually the best bets, as long as they aren't fried or drowned in butter or rich sauces. If everything comes with a sauce, ask for yours on the side. Often chefs will accommodate your request for fish broiled with little or no fat – wine is a good substitute (the alcohol evaporates).

☆ As side dishes, white or sweet potatoes (in any form but fried or heavily buttered), brown rice, kasha or groats, plus lightly cooked fresh vegetables are all appropriate.

☆ Desserts should be limited to unsweetened fresh or cooked fruits when you're eating out. (Indulge in sugar-free Best Odds treats when you get home: see pages 93–96.) Fruit or berries can be garnished with a dollop of unsweetened whipped cream or sour cream, but shouldn't be sugared or soaked in liqueurs.

Motherhood

'Will I be happy with the baby once I have it?'

Most people approach any major change in their lives – marriage, a new career, or an impending birth – wondering whether it will be a change they'll be happy with. And if they start out with unrealistic expectations, they may very well end up disappointed. If your visions of motherhood are filled with nothing

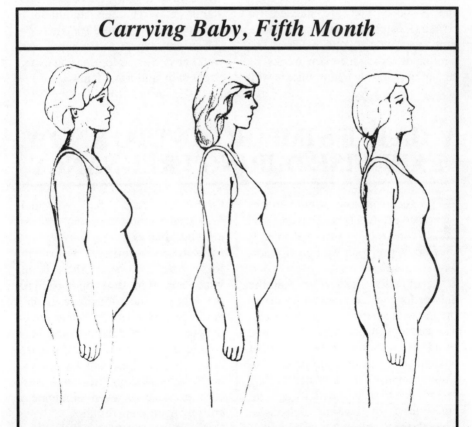

Carrying Baby, Fifth Month

Here are just three of the very different ways that a woman may carry near the end of her fifth month. The variations on these are endless. Depending on your size, your shape, the amount of weight you've gained, and the position of your uterus, you may be carrying higher, lower, bigger, smaller, wider, or more compactly.

but leisurely morning walks through the park, sunny days at the zoo, and hours coordinating a wardrobe of miniature, sparkling clean clothes, you're in for a heavy dose of reality shock. There'll be many morning that will turn into evenings before you and your baby ever have the time to see the light of day, many sunny days that will be spent largely in the laundry room, and few tiny outfits that will escape unstained by spat-up puréed bananas and baby vitamins. And if you have images of bringing a cooing, enchanting Gerber baby home from the hospital, you are headed for certain postpartum disillusionment. Not only won't your newborn be smiling or cooing for many weeks, he or she may hardly communicate with you at all, except to cry – most particularly when you're sitting down to dinner, starting to make love, have to go to the bathroom, or are so tired you can't move.

What you *can* expect realistically, however, are some of the most wonderous, miraculous experiences of your life. The joy you will feel when cuddling a warm, sleeping bundle of baby (even if that cherub was a colicky devil moments before) is incomparable. That – along with that first toothless smile meant just for you – will be well worth all the sleepless nights, delayed dinners, mountains of laundry, and frustrated romance.

Can you expect to be happy with your baby? Yes, as long as you expect a real baby and not a fantasy.

WHAT IT'S IMPORTANT TO KNOW: EXERCISE DURING PREGNANCY

Executives do it. Senior citizens do it. Doctors, lawyers, and construction workers do it. If they do it, pregnant women wonder, why shouldn't we?

'It,' of course, is exercise. And the answer for most women with normal pregnancies seems to be: you should. The concept of pregnancy as a state of ill health, and of the pregnant woman as an invalid, too delicate to climb a flight of stairs or carry a bag of groceries, is as dated as general anaesthesia in routine deliveries. Though there still isn't a vast body of research on the subject of exercise during pregnancy, moderate physical activity is now considered not only thoroughly safe, but extremely beneficial for most expectant mothers and their babies.

As anxious as you might be to hit the jogging trail, however, there is one vitally important stop you must make first – at your doctor's office. Even if you're feeling terrific, you must obtain medical clearance before you start suiting up in your husband's extra-large tracksuit. Pregnant women who are in high-risk categories may have to curb exercise or even eliminate it entirely from their routines.

But if yours is among the great majority of normal pregnancies, and your doctor has given you the go ahead, suit up and read on.

Basic Position and Kegel Exercises

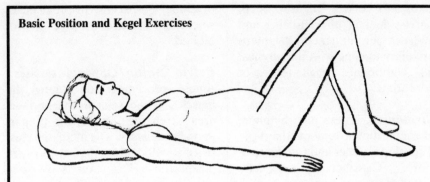

Lie on your back, knees bent, feet about 12 inches apart, soles flat on the floor. Your head and shoulders should be supported by cushions, and your arms resting flat at your sides. To do Kegels, firmly tense the muscles around your vagina and anus. Hold for as long as you can (working up to 8 to 10 seconds), then slowly release the muscles and relax. These also can be done in a standing position or while urinating (see page 323). Do at least 25 repetitions at various times during the day.

The Benefits of Exercise

It appears that women who don't get any exercise during pregnancy become progressively less fit as the months pass by – particularly because they are becoming heavier and heavier. A good exercise programme (which can be built right into your daily lifestyle) can counteract this trend toward decreasing fitness.

There are four kinds of exercise that can be useful during pregnancy: aerobics, specially-designed-for-pregnancy calisthenics, relaxation techniques, and Kegel exercises.

Aerobics. These are rhythmic, repetitive activities strenuous enough to demand increased oxygen to the muscles, but not so strenuous that demand exceeds supply (walking, jogging, bicycling, swimming, tennis singles). Aerobic exercises stimulate the heart and lungs, and muscle and joint activity – producing beneficial overall body changes, especially an increase in the ability to process and utilize oxygen, which is very important for you and your baby. Exercise too strenuous to be sustained for the 20 to 30 minutes necessary to reach this 'training effect' (sprinting), or not strenuous enough (tennis doubles), is not considered aerobic.

Aerobic exercise improves circulation (enhancing the transport of oxygen and nutrients to your foetus while decreasing the risk of varicose veins, haemorrhoids, and fluid retention); increases muscle tone and strength (often relieving backache and constipation, making it easier to carry the extra weight of pregnancy, and facilitating delivery); builds endurance (making you more likely to be able to cope with a lengthy labour); burns calories (allowing you to eat more of the good food you and your baby need without gaining excessive weight, and promising a better postpartum figure); lessens fatigue and promotes a better night's sleep; imparts a feeling of well-being and confidence; and in general heightens your ability to cope with the physical and emotional challenges of childbearing.

Calisthenics. These are rhythmic, light gymnastic movements that tone and develop muscles and can improve posture. Calisthenics especially designed for pregnant women can be very useful in relieving backache, in improving physical and mental well-being, and in preparing your body for the arduous task of childbirth.

Relaxation Techniques. Breathing and concentration exercises (which relax mind and body) help conserve energy for when it's needed, assist the mind to focus on the task at hand, and increase body awareness – all of which help a woman better meet the challenges of childbirth. Relaxation techniques are valuable in combination with more physical routines,

or alone – especially in pregnancies when more active exercise is prohibited.

Pelvic Toning. Or Kegel exercise: a simple procedure for toning the muscles in the vaginal and perineal area, strengthening them in preparation for delivery. The increased elasticity will also aid recovery postpartum. This exercise is one virtually every pregnant woman can perform any time, any place.

Developing a Good Exercise Programme

Get Started. The best time to get fit is before you get pregnant. But it's never too late to start – even if you're already pushing nine months.

Get Off to a Slow Start. Once you've decided to start exercising (and you've invested your money in running shoes and leotards), it's

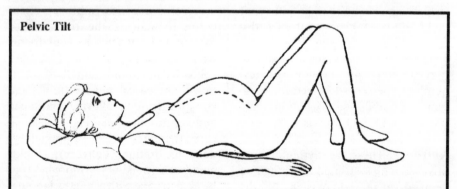

Pelvic Tilt

Assume the basic position (see page 167). Exhale as you press the small of your back against the floor. then inhale and relax your spine. Repeat this several times. The tilt can also be done standing up straight, with your back against a wall (inhale while pressing the small of your back into the wall). The standing version is an excellent way to improve your posture and a good alternative if your practitioner recommends that you do not lie on your back after the fourth month.

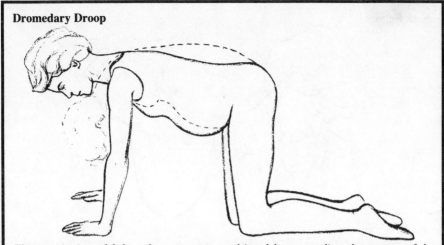

Dromedary Droop

This exercise is useful throughout pregnancy and into labour, to relieve the pressure of the enlarged uterus on your spine. Get down on your hands and knees, with your back in a naturally relaxed position (don't let your spine sag). Keep your head straight, your neck aligned with your spine. Then bump your back, tightening your abdomen and buttocks, allow your head to drop all the way down. Gradually release your back and raise your head to the original position. Repeat several times.

always tempting to start off with a bang, running three miles the first morning or doing Jane Fonda's workout twice the first afternoon. But such enthusiastic beginnings lead not to fitness but to sore muscles, sagging resolve, and abrupt endings. They can also be hazardous.

Of course, if you've been following an exercise programme before pregnancy, you can probably continue it – though possibly in a modified form (see Playing It Safe, page 172). If you're a fledgling athlete, however, build up slowly. Start with 10 minutes of warm-ups followed by 5 minutes of more strenuous workout. Stop sooner if you begin to tire. After a few days, if your body has adjusted well, increase the workout by a couple of minutes a day.

Get Off to a Slow Start Every Time You Start. Warm-ups can be tedious when you're anxious to get your workout started (and over with). But as every athlete knows, they're an essential part of any exercise programme. They ensure that the heart and circulation won't be taxed suddenly, and that the muscles and joints, which are more vulnerable when 'cold' – and particularly vulnerable during pregnancy – won't be injured. Walk before you run, stretch before you begin calisthenics, swim slowly before you start your laps.

Finish as Slowly as You Start. Collapse seems like the logical conclusion to a workout, but it isn't physiologically sound. Stopping abruptly traps blood in the muscles, reducing blood supply to other parts of your body and to your baby. Dizziness, faintness, extra heart-beats, or nausea may result. So finish your exercise with exercise: about 5

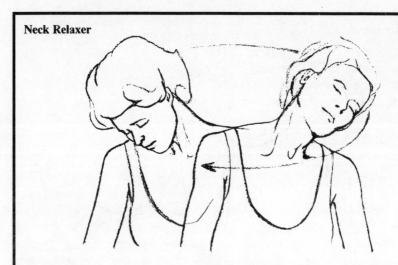

Neck Relaxer

The neck is often a focus of tension, tightening under stress. This exercise can help to relax both your neck and the rest of you: Sit in a comfortable position (Tailor Sit might be best) with your eyes closed. Gently roll your head around, making a full circle, and inhaling as you do. Exhale and relax, letting your head drop forward comfortably. Repeat 4 or 5 times, alternating the direction of the roll and relaxing between rolls. Do this exercise several times a day.

minutes of walking after running, paddling after a vigorous swim, light calisthenics or limbering exercises after almost any activity. Top off your cool-down with a few minutes of relaxation.

Watch the Clock. Too little exercise is not effective; too much can be debilitating. A full workout, from warm-up to cool-down, can take anywhere from 30 minutes to an hour. If you want to get the benefits of aerobic activities, you need to get your pulse (heart rate) to 140 beats for 20 minutes, 130 beats for 45 minutes, or 120 beats for an hour and a half. For healthy women who were entirely sedentary before pregnancy, working up to between 15 and 40 minutes every other day is a realistic and safe goal. Never exercise very vigorously for more than 15 minutes.

Keep It Up. Exercising erratically (four times one week and none the next) won't get you in shape. Exercising regularly (three or four times a week, every week) will. If you're too tired for a strenuous workout, don't push yourself; but do try to do the warm-ups so that your muscles will stay limber and your discipline won't dissolve. Many women find that they feel better if they exercise every day.

Work Exercise into Your Schedule. The best way to be sure of doing your exercise is to allot a specific time for it: first thing in the morning; before going off to work; during a coffee break, if you have the place for it; or before dinner. If you have no regular block of free time for an exercise session, you can build exercise into your daily activities. Walk to work, if you can, or park your car or get off the bus a distance from the job and walk part of the way. Or walk an older child to school (or to a friend's) instead of driving. Do your vacuuming in a steady, 20-minute stretch after a few warm-ups, and you will exercise your body and clean the carpets at the same time. Instead of flopping down in front of the TV with your spouse after the dinner dishes are done, ask him to join you for a walk. No matter how busy your day, if there's the will, there's always a way to fit in some form of exercise.

Compensate for the Calories You Burn.
Probably the best part of an exercise programme is the extra eating you'll have to do. As always, make those calories count. Take this opportunity to add even *more* good-for-baby nutrients to your diet. You'll have to consume about 100 to 200 additional calories for every half hour of strenuous exercising, and at least a full glass of extra liquid to compensate for fluids lost through perspiration. You will need more in warm weather, or when you are perspiring profusely: drink before, during, and after exercising. The scale can give you a clue to how much fluid you need to replace: 2 cups for each pound lost during exercise.

If You Choose the Group Approach:
Take a class or join a health club programme that is specifically designed for pregnant women. Be aware that not everyone who claims to be an expert, is; ask for the instructor's credentials before enrolling. Classes work better for some women than solo exercising (particularly if self-discipline is lacking) and provide support and feedback. The best programmes maintain moderate

Tailor Sit, Tailor Stretch

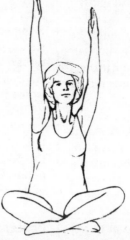

Sitting cross-legged is particularly comfortable during pregnancy. Sit this way often and do arm stretches. Place your hands on your shoulders, then lift both arms above your head. Stretch one arm higher than the other, reaching for the ceiling, then relax it and repeat with the other arm. Repeat 10 times on each side.

intensity; meet at least three times weekly; individualise, and don't insist that every woman do the same routine; don't use fast-tempoed music, which may push participants into working too hard; have a network of medical specialists available for questions.

Playing it Safe

Don't Work Out on an Empty Stomach. Mother's rule about not swimming after a meal was valid. But exercising on an empty stomach could be just as hazardous. If you haven't eaten for hours, it's a good idea to have a light snack and a drink 15 to 30 minutes before beginning your warm-ups. If you're uncomfortable eating that close to exercising, have your snack an hour before.

Dress for the Occasion. Wear clothes that are loose or stretch when you're exercising. Fabrics should let your body breathe – right down to your underwear, which should be cotton. Well-fitting running shoes or well-cushioned sneakers will protect your joints when you're jogging or walking.

Do Everything in Moderation. *Never* exercise to the point of exhaustion when you're pregnant; the chemical by-products of over-exertion are not good for the foetus. (If you're a trained athlete, you shouldn't even exercise to your fullest capacity, whether it exhausts you or not.) There are several ways of checking to see whether you're overdoing it. First, if it feels good, it's prob-

ably okay. If there's any pain or strain, it's not. A little perspiration is fine; a drenching sweat is a sign to slow down. A pulse that is still over 100 five minutes after completing a workout means you've worked too hard. So does needing a nap when you're finished. You should feel exhilarated, not depleted.

Know When to Stop. Your body will signal you when it's time. Signals include: pain of any kind; a cramp or stitch; uterine contractions; light-headedness or dizziness; severe breathlessness; bleeding; loss of muscle control; nausea; or headache. If symptoms aren't relieved by rest, check with your doctor (but call immediately if you have any bleeding). In the second and third trimester, you may notice a gradual decrease in performance and efficiency. It's best to take a clue from your body and slow down.

Stay Cool. Don't exercise in very hot or humid weather; don't use saunas, steam rooms, or hot tubs. Until research shows otherwise, exercise or environments that raise a pregnant woman's temperature more than 1½ to 2 degrees Fahrenheit should be considered dangerous (blood is shunted away from the uterus to the skin as the body attempts to reduce its temperature). So exercise at a cool time of day or in a cool setting.

Proceed with Caution. Even the most skilled sportswoman may lack grace when she's pregnant. As your centre of gravity shifts forward with your uterus, a fall becomes an ever-

Choosing the Right Pregnancy Exercise

Select the type of exercise that's right for you. Though you can probably continue a sport or exercise you are already proficient at, it's not advisable to undertake a new one during pregnancy. It is particularly important that you have a *high* degree of proficiency if you attempt such potentially dangerous sports as downhill skiing and horseback riding.

Exercises even a novice can embark on during pregnancy include:

☆ Walking, preferably at a brisk pace

☆ Swimming in shallow water

☆ Cycling on a stationary bike

☆ Calisthenics designed especially for pregnancy

☆ Pelvic toning

☆ Relaxation routines

Those that even an expert should avoid because of greater risks include:

☆ Scuba diving (diving gear may restrict circulation; decompression sickness is hazardous to foetus)

☆ Water skiing (water could be forced into the vagina in a fall)

☆ Diving and jumping into pools (this can force water into the vagina and cause injuries)

☆ Sprinting (too much oxygen is demanded too quickly)

☆ Skiing above 10,000 feet (the high altitude deprives both mother and foetus of oxygen)

☆ Bicycling on wet pavement or winding paths (falls are likely), and cycling in racing posture, leaning forward (which can cause backache)

☆ Contact sports, such as football and wrestling (they carry a high risk of injury)

☆ Calisthenics not designed for pregnancy, including those that pull on the abdomen (such as sit-ups or double straight leg lifts); that might force air into the vagina (such as upside-down 'bicycling'); that, stretch inner thigh or adductor muscles; that call for holding the soles of the feet together while sitting on the floor and bouncing or pressing down on your knees; that cause lordosis (an exaggerated inward curving of the spine); that require contortions or bridging; that call for knee-chest positions (these need be avoided in the first half of pregnancy only).

increasing possibility. Be aware, and be careful. Late in pregnancy, avoid sports that require sudden moves or a good sense of balance, such as tennis.

Stay Off Your Back, and Don't Point Your Toes. After the fourth month, don't exercise flat on your back, as your enlarging uterus could compress a major blood vessel. Pointing your toes – at any point – may lead to cramping. Flex instead.

Taper Off in the Last Trimester. Though everybody has heard stories of pregnant athletes who have stayed in the pool or on the slopes right up until delivery, it is wise for most women to slack off during the last three months. This is especially true during the ninth month, when stretching routines and walking should provide adequate exercise. Serious athletics can be resumed at about six weeks postpartum.

If You Don't Exercise

Exercising during pregnancy can certainly do you a lot of good. It can relieve backaches, prevent constipation and varicose veins, and give you a general sense of wellbeing during gestation, make childbirth a little quicker and easier, and leave you in better physical shape postpartum. But sitting it out (whether by choice or by a doctor's prescription), getting most of your exercise from opening and closing your car door, won't do you or your baby any harm. In fact, if you're abstaining from exercise on doctor's orders, you're helping, not hurting, your baby and yourself.

10
The Sixth Month

WHAT YOU CAN EXPECT AT THIS MONTH'S CHECKUP

This month you can expect your doctor or midwife to check the following, though there may be variations depending upon your particular needs and upon his or her style of practice:[1]

☆ Weight and blood pressure

☆ Urinalysis

☆ Foetal heartbeat

☆ Height of fundus (top of uterus)

☆ Size of uterus and position of foetus, by abdominal palpation

☆ Blood test for haemoglobin if indicated

☆ Feet, hands and legs for oedema (swelling due to fluid retention); legs and vulva for varicose veins

☆ Inquiry into whether the baby is moving well

☆ Symptoms you may have been experiencing, especially unusual ones

☆ Questions and problems you want to discuss – have a list ready

WHAT YOU MAY BE FEELING

You may feel all of these symptoms at one time or another, or only a few of them. Some may have continued from last month, others may be new. Still others may hardly be noticed because you've become so used to them. You may also have other, less common symptoms.

Physically:

☆ More definite foetal activity

☆ Whitish vaginal discharge (leukorrhoea)

1. See appendix for an explanation of the procedures and tests performed.

☆ Lower abdominal achiness (from stretching ligaments)

☆ Constipation

☆ Heartburn and indigestion, flatulence, and bloating

☆ Occasional headaches, faintness or dizziness

☆ Nasal congestion and occasional nosebleeds; ear stuffiness

☆ Hearty appetite

☆ Leg cramps

☆ Mild oedema (swelling) of ankles and feet, and occasionally hands and face

☆ Varicose veins of legs and/or haemorrhoids

☆ Itchy abdomen

☆ Backache

☆ Skin pigmentation changes on abdomen and/or face

Emotionally:

☆ Fewer mood swings; continued absentmindedness

☆ A beginning of boredom with the pregnancy ('Can't anyone think about anything else?')

What You May Look Like

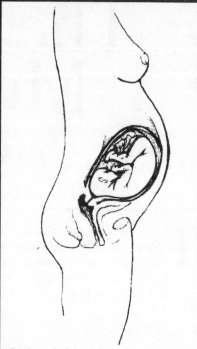

By the end of the sixth month, the foetus is about 13 inches long and weighs about 1¼ pounds. Its skin is thin and shiny, with no underlying fat; its finger and toe prints are visible. Eyelids begin to part, and the eyes open. With intensive care, the foetus may survive if born now.

☆ Some anxiety about the future

WHAT YOU MAY BE CONCERNED ABOUT

Pins and Needles

'I frequently get a tingling sensation in my hands and feet. Does this indicate a problem with my circulation?'

As if it weren't enough to be on tenterhooks during pregnancy, some women occasionally experience the disconcerting tingling sensation of pins and needles in their extremities.

Although it may feel as if your circulation is being cut off, this isn't the case. No one knows why this condition occurs or how to eliminate it, but it is known that it doesn't indicate anything serious. Changing your position may help.

If you are experiencing a great deal of swelling of your hands, you may also develop carpal tunnel syndrome, in which pressure on a nerve in the wrist causes burning of the palm next to your thumb and first two fingers. The pain and burning (and sometimes numbness and tingling) can radiate up your arm. The symptoms may worsen at night because, thanks to gravity, fluids have accumulated in your hands all day, making the swelling more severe. Ask your doctor about splinting and other possible treatment.

Baby Kicking

'Some days the baby is kicking all the time; other days he seems very quiet. Is this normal?'

Foetuses are only human. Just like us, they have 'up' days, when they feel like kicking up their heels (and elbows and knees), and 'down' days, when they'd rather take it easy. Most often, their responses are based on what you've been doing. Like babies out of the womb, foetuses are lulled by rocking. When you're on the go all day, your baby is likely to be pacified by the rhythm of your routine, and you're likely not to notice much kicking – partly because baby's slowed down, partly because you're so busy you overlook what movements there are. When you're relaxing, he or she is bound to start acting up. That's why

most expectant mothers feel foetal movement more often in bed at night, or in the morning before rising. Some pregnant women report increased foetal activity when they're excited or nervous: The baby may be stimulated by the increased adrenaline in mother's system.

Don't compare baby-movement notes with other pregnant women. Each foetus, like each newborn, has an individual pattern of activity and development. Some seem always active; others mostly quiet. The kicking of some is as regular as clockwork; that of others may exhibit no discernible pattern. As long as there is no radical slowdown in activity, all are normal.

After the 30th week, any 24-hour stretch of a significant decrease or of no noticeable activity should be reported to your doctor immediately – though it is not necessarily an ominous sign. Until then, even if a full day goes by without your hearing from your baby, don't worry. Considering the often over-active imagination of the expectant mother, that may be easier for us to say than for you to do. If that's the case, you can try to elicit a foetal response by lying down (with a good book, not with your worries) for an hour or two. You might even poke your abdomen *gently*. Be aware, however, that this does not always work. Sometimes, you just have to wait until your baby's good and ready to communicate.

'Sometimes the baby pushes so hard it hurts.'

As your baby matures in the uterus, he or she becomes stronger and stronger, and those once butterfly-like foetal movements pack more and more power. Don't be surprised if you get kicked in the ribs or poked in the abdomen or cervix with such force it hurts. When you seem to be under a particularly fierce attack, try changing your position. It may knock your little wing forward off balance and temporarily stem the assault.

'The baby seems to be kicking all over, and I'm very large. Could I be carrying twins?'

At some point in her pregnancy, just about every woman begins to think that she's carrying either twins or a human octopus. For most, of course, neither is true. Until a foetus becomes so large that his movements are restricted by the confines of his uterine home (usually at about 34 weeks), he's able to perform numerous acrobatics. So, while it may sometimes feel as if you're being pummeled by a dozen fists, it's more likely to be two fists that get around – along with tiny knees, elbows, and feet.

If your abdomen is unusually large and/or if there are fraternal twins in the family, if you have taken a fertility drug, or if you are over 35, your doctor may have already considered the possibility of twins. Sometimes twins are diagnosed when the examiner identifies two heartbeats; though in early pregnancy, ultrasound is more often needed to make the diagnosis. Later, the examiner may be able to palpate two or more foetuses through the abdomen with his or her hands. It does happen, however, that because of one foetus lying over the other or some other unusual posi-tioning, twins occasionally arrive unannounced and unanticipated at delivery. To avoid such a surprise package, if you're suspicious that you're carrying twins, ask your practitioner about an ultrasound examination to explore the possibility ahead of time.

Leg Cramps

'I have leg cramps at night that interfere with my sleep.'

Between your racing mind and your bulging belly, you probably have enough trouble sleeping without having to suffer from leg cramps. Unfortunately, these painful spasms, which occur most often at night, are very common among pregnant women in the second and third trimesters. Fortunately, however, there are ways of both preventing and alleviating them.

Since most leg cramps are believed to be caused by an excess of phosphorus and a shortage of calcium circulating in the blood, taking calcium tablets which do not contain phosphorus (calcium carbonate is most absorbable) is generally effective in alleviating them. It may be necessary – but only on your doctor's advice – to reduce phosphorus intake by cutting down on milk and meat. (But be sure that you are getting your calcium and protein elsewhere. See the Best-Odds Diet, page 89, for substitutes.) Because fatigue and the pressure of the enlarging uterus on certain nerves are also thought to be possible contributing factors, wearing support hose during the day and alternating periods of rest with periods of physical activity may also be helpful in eliminating the problem of leg cramps.

If you do get a cramp in your calf, straighten your leg and flex your ankle and toes slowly up toward your nose. This should soon lessen the pain. (Doing this several times before retiring at night may even help ward off the cramps.) Standing on a cold surface is sometimes useful, too. If either technique reduces the pain, massage or local heat can then be used for added relief. If neither reduces it, don't massage your calves or apply heat. Do contact your doctor if the pain continues, as there is a slight possibility that a thrombus (blood clot) may have developed.

Rectal Bleeding and Haemorrhoids

'I'm concerned about the rectal bleeding I've been having.'

Bleeding is always a frightening symptom, especially during pregnancy – and particularly in an area so close to your birth canal. But unlike vaginal bleeding, rectal bleeding doesn't signal a possible threat to your baby. During pregnancy it's frequently due to external and, less often, internal haemorrhoids. Haemorrhoids, which are varicose veins of the rectum, afflict between 20% and 50% of all pregnant women. Just as the veins of the legs are more susceptible to varicosities at this time, so are the veins of the rectum. Constipation often causes or compounds the problem.

Haemorrhoids (also called piles because of the resemblance these swollen veins sometimes bear to a pile of grapes or marbles) can cause itching and pain as well as bleeding. Rectal bleeding may also stem from fissures – cracks in the anus caused by constipation, which can accompany haemorrhoids or appear independently. They are generally extremely painful.

Don't try to self-diagnose haemorrhoids. Rectal bleeding is occasionally a sign of serious disease and should always be evaluated by a doctor. But if you do have haemorrhoids and/or fissures, your role will be the most important in treating them. Good self-care can usually eliminate the need for more radical medical therapy.

☆ Avoid constipation. It is *not* a necessary component of pregnancy; see page 126. (Preventing constipation is, incidentally, frequently an excellent way to prevent haemorrhoids completely.)

☆ Sleep on your side to avoid putting extra pressure on the rectal veins; avoid long hours of standing or sitting.

☆ Don't strain at the lavatory. Sitting with your feet on a stepstool may make evacuation easier.

☆ Do Kegel exercises: they improve circulation in the region. (See page 323.)

☆ Take warm baths twice a day.

☆ Apply witch hazel soaks or ice packs to the area.

☆ Use topical medications or suppositories *only* if prescribed by the doctor. Do not take mineral oil.

☆ Keep the perineal area (from vagina to rectum) scrupulously clean. Wash the area with water after bowel movements, always wiping from front to back. Use only white toilet paper.

☆ If sitting is painful, get a special inflatable seat (it's shaped like an inner tube).

☆ Lie down several times a day – if possible, on your side. Watch TV, read, talk to your husband in this position.

☆ With good care, haemorrhoids can be kept from becoming chronic and should disappear after delivery.

Urinary Tract Infection

'I'm afraid I have a urinary tract infection.'

Urinary tract infections (UTIs) are so common in pregnancy that 10% of pregnant women can expect to contract at least one. Most often it will be cystitis, a simple bladder infection. Even in cystitis, the symptoms (an urge to urinate frequently, and a burning sensation when the urine – often only a drop or two – is passed) can become quite uncomfortable. There may also be sharp lower abdominal pain. Cystitis should be treated promptly by a doctor, with one of the antibiotics approved for use during pregnancy. Do not take medication previously prescribed for you or anyone else, even if it was prescribed for a urinary tract infection.

Untreated bladder infection may progress to kidney infection (pyelonephritis), which is more threatening to mother and baby. Symptoms are similar to those of cystitis but may also be accompanied by fever (often as high as 103 degrees), chills, blood in the urine, and backache (in the midback or on one or both sides). Should you experience these symptoms, notify your doctor *immediately*. Antibiotics can generally bring relief, but hospitalization for intravenous administration will probably be necessary.

Many doctors today try to head off kidney infection by screening pregnant women, at their first visit, for susceptibility. If a culture of the urine turns up bacteria (and it does in about 5% of pregnant women) antibiotics are administered to effectively prevent the development of cystitis or pyelonephritis.

There are some home remedies and preventives that may also help ward off UTI; used in conjunction with medical treatment, they may help speed recovery when infection occurs.

☆ Drink plenty of fluids, particularly water. Unsweetened citrus and cranberry juices may also be beneficial. But avoid coffee, tea (even the decaffeinated varieties), and alcohol.

☆ Empty your bladder just before and after intercourse.

☆ Every time you urinate, take time to be sure your bladder is thoroughly emptied.

☆ Wear cotton-crotch underwear

and pantyhose, and avoid wearing tight under or outer pants. Don't wear pantyhose under slacks. And sleep without panties on.

☆ Keep the vaginal and perineal areas meticulously clean. Wash daily and avoid perfumed soaps, sprays, and powders in the area. Always wipe from front to back after using the toilet.

☆ Eat plain yogurt containing active cultures when taking antibiotics to help restore bacterial balance in your intestines.

☆ Keep your resistance high by eating a nutritious low-sugar diet (see Best-Odds Diet, page 82), getting plenty of rest, not working to the point of fatigue, and not letting your life get too stressful.

Itchy Abdomen

'My belly itches constantly. It's driving me crazy.'

Join the club. Pregnant bellies are itchy bellies, and they can become progressively itchier as the months pass. Your skin is stretching, being pulled taut across your abdomen, and the result is dryness (more pronounced in some women than others) and itching. Try not to scratch, or at least keep scratching to a minimum. Keeping the area well softened with lotion may ease the itch but probably won't cure it.

Pre-eclampsia and Eclampsia

'Recently a friend of mine was hospitalized for pre-eclampsia. How can you tell if you have it?'

Pre-eclampsia is always characterized by a precipitate rise in blood pressure and generalized oedema and or protein in the urine. If untreated, it will result in the development of its more severe successor, eclampsia, in which convulsions occur.

Fortunately, even in its mildest form the condition is rare, occurring in only 7% of pregnant women, two-thirds of whom come into pregnancy with chronic hypertension (high blood pressure). It is most common beyond the 20th week, and in first pregnancies. In women who are receiving regular prenatal care, it is diagnosed and treated early, preventing needless complications. Though routine check-ups sometimes seem a waste of time in a healthy pregnancy, it is at such visits that the earliest signs of pre-eclampsia can be picked up.

If you are seeing your doctor or midwife regularly, haven't had a sudden rapid weight gain, severe swelling of your hands and face, headaches, or vision disturbances or protein in your urine you needn't worry about pre-eclampsia. See page 136 for tips on preventing and dealing with high blood pressure in pregnancy. For further advice consult the Pre-eclamptic Toxaemia Society, 88 Plumberow Lee, Chapel North, Basildon, Essex.

Staying on the Job

'I stand a lot on my job. I was plann-ing to work up until I deliver, but is that safe?'

These days, when more first-time expectant mothers are working than are not, the question of how a mother-to-be's working affects an unborn foetus is an important one. The answer, at this point, however, isn't all that clear. We all know women who went from the office or the studio or the shop right to the hospital and delivered perfectly healthy babies. Some studies, on the other hand, are beginning to show that steady stre-nuous or stressful activity during the last half of pregnancy may result in babies that are smaller than average, and in placentas that have damaged areas in them. In a study of African women, hard physical labour during pregnancy retarded foetal growth and increased foetal and neonatal morta-lity – probably because the amount of exercise and the body positions assumed during work reduced blood flow to the placenta.

Whether this has any significance for western women, however, is not known because such heavy labour isn't common for females here. Stu-dies do suggest that women who stand on the job after the 28th week – especially if they also have other children at home to care for – develop elevated blood pressure and deliver babies who weigh somewhat less than average. The risk increases if women stand at their work until term. No one yet knows, however, whether low birth weight and placental damage will later translate into physical or mental problems for the offspring. At the moment, it is believed they don't.

Should women who stand on the job – salespeople, cooks, waitresses, nurses, and so on – work past the 28th week? If they have hypertension, or have children at home to care for without help (and if they have the choice), probably not. But many doctors will permit women who feel fine to work a little longer. Standing on the job all the way to term, however, is not a good idea – espec-ially considering the added dis-comfort of backache, varicose veins, haemorrhoids, and so on that may accrue.

It's also recommended that women not stay at jobs which require lifting, climbing (stairs, poles, or ladders), or bending below waist level past the 20th week if this kind of work is intensive, and past the 28th week if it is moderate.

On the other hand, you can prob-ably plan on going straight from a desk job to the delivery room without any threat to you or your baby. A sedentary job that isn't particularly stressful may actually be less of a strain to you both than staying at home with a vacuum cleaner and mop. And doing a small amount of walking – up to an hour or two daily – on the job or off, is not only harmless, but may be beneficial (assuming you aren't carrying heavy loads).

A number of organisations and groups have been concerned about the working conditions of pregnant women in this country. The Women's Health Information Centre, 52 Featherstone Street, London EC1 (01–251 6580) is a useful source of information on the subject.

☆ Maternity Alliance, 309 Kentish Town Road, London NW5 2TJ campaigns for improved maternity rights and provides information on rights at work.

No matter how long you keep working, there are ways of reducing on-the-job stress during pregnancy:

☆ Wear support hose.

☆ Take frequent breaks. Stand up and walk around if you've been sitting; sit down with your feet up if you've been standing. Do some strething exercises, especially for your back and legs.

☆ Stop working when you're fatigued.

☆ At your desk, keep your legs elevated (on a stool or carton) when possible.

☆ If you are standing for long stretches, keep one foot on a low stool, knee bent, to take pressure off your back. (See illustration, page 156.)

☆ Rest a lot when you are not working; cut down on strenuous activities such as running, tennis, climbing, and so on. The more strenuous your job, the more you need to cut down on other activities.

☆ Rest on your left side during your lunch hour, if possible. Sleep on your left side at night.

☆ Stay out of smoke-filled areas; they are not only bad for the baby, but can increase your fatigue.

☆ Avoid noxious fumes and chemicals.

☆ Avoid extremes in temperature.

☆ Empty your bladder at least every two hours.

☆ If you must stand or walk on the job, cut down on your hours, if possible, and increase your nap period.

Pain of Childbirth

'Now that pregnancy has become an unavoidable reality, I'm worrying about whether I will be able to tolerate the pain of childbirth.'

Though almost every expectant mother eagerly awaits the birth of her child, very few look forward to the labour and delivery that precede it. Especially for those who've never experienced significant discomfort, the fear of this unknown is very real – and very natural. Unhappily, it's often compounded for these women by the horror tales of mothers, aunts, and friends whose footsteps to the labour room they dread to follow.

There's no point in dreading the pain – which may end up being worse than you bargained for or not so bad after all. But there's a lot to be said for being prepared for it. When women who anticipate that labour will be an incomparable, exhilarating, and ultimately fulfilling experience end up with 24 hours of excruciating back labour, they suffer as much from disappointment as from pain. And because the pain is unexpected, they have trouble dealing with it.

In general, both women who fear the worst pain and those who expect the least pain end up fearing and fighting the contractions of labour and are less well off during labour and delivery than women who are realistic in their expectations and prepared for any eventuality.

If you prepare both your mind and your body, you should be able to reduce your anxiety now, and at the same time help make your actual labour more comfortable and easier to tolerate.

Get Educated. One reason earlier generations of women found labour so unbearable was that they didn't understand what was happening to their bodies. Take a good childbirth education class with your partner if it's at all possible (see Childbirth Education, page 185); if it isn't, read as much on the subject of labour and delivery as you can (try to touch on all the major schools of thought), including the description beginning on page 243. What you don't know can hurt you more than it should.

Get Moving. You wouldn't think of running a marathon without the proper physical training. Neither should you consider going into labour (which is no less a Herculean feat) untrained. Work out faithfully with all the breathing and toning-up exercises your practitioner and/or antenatal teacher recommends. (If they haven't recommended any, see page 166 for several basic exercises.)

Put Pain in Perspective. There are at least two good things to be said about the pain of childbirth, no matter how intense. First, it has a definite time limit. Though it may be difficult to believe at the time, you will not be in labour forever. Average labour

with a first child is between 12 and 18 hours – and only a few of those hours are likely to be very uncomfortable. Second, it's a pain with a positive purpose: Contractions progressively thin and open your cervix, each contraction bringing you closer to the birth of your baby. Don't feel guilty, however, if you lose sight of that purpose during very hard labour and care little about anything but getting it over with. A low tolerance for pain does not reflect on the quality of your maternal love.

Don't Plan on Going Through It Alone. Even if you don't feel like holding hands with your partner during labour, it will be comforting to know he (or a close friend or relative) is there to mop your brow, to feed you ice chips, to massage your back or neck, to coach you through contractions, or just for you to curse at. Your partner should go through childbirth classes with you if possible, or if it's not, read up on the partner's role, starting on page 260.

Be Ready to Ask for Pain Relief If It's Needed. Asking for or accepting medication is a sign neither of failure nor of weakness, and it is sometimes absolutely necessary for you to be at your most effective. Keep in mind that you don't have to be a martyr to be a mother. (See page 203 for more on pain relief during labour and delivery.)

Labour and Delivery

'I'm getting very anxious about labour and delivery. What if I fail?'

Childbirth education has probably

done as much as any of the miraculous medical advancements in the past decade to improve the experience of women in labour. However, by creating a mystique of the perfect labour and delivery, it has left some parents-to-be feeling pressured to achieve that ideal experience (much as the sexual revolution made multi-orgasmic sex obligatory). Childbirth becomes, in effect, the final exam for 'prepared' parents, one in which they are expected to excel. It's not surprising many are afraid of failing, and of thereby letting down not only themselves, but also their doctors, nurse-midwives, and antenatal teachers.

But childbirth is not a test that you pass or fail. Nor is there one right way to experience it. Even forgetting, in the excitement, everything you're 'supposed' to do won't change the outcome of the delivery.

Learn everything you can in your classes and from your reading, but don't become so obsessed with 'natural childbirth' that you forget that childbirth is a natural process – one that women managed to stumble through successfully for thousands of years before Mrs. Lamaze gave birth to her son, the doctor.

'I'm afraid I'll do something embarrassing during labour.'

The prospect of screaming or crying out, or of involuntarily emptying your bladder or bowel might seem embarrassing now. During labour, however, avoiding humiliation will be the farthest thing from your mind. Besides, nothing you can do or say during labour will shock or disgust your birth attendants, who've doubtless seen and heard it all before. The important thing is to be yourself, to do what makes you feel most comfortable. If you are ordinarily a vocal, emotive person, don't try to hold in your moans. On the other hand, if you're normally very inhibited and would rather whimper quietly into your pillow, don't feel under an obligation to out-yell the woman in the next room.

'I dread losing control during labour and delivery.'

To members of the take-charge-of-your-life generation, the thought of relinquishing control of your labour and delivery to the medical staff can be a little unnerving. Of course you want the doctors and midwives to take the best possible care of you and your baby. But you'd still like to maintain a modicum of control. And you can – by working hard now at your childbirth preparation exercises, becoming familiar with the birth process step by step (see page 259), and by having good rapport with a practitioner who respects your opinions.

WHAT IT'S IMPORTANT TO KNOW
CHILDBIRTH EDUCATION

When your parents were expecting you, being prepared for childbirth meant that the baby's room was painted, the layette was ordered, and a suitcase packed with pretty nightgowns for the hospital was waiting at the door. It was the arrival of the child – not the childbirth experience – that was anticipated, planned for, and looked forward to. Women knew little of what to expect from labour and delivery; husbands knew even less.

Now that general anaesthesia is relegated mainly to emergency caesareans, waiting rooms are for nervous grandparents, and mother and father can go through childbirth together – ignorance is neither wise nor acceptable. Preparing for childbirth has come to mean preparing for the labour and delivery experience as much as for the new baby. Expectant couples devour stacks of books, magazine articles, and pamphlets. They participate fully in their antenatal visits, seeking answers to all their questions, reassurance for all their worries. And more and more often, they attend childbirth education classes.

Just what are these classes about, and why are they proliferating faster than stretch marks in the sixth month? The original pioneering classes were intended to explain a new approach to childbirth – without medication and without fear – and were commonly known as classes in 'natural childbirth'. Since then, there has been a shift in emphasis from natural childbirth (though it's still considered the ideal) to education and preparation for all the possible eventualities of labour and delivery. So that whether the birth turns out to be natural or complicated, vaginal or surgical, with an episiotomy or without one, parents will understand what is happening and will be able to participate as fully as possible.

Most curricula are based on the following:

☆ The imparting of accurate information, intended to reduce fears, improve the ability to cope with pain, and enhance decision-making skills.

☆ The teaching of specially designed techniques of relaxation, distraction, muscular control, and respiratory activity – all of which can increase a couple's sense of being in control, while contributing to the woman's endurance and a reduction in her perception of pain.

☆ The development of a productive working relationship between the labouring mother and her partner, which, if maintained during labour and delivery, may serve to provide a supportive environment which can, in turn, help her to minimize her anxieties and maximize her efforts during labour.

Benefits of Taking a Childbirth Class

Just how much a couple benefits from a childbirth course depends on the course, on the teacher, and on their own attitudes. These classes work better for some couples than for others. Some thrive in group situations and find sharing feelings natural and useful; others are uncomfortable in groups and find sharing difficult and unproductive. Some enjoy learning relaxation and breathing techniques and ultimately find them effective in the control of pain during labour;

others feel that the rhythmic repetition of such exercises is forced and intrusive (tension-producing rather than tension-alleviating) and end up not using them. Just about every couple, however, stands to gain something from taking a *good* childbirth class – and certainly has nothing to lose. Some benefits include:

☆ The opportunity to spend time with other expectant couples: to share pregnancy experiences, compare progress, and swap tales of woes, worries, aches and pains. It'll also give you the chance to make friends-with-babies, for later. Some classes hold 'reunions' once everyone has delivered.

☆ Increased involvement of the father in the pregnancy, particularly important if he isn't able to attend antenatal visits. Classes will familiarize him with the process of labour and delivery so that he can be a more effective partner and allow him to meet other expectant fathers. Some courses even include a special session for fathers only, which gives them the chance to express and find relief for the anxieties they're reluctant to burden their wives with.

☆ A weekly chance to ask questions that come up between antenatal visits, or that you don't feel comfortable asking your doctor.

☆ An opportunity to get hands-on instruction in breathing, relaxation, and coaching techniques, and to have an expert check how well you're performing them.

☆ An opportunity to develop confidence in your ability to meet the strenuous demands of labour and delivery, through increased knowledge (which helps banish fear of the unknown) and the acquisition of coping skills, which may enable you to feel more in control.

☆ A chance to learn coping strategies that may help to decrease your perception of pain, and hence increase your tolerance for it during labour and delivery – which may translate into less need for medication.

☆ The possibility of an improved, less stressful labour, thanks to better understanding of the birthing process and the development of coping skills. Couples who've had childbirth preparation generally rate their childbirth experiences as more satisfying overall than those who haven't.

☆ Possibly, a slightly shorter labour. Studies show that the average labour of women who have had childbirth education is somewhat shorter than that of women who haven't, probably because the training and preparation enables them to work with, instead of against, the work of the uterus. (There is no guarantee of a short labour, only the possibility of a *shorter* one.)

Choosing a Childbirth Class

In some communities where childbirth classes are few and far between, the choice is a relatively simple one. In others, the variety of offerings can be overwhelming and confusing. There are courses run by hospitals, by private instructors, by doctors or midwives at local clinics and surgeries. There are 'earlybird' prenatal classes – taken in the first or second trimester – which cover such concerns of pregnancy as nutrition, exercise, foetal development, hygiene, sexuality, dreams and fantasies; and there are down-to-the-wire 6- to 10-week childbirth classes, usually begun in the seventh or eighth month, which concentrate on labour, delivery, and postpartum mother and baby care.

If the pickings are slim, taking any childbirth class is probably better than taking none at all – as long as you keep your perspective and don't accept every word spoken in class as gospel. If there is a selection of courses where you live, it may help to consider the following when making your decision.

☆ Taking a class which is run either by your doctor or in conjunction with your doctor, or is recommended by him or her, often works out best. If the labouring and delivering philosophies of your antenatal teacher vary greatly from those of the person who'll be assisting you during labour and delivery, you're bound to run into confusing contradictions and conflicts. If differences of opinion do arise, make sure you air them with your doctor well before delivery.

☆ Small is best. Five or six couples to a class is ideal; more than 10 isn't recommended. Not only can a teacher give more time and individualized attention to an intimate group – particularly important during the breathing and relaxation technique practice sessions – but the camaraderie in a small group is more satisfying.

☆ Classes which set up unrealistic expectations can work against you. (If you're guaranteed that taking the class will make labour short or painless or glorious, for instance, beware.) There's no way to know for sure what a teacher's philosophy of childbirth will be until you take the class – unless you're able to sit in on one in advance – but talking to him or her before signing up can give you some idea.

☆ What is the rate of drug-free labours among class 'graduates'? This may be helpful information, but it can also be misleading. Does a low rate indicate that students were so well prepared in the various natural pain-reducing strategies that they rarely needed medication? Or were they so convinced that asking for medication was a sign of failure that they stoically withstood severe pain? Perhaps the best way to find the answer is to talk to some of the graduates.

☆ What is the curriculum like? Ask for a course outline, and if you can, sit in on a class. A good course will include a discussion of caesarean section (recognizing that about 1 in 9 of students may end up having one) and of medication (recognizing that some will also need this, too). It will deal with feelings, as well as procedures.

☆ How is the class taught? Are films

of actual childbirths shown? Will you hear from mothers and fathers who've recently delivered? Is there discussion, or just lecture? Will there be an opportunity for parents-to-be to ask questions? Is adequate time provided during class for practising the various techniques that are taught? Is one particular philosophy followed – Lamaze or Bradley, for example?

The Most Common Schools of Thought

There are several major childbirth education philosophies, though many instructors combine elements of each.

Grantly Dick-Read. This psycho-physical approach dates back to the '40s and '50s and was the first organized approach to childbirth preparation in the United States. Combining relaxation techniques and prenatal education to break the fear-tension-pain cycle of labour and delivery, it was the first to include fathers in the education process and to bring them into the labour room.

Lamaze. Also called the psycho-prophylactic method, this approach is similar in some ways to the psycho-physical approach in that its major weapons against pain are knowledge and relaxation techniques. In addition, Lamaze depends on conditioning, à la Dr Pavlov, who conditioned dogs to salivate at the sound of a bell. The expectant mother is conditioned, through intensive training and practice, to substitute

useful responses to the stimulus of labour contractions in place of counterproductive ones. In recent years, the father or other coach has trained with the mother to assist her during both labour and delivery.

Bradley. This approach, which originated the husband-coached delivery, emphasizes good diet and uses exercise to ease the discomforts of pregnancy and prepare muscles for birth and breasts for nursing. Women learn to imitate their sleeping position and breathing (which is deep and slow) and to use relaxation to make the first stage of labour more comfortable. Rather than the usual panting and contrived breathing patterns, the Bradley method employs deep abdominal breathing; instead of using distraction and a focus of concentration outside the body to take the mind off discomfort. Bradley recommends that the labouring woman concentrate within and work with her body. Medication is reserved for complications and caesareans, and about 94% of Bradley graduates go without it. Bradley-based classes begin as soon as pregnancy is confirmed and continue into the postpartum period in the belief that it takes a full nine months to get physically and emotionally prepared for labour and delivery. However, classes are not usually available in the UK.

National Childbirth Trust. In the UK, the National Childbirth Trust (NCT) offers the most widespread alternative to the National Health Service antenatal classes, although in some urban areas, particularly London, more choice is available. This choice includes the classes run by the Birth Centres.

Most NCT classes are small groups, held in private homes. Many classes are held in the evening, giving both you and your partner the opportunity to attend together. By helping you both to gain confidence in your own active participation in the experience of childbirth and parenthood, the classes will offer you the opportunity to learn more about labour and childbirth. The skills of relaxation, breathing techniques and massage will be introduced, and the medical procedures in practice in your local area will be discussed. You will also be put in touch with a network of post-natal support, through breastfeeding counsellors and informal links with other NCT members.

11
The Seventh Month

WHAT YOU CAN EXPECT AT THIS MONTH'S CHECKUP

From 28 to 36 weeks you will be seen by a midwife or doctor every fortnight. In this month you can expect to be checked for the following, though there may be variations depending upon your particular needs and upon your doctor or midwife's style of practice:[1]

☆ Weight and blood pressure

☆ Urinalysis

☆ Foetal heartbeat

☆ Blood test for haemoglobin, if indicated

☆ Height of fundus (top of uterus)

☆ Size and position of foetus, by abdominal palpation

☆ Feet, hands and legs for oedema (swelling); legs and vulva for varicose veins

☆ Symptoms you have been experiencing, especially unusual ones

☆ Inquiry into any unusual vaginal discharge or bleeding

☆ Questions and problems you want to discuss – have a list ready

WHAT YOU MAY BE FEELING

You may feel all of these symptoms at one time or another, or only a few of them. Some may have continued from last month, others may be new. Still others may hardly be noticed because you've become so used to them. You may also have other, less common symptoms.

Physically:

☆ Stronger and more frequent foetal activity

---

1. See appendix for an explanation of the procedures and tests performed.

☆ Increasingly heavy whitish vaginal discharge (leukorrhoea)

☆ Lower abdominal achiness

☆ Constipation, heartburn and indigestion, flatulence and bloating

☆ Occasional headaches, faintness or dizziness

☆ Nasal congestion and occasional nosebleeds; ear stuffiness

☆ Leg cramps

☆ Backache

☆ Mild oedema (swelling) of ankles and feet, and occasionally hands and face

☆ Varicose veins of legs and/or haemorrhoids

☆ Itchy abdomen

☆ Shortness of breath

☆ Difficulty sleeping

☆ Scattered Braxton Hicks contractions, usually painless (the uterus hardens for a minute, then returns to normal)

☆ Clumsiness (which makes it easier to take a fall – be careful)

☆ Colostrum, either leaking or expressed, from breasts

Emotionally:

☆ Increasing apprehension about the baby, and about labour and delivery

☆ Continued absentmindedness

☆ Increased dreaming and fantasizing about the baby

What You May Look Like

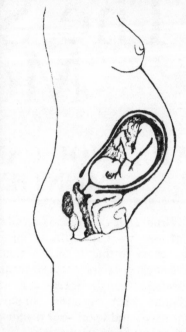

By the end of the seventh month, fat begins to be deposited. The foetus may suck its thumb, hiccup, cry; can taste sweet or sour; responds to stimuli, including pain, light, and sound. Placental function begins to diminish, as does the volume of amniotic fluid, as the 3-pounder fills the uterus. Good chance of survival if born now.

☆ Increased boredom and weariness with the pregnancy, the beginning of anxiousness to be over with it

WHAT YOU MAY BE CONCERNED ABOUT

Increasing Fatigue

'I've heard women are supposed to feel terrific in the last trimester. I feel tired all the time.'

'Supposed to' is a phrase that ought to be stricken from a pregnant woman's vocabulary. There's no one way you're supposed to feel at any time in pregnancy. Though some women may feel less tired in the third trimester than in the first and second, it can be perfectly normal to continue feeling fatigued or to feel even more fatigued. Actually, there are probably more reasons to feel tired in the last trimester than to feel terrific. First of all, you're carrying around a lot more weight than you were earlier. Second, because of your bulk, you may be having trouble sleeping. You may also be losing sleep to a constantly racing mind. Taking care of other children, a job, or both may be taking a toll on you – and so may preparing for the baby.

Just because your fatigue is a normal part of pregnancy doesn't mean you should ignore it. As always, it's a signal from your body that you should slow down. Take the hint: Rest and relax as much as you can. You'll need every bit of strength you can save up for labour, delivery, and – more important – what follows them.

Extreme fatigue that doesn't ease up when you get more rest should be reported to your doctor. Anaemia sometimes strikes at the beginning of the third trimester, and many doctors do a routine blood test for it in the seventh month. (See page 139.)

Concern About the Baby's Well-Being

'I worry all the time that something is wrong with my baby.'

There probably isn't an expectant mother (or father) who hasn't been haunted by this same fear. Some will even put off buying baby clothes and furniture, or choosing the baby's name, until toes and fingers have been counted, the Apgars have been calculated, and the doctor/midwife has congratulated them on a healthy baby.

But the odds of having a completely normal baby have never been better. The UK infant mortality rate is the lowest in history, down to between 10 and 11 per 1,000 births. And most of the perinatal deaths occur in the newborns of indigent women living in inner cities and depressed rural areas who receive medical care late or not at all and who are inadequately nourished. A majority of the remainder occur in infants of high-risk women: those with a family history of genetic disease; with uncontrolled chronic illnesses; who drink heavily and/or smoke or take drugs; or who are carrying multiple foetuses. Even for these women, close medical supervision and good prenatal care has recently greatly increased the chances of having healthy babies.

Some experts had forecast that as the death rate fell – because more babies with birth defects would be saved by medical miracles – the rate of children with handicaps would rise. This hasn't happened; the percentage of birth defects, in fact, appears to be declining. And, again, these defects are more likely to occur in children born to high-risk women. Even when a child is born with a birth defect, he or she isn't necessarily permanently handicapped. Most minor, and many serious defects are now correctable. If diagnosed in utero some can be treated before birth through surgery or medication. Heart defects and other internal abnormalities can be mended with microsurgery shortly after birth; cleft palates and bone or limb abnormalities can be surgically repaired. Children who are intellectually disabled can, with early intervention, make remarkable strides.

So when worry strikes, strike back – with the knowledge that your baby couldn't have picked a better time to be born (and grow up) healthy.

Oedema (Swelling) of the Hands and Feet

'My ankles seem to be swollen, especially when the weather is warm. Is this a bad sign?'

Any degree of oedema (swelling due to excessive accumulation of fluids in the tissues) was once considered a potential danger sign in pregnancy. Now doctors recognize that mild oedema is related to the normal and necessary increase in body fluids in pregnancy. Some swelling of the ankles and legs without accompanying symptoms to suggest the development of pre-eclampsia (see below) is considered completely normal. In fact, 75% of women develop such oedema at some point in their pregnancies.[2] It's particularly common late in the day, in warm weather, or after standing or sitting a lot. Much of it should disappear however, after a good night's sleep.

Generally, oedema is nothing but a little uncomfortable. To ease discomfort, elevate your legs or lie down when you can, preferably on your left side; wear comfortable shoes or slippers; avoid elastic-top socks or stockings. If the oedema is really bothersome, put support panty-hose on before you get up in the morning, while the swelling is down. Help your excretory system to flush out waste products and excess fluids by drinking at least eight to ten eight-ounce glasses of liquids daily. Though it's no longer believed that salt restriction is wise during pregnancy, excessive salt intake isn't any smarter and could increase fluid retention.

If your hands and/or face become puffy, or if the oedema persists for more than 24 hours at a time, you should notify your doctor. Such swelling may be insignificant, or – if accompanied by rapid weight gain, a rise in blood pressure, and protein in the urine – it could signal the beginning of pre-eclampsia. (See page 136.)

Overheating

'I feel so warm most of the time, and I sweat a lot. Is this normal?'

---

2. One in four pregnant women never experience oedema, and this can be completely normal, too. Others may not notice swelling.

With your basal metabolic rate (the rate at which your body expends energy at total rest) up about 20% during pregnancy, the heat's on. Not only are you likely to feel too warm in warm weather, you may even feel overheated in the winter – when everyone else is cool. You will also probably perspire more, especially at night. This is a mixed blessing. While it helps to cool you off and rids your body of waste products, it is admittedly unpleasant.

To minimize discomfort: bathe often; use a good antiperspirant; and dress in layers – especially in the winter – so you can peel down to shirt-sleeves when you start heating up. And don't forget to take extra fluids to replace those lost through your pores.

Making Love and the Baby

'After I have an orgasm my baby usually stops kicking for about half an hour. Is sex harmful to him or her at this stage of pregnancy?'

Babies are individuals even while they're still in the womb. And their reactions to their parents' lovemaking vary. Some, like your baby, are rocked to sleep by the rhythmic motion of coitus and the uterine contractions that follow orgasm. Others, stimulated by the activity, may become more lively. Both reactions are normal; neither indicates any awareness of the proceedings on the foetus's part, or any kind of foetal distress.

Whether sexual intercourse is totally safe during the last two months of pregnancy, even in a normal pregnancy, is a matter of increasing controversy in the obstetrical community. Acquitted several years ago as an accessory to premature labour and perinatal infection, coitus in the final weeks of gestation is once again being implicated in such complications by researchers. To learn what is believed safe in sexual relations for expectant parents, see Making Love During Pregnancy, page 145.

Premature Labour

'Is there anything I can do to ensure that my baby won't be born prematurely?'

Far more babies are born late than early. Only about 7 in 100 deliveries are premature or preterm; that is, take place before the 37th week of pregnancy. And about three fourths of these involve women who are at high risk for premature delivery. The rate is lower for white women (fewer than 6 in 100) and higher for black women (nearly 13 out of 100), partly for socioeconomic reasons. Dramatic advances in preventing preterm labour, combined with better care, should go a long way in reducing the incidence of prematurity.

There are a wide variety of factors that are believed to be related to increased risk of preterm delivery. The more risk factors in a woman's history, the greater the chance that she will deliver prematurely. The risk factors that follow can be controlled, either partially or completely, greatly increasing the odds that a woman will carry to term.

Smoking. Quit as early as possible in pregnancy, or before.

Alcohol Consumption. Avoid regular drinking of beer, wine and liquor (no one yet knows how much is too much, so it's safer to abstain).

Drug Abuse. Don't use unprescribed drugs during pregnancy.

Inadequate Weight Gain. If your prepregnant weight was normal, gain a minimum of 20 pounds; if you were significantly underweight before conceiving, gain closer to 30 pounds. (Overweight women, with excellent nutrition and their doctor's permission, may be able to gain less safely.)

Inadequate Nutrition. Follow a well-balanced diet (See the Best-Odds Diet, page 82) throughout pregnancy. Be sure that your vitamin supplement contains zinc; some recent studies have linked zinc deficiency with preterm labour.

Standing, or Heavy Physical Labour. If your job alone or your job plus housework require you to stand for several hours each day, stop working or cut down.

Sexual Intercourse (for Some Women). Expectant mothers who are at high risk for premature delivery are generally advised to abstain from intercourse and/or orgasm during the final two or three months of pregnancy. Or, to use a condom to prevent infection of the amniotic sac, which it is believed might trigger early labour.

Hormonal Imbalance. Just as it can trigger late miscarriage, an imbalance of hormones can sometimes trigger premature delivery; hormone replacement may prevent both.

Other risk factors are not always possible to eliminate, but their effects can sometimes be modified:

Infections (such as venereal disease, urinary tract and vaginal infections, and rubella). Avoid exposure whenever possible (see individual diseases), and seek prompt treatment if you do contract infection. In general, it helps to keep yourself in good health through adequate rest, optimal nutrition, exercise and regular prenatal care.

Incompetent Cervix. This condition, in which a weak cervix opens prematurely, is often undiagnosed until after at least one instance of miscarriage or premature labour. When diagnosed, premature delivery can be avoided by suturing the cervix after the 14th week.

Placenta Previa (when the placenta is located low in the uterus, near or over the cervix). This condition may be diagnosed early through the use of ultrasound, or may be signalled by bleeding in mid or late pregnancy. Premature labour may be headed off by complete bed rest.

Chronic Maternal Illness (high blood pressure; heart, liver, or kidney disease; diabetes). Good medical care, sometimes necessitating bed rest, can often prevent premature delivery. (Premature babies of diabetic mothers, however, are rarely born with a low birth weight.)

Stress. Sometimes the cause can be controlled (by quitting a stressful job, getting counselling if your marriage is floundering); sometimes it cannot (as when your husband loses his job, you lose your husband through divorce or death, or you are pregnant and alone). But all kinds of stress can be reduced through education, relaxation techniques, good nutrition, a balance of exercise and rest, and talking out your problem – often in a self-help group.

Age Under 17. Optimal nutrition and antenatal care can help compensate for the fact that the mother, like her foetus, is still growing.

Age Over 35. Optimal nutrition, good antenatal care, reduction of stress, and antenatal screening for obstetrical problems specific to older women all reduce risk.

Low Educational or Socioeconomic Level. Again, good nutrition and medical care, and the elimination of all possible risk factors, can decrease the risk.

Structural Abnormalities of the Uterus. Once the problem has been diagnosed, surgical repair can frequently prevent future preterm births.

Multiple Gestations. Women carrying more than one foetus deliver an average of three weeks early.

Meticulous prenatal care, bed rest and restrictions on activity as needed in the last trimester, and elimination of all other risk factors may help prevent a too-early birth.

History of Premature Deliveries. A diagnosed cause can be corrected; top-notch prenatal care, reduction of other risk factors, and limitations on activities may help to prevent a repeat.

When the cause of preterm labour cannot be prevented or modified, often the threatened labour itself can be postponed. Even a brief delay can be beneficial; each additional day the baby remains in the uterus (until term) improves its chance of survival. Only when the mother and/or child are endangered, such as when the placenta separates prematurely from the uterus (abruptio placenta), or there is foetal or maternal distress, is no attempt made to postpone early delivery.

Postponement (or the prevention of the onset of premature labour) can often be achieved through limitations on sexual intercourse and other physical activities, bed rest, and, if necessary, hospitalization and the administration of tocolytic agents (drugs which relax the uterine muscles and halt contractions). When treatment has successfully delayed labour, the expectant mother may be able to return home on oral medication and with orders to rest in bed.

But it is possible to postpone premature labour only if it is diagnosed early, before the cervix has effaced and dilated significantly and/or the membranes have ruptured. Since a premature baby is smaller than one at full term, the cervix does not have to dilate a full 10 centimetres before expulsion of the foetus; as a result, premature labour progresses quickly.[3]

So you can see it's important to be familiar with the signs of early labour, which follow, and to alert your doctor or midwife if you've the slightest suspicion that labour is beginning. *Don't worry about bothering your doctor or midwife* – no matter what the day or hour.

☆ Menstrual-like cramps, with or without diarrhoea, nausea, or indigestion.

☆ Lower back pain, or a change in the nature of lower backache.

☆ An achiness or feeling of pressure in the pelvic floor, the thighs, or the groin.

☆ A change in your vaginal discharge, particularly if it is watery or tinged or streaked pinkish or brownish with blood. The passage of a thick, gelatinous mucous plug may or may not precede this 'bloody show'.

☆ Rupture of membranes (you feel a trickle or rush of fluid from your vagina).

You can have all these symptoms and not be in premature labour, but only your doctor can tell you for sure. If he or she suspects you're in labour,

you will probably be examined promptly.

If premature labour does take place – despite steps to prevent or postpone it – your chances of taking a healthy, normal baby home from the hospital are excellent. (Of course, that trip home with the baby may have to be delayed days, weeks, or even months.) Top-grade medical care, utilizing the latest advances in neonatology (care of the newborn), often begins during labour with administration of the drug betamethasone, which speeds the maturity of the foetal lungs. Sometimes a woman will be moved early in labour into a regional perinatal centre, so that the baby can be delivered directly into a special care baby unit (SCBU). With continued care in such units, even 2- and 3-pound premies have a nearly 100% chance of survival, and a very good chance of growing up without any handicapping after effects.

Approaching Responsibility

'I'm beginning to worry that I won't be able to manage my job, my house, my marriage – and the baby, too.'

You probably won't be able to manage if you attempt to be a full-time career woman, housekeeper, wife, and mother – seeking perfection in each. Many new mothers have tried to be 'superwomen'; few have succeeded without sacrificing their health and sanity.

But it will be possible to survive if you reconcile yourself to the reality that you can't do it all – at least in the

---

3. If premature labour threatens and/or membranes rupture before significant dilatation occurs, and tests show the foetal lungs are immature, some physicians try to postpone delivery for two to three days. During that time, they administer a steroid drug to spur foetal lung maturation. Doctors differ on whether or not this is an effective course.

beginning. If job, husband, and baby are important, perhaps keeping the house immaculate will have to give way. If full-time motherhood appeals to you and you can afford to stay at home for a while, maybe you can shelve your career temporarily. Or work part-time, as a compromise. It's just a matter of deciding in advance what your priorities are.

Whatever decision you make, your new life will be easier if you don't have to go it alone. Behind the most successful mother there's usually a cooperative father, willing to share the workload. Don't feel guilty about asking him to change nappies and bath the baby after a long day at the office. There's probably no better way for him to unwind and, at the same time, to get to know his child. If father isn't available (all or part of the time), then you are going to need to think about other sources of assistance: mothers or other relatives, childcare or household workers, playgroups, day care centres.

Accidents

'I missed the curb today when I was out walking and fell belly-first on the pavement. I'm not worried about my skinned knees and elbows, but I'm terrified that I've hurt the baby.'

A woman in the last trimester of pregnancy isn't exactly the most graceful creature on earth. A poor sense of balance, due to a shifting forward of her centre of gravity, and looser, less stable joints contribute to her awkwardness and make her prone to minor falls – particularly belly-flops. So does her tendency to tire easily,

her predisposition to preoccupation and daydreaming, and the difficulty she may be having seeing past her belly to her feet.

But while a curb-side spill may leave you with multiple scrapes and bruises (particularly to the ego), it's extremely rare for a foetus to suffer the consequences of its mother's clumsiness. Your baby is protected by the world's most sophisticated shock-absorption system, comprised of amniotic fluids, tough membranes, a muscular uterus, and a sturdy abdominal cavity girded with muscles and bones. For this system to be penetrated, and for your baby to be hurt, you'd have to sustain very serious injuries – the kind that would very likely land you in the hospital.

Even though there's probably no harm done, you should let your doctor know about a fall. You may be asked to come in so that your baby's heartbeat can be checked – mostly to set your mind at ease. Should you notice vaginal bleeding, a leaking of amniotic fluid, or that your baby is unusually inactive, however, medical attention should be sought immediately. Have someone take you to a maternity hospital or casualty department, if you can't reach your doctor.

Back and Leg Pain

'I've been having pain on the right side of my back, that runs right down my hip and leg. What's happening?'

This is just another one of those occupational hazards of expectant motherhood. The pressure of the enlarging uterus, which has caused so many other discomforts, can also extend to the sciatic nerve – causing lower back, buttock, and leg pain. Rest, and a heating pad applied locally, may help.

Foetal Hiccups

'I sometimes feel regular little spasms in my abdomen. Is this kicking, or a twitch, or what?'

Believe it or not, your baby's got hiccups. The phenomenon is very common in foetuses in the last half of pregnancy. Some get hiccups several times a day, every day. Others never get them at all. The same pattern may continue after birth.

But before you start holding a paper bag over your belly, you should know that hiccups don't cause the same discomfort in babies (in or out of the uterus) as they do in adults – even when they last as long as 20 minutes or more. So just relax and enjoy this little entertainment from within.

Dreams and Fantasies

'I've been having so many vivid dreams about the baby that I'm beginning to think I'm going mad.'

Though the many night- and day-dreams (both horrifying and pleasant) a pregnant woman can experience in the last trimester may make her feel as though she's losing her sanity, they're actually helping to keep her sane. Dreams and fantasies are both healthy and normal, and help

expectant women to sort out worries and fears in a non-threatening way.

Each of the dream and fantasy themes commonly reported by pregnant women expresses one or more of the deep feelings and concerns that might otherwise be suppressed:

☆ Being unprepared, forgetting or losing things – not feeding the baby; missing a doctor's appointment; going out to shop and forgetting you have a baby; being unprepared for the baby when it arrives; losing car keys, or even the baby – can express fear of not being adequate to the task of motherhood.

☆ Being attacked or hurt – by intruders, burglars, animals; falling down the stairs after a push or a slip – may indicate a sense of vulnerability.

☆ Being enclosed or unable to escape – trapped in a tunnel, car, a small room; drowning in a pool, a lake of snowy slush, a car wash – can signify fear of being tied down and deprived of freedom by the baby.

☆ Going off the diet – gaining too much weight, or gaining a lot of weight overnight; overeating; eating or drinking the wrong things (two hot fudge sundaes or a bottle of wine) or not eating the right things (forgetting to drink milk for a week) – is common among those trying to adjust to a restricted diet.

☆ Losing appeal – becoming unattractive or repulsive to her husband, her husband finding another woman – expresses nearly every woman's fear that pregnancy will destroy her looks forever and drive her husband away.

☆ Sexual encounters – either positive or negative, pleasure- or guilt-provoking – may be an indication of the sexual confusion and ambivalence often experienced during pregnancy.

☆ Death and resurrection – lost parents or other relatives reappearing – may be the subconscious mind's way of linking old and new generations.

☆ Family life with the new baby – getting ready for the baby; loving and playing with the baby – is practice parenting, bonding mother with the baby prior to birth.

☆ What the baby will be like – can represent a wide variety of concerns. Dreams about the baby being deformed or unusual in size express anxiety about the health of the baby. Fantasies about the infant having unusual skills (like talking or walking at birth) may indicate concern about the baby's intelligence and ambition for his or her future. Premonitions that the baby will be a boy or a girl could signal a problem – your heart may be too set on one or the other. So could dreams about the baby's hair or eye colour or resemblance to one parent or the other. Nightmares of the baby being born fully grown could be signalling another problem – your fear of having to handle a tiny baby.

Though dreams and fantasies in pregnancy are much more anxiety-provoking than they are at other times, they are also more useful. If you listen to what your motherhood fantasies are telling you – and heed their warnings – you can make the transition into real-life motherhood more easily.

WHAT IT'S IMPORTANT TO KNOW: ALL ABOUT CHILDBIRTH MEDICATION

On January 19, 1847, Scottish physician James Young Simpson splashed a half teaspoonful of chloroform on a handkerchief and held it over the nose of a labouring woman. Less than half an hour later, she became the first woman to deliver while under anaesthesia. (There was only one complication: When the woman – whose first baby had been born after three days of painful labour – awoke, Dr Simpson was unable to convince her that she'd actually given birth.)

This revolution in obstetrical practice was welcomed by women, but fought by both the clergy and some members of the medical profession, who believed that pain in childbirth (woman's punishment for Eve's indiscretions in Eden) was a burden that women were born to carry. Relief of the pain would be immoral.

But opponents were doomed to

failure. Once word got around that childbirth didn't have to hurt, obstetrical patients wouldn't take 'no pain relief' for an answer. No longer was it a question of whether anaesthesia had a place in obstetrics, but what kind of anaesthesia would fill that place best.

The search for the perfect pain relief – a drug that would eliminate pain without harming either mother or child – was on. Enormous progress was made (and is still being made); analgesics and anaesthetics became safer and more effective every year.

And then, in the 1950s and 1960s, the love affair between childbirth medication and obstetrical patients began to get shaky. Women wanted to be awake for their deliveries and to experience every sensation, in spite of the discomfort. And they wanted their babies to arrive as alert as they were – instead of drugged from the effects of anaesthesia.

In the 1980s, enlightened practitioners and patients alike are recognizing that, used prudently, childbirth medication plays a vital role in obstetrics. Though an unmedicated birth is considered the ideal, it's understood that there are times when it's not in the best interest of mother and/or child. This is particularly true when labour is long and complicated; when the pain is more than the mother can tolerate, or is interfering with her ability to push; in breech deliveries, and when outlet forceps are used; or, rarely, to slow down a precipitous (too rapid) labour. It can also be used to calm a woman who is so agitated that she is hindering the progress of labour.

Prudent use of any type of medication always requires a careful weighing of risk against benefit. In the case of obstetrical drugs, risks and benefits must be examined for both mother and baby, making the equation a more complicated one. In some instances, the risks of medications clearly outweigh the benefits they offer – as when the foetus doesn't appear strong enough to cope with the stresses of both labour and drugs because of prematurity or other factors.

Most experts agree that when childbirth medication is used, benefits can be increased and risks reduced by:

☆ Selecting a drug that has the fewest potential side effects or risks to mother and child and still provides effective pain relief (the goal, except in surgical deliveries, is not *total* elimination of pain), giving it in the smallest possible effective doses and at the optimum time.

☆ Having an expert anaesthetist administer anaesthesia. (You have the right to insist on this if you are to have general or spinal anaesthesia.)

A major concern of careful medicating in obstetrics is not only the safety of the person receiving the medication (the mother), but that of an innocent bystander (the baby). Babies whose mothers have medication during delivery may be born drowsy, sluggish, unresponsive, and sometimes with breathing and sucking difficulties and an irregular heartbeat. Studies show, however, that when drugs have been properly used, these adverse effects largely disappear soon after birth. A foetus can handle a certain degree of the hypoxia (oxygen deprivation) that sometimes results from too much medication in labour or too much anaesthesia during delivery; only very extreme cases of deprivation are hazardous. If a baby is so drugged that he doesn't breathe spontaneously at birth, quick resuscitation (a simple procedure) will prevent long-term damage. The problem is usually avoided in surgical deliveries by extracting the foetus very soon after anaesthesia is administered, before the drug has a chance to cross the placenta and affect him or her.

What Kinds of Pain Relief Are Most Commonly Used?

A variety of analgesics (pain relievers), anaesthetics (substances that produce loss of sensation), and ataraxics (tranquillizers) may be given during labour and delivery. Which drug, if any, will be administered will depend on the situation, as well as upon the obstetrician's and/or anaesthetist's preference and expertise, and – except in emergencies – the wishes of the mother. The efficacy will depend upon the woman, the dosage, and other factors. (Very rarely, a drug won't produce the desired effect, and will give little or no pain relief.) Obstetrical pain relief is most commonly accomplished with the following drugs:

Analgesics. Pethidine is a frequently used obstetrical analgesic. It is used intramuscularly (one shot, usually in the buttocks). Pethidine does not usually interfere with the contractions or their work, though with larger doses the contractions may appear to be less frequent. It may actually help normalize contractions in a dysfunctional uterus (one that is functioning abnormally). Like other analgesics, Pethidine is not generally administered until labour is well established and false labour has been ruled out, but at least two to three hours before delivery is expected. A mother's reaction to the drug and the degree of pain relief achieved vary widely. Some women find it relaxes them and makes them better able to cope with contractions. Others very much dislike the drowsy feeling and find they are less able to cope. Side effects may, depending on a woman's sensitivity, include nausea, vomiting, depression, and a drop in blood pressure. The effect Pethidine will have on the newborn depends on the dose and how close to delivery it is administered. If it is given too close to delivery, the baby may be sleepy and unable to suck; less frequently, respiration may be depressed and supplemental oxygen may be required. These effects are generally short-term and, if necessary, can be counteracted. Pethidine may also be given postpartum, to relieve the pain of a caesarean.

Tranquillizers. These drugs (such as Phenergan, Chlorpromazine and Valium) are used to calm and relax an anxious woman so that she can participate more fully in childbirth. Tranquillizers can also enhance the effectiveness of analgesics, such as Pethidine. Like analgesics, tranquillizers are usually administered once labour is well established, and considerably before delivery. But they are occasionally used in early labour if a first-time mother is extremely nervous. Women's reactions to the effects of tranquillizers vary. Some welcome the gentle drowsiness; others find it interferes with their control. A small dose may serve to relieve anxiety without impairing alertness. A larger dose may cause slurring of speech and dozing between contraction peaks – making use of prepared childbirth techniques impossible. Though the risks of a foetus from tranquillizers are minimal (except in cases of foetal distress), it's a good idea for you and your partner to try non-drug relaxation techniques before asking for medication.

Inhalants. Entenox is the inhalant analgesic which is most widely used in Britain. It is a mixture of 50% nitrous oxide (laughing gas) and 50% oxygen. It comes ready mixed in a cylinder with a rubber mask or mouthpiece which a woman controls herself, taking deep breaths at the beginning of a contraction, and then putting it down. It reduces the sensation at the height of a contraction and can be used effectively towards the end of the first stage for transition and second stage.

Regional Nerve Blocks. Anaesthetics injected along the course of a nerve or nerves may be used to deaden sensation in that region. In childbirth, anaesthetics may completely numb the area from the waist down for surgical delivery, or numb a smaller area partially or totally for a vaginal one. Regional blocks have an advantage over general anaesthesia for surgical delivery, in that the mother is awake during the birth and is alert afterward. In a vaginal delivery, they have the possible disadvantage of inhibiting the urge to push. Occasionally, oxytocin may be administered to rev up contractions that have become sluggish because of the anaesthetic effect. Often a catheter (tube) is inserted into the bladder to drain urine (because the urge to urinate is also suppressed). The most frequently used blocks are: pudendal, epidural, spinal, caudal, and paracervical.

A pudendal block, occasionally used to relieve early second-stage pain, is usually reserved for the vaginal delivery itself. Administered through a needle inserted into the perineal or vaginal area (while the mother lies on her back with her feet in stirrups), it reduces pain in the region, but not uterine discomfort. It is useful when outlet forceps (forceps used to ease the baby out once its head is visible at the vaginal outlet) are used, and its effect can last through episiotomy and repair.

The epidural block (or lumbar epidural) is becoming increasingly popular for both vaginal and caesarean deliveries, as well as for the relief of labour pain and to slow down very intense contractions. The major reason is its relative safety (less drug is needed to achieve the desired effect) and its ease of administration. The drug (usually bupivacaine) is administered as needed during labour and/or delivery, through a fine tube which has been inserted through a needle in the back (after a local anaesthetic numbs the area), into the epidural space between the spinal cord and the outer membrane, usually while the mother lies on her left side or leans over a table to steady herself. Blood pressure is checked frequently because the procedure can cause it to drop suddenly. Intravenous fluids will be given to counteract this reaction. Leaning the uterus to the left may also help. Because of the risk of a blood pressure drop, an epidural is generally not used when there is a bleeding complication, such as placenta praevia, severe pre-eclampsia or eclampsia, or foetal distress.

Spinal blocks (for caesarean) and low spinal, or saddle, blocks (for vaginal delivery) are administered in a single dose just prior to delivery but are rarely used in the UK. The mother lies on her side (back arched, neck and knees flexed) and an anaesthetic is injected into the fluid surrounding the spinal cord. There may be some nausea and vomiting while the drug is in effect, about 1 to 1½ hours. As with an epidural, there is a risk of a drop in blood pressure. Elevation of the legs, leaning the uterus to the left, intravenous fluids, and, occasionally, medication may be used to prevent or counteract this complication. After delivery, spinal-block patients must usually remain flat on their backs for about eight hours, and a few may experience post-spinal headache. As with epidurals, spinals are not usually used when there is placenta praevia, pre-eclampsia or eclampsia, or foetal distress.

The caudal block is similar to the epidural, except that it blocks sensation in a more limited area, takes a larger dose to be effective, and requires greater skill on the part of the anaesthetist. It also inhibits labour. Because of these potential risks, it is used less frequently today than it was in the past.

The paracervical block relieves the pain of labour, but not that of delivery. Because of potential hazard to the foetus, it is rarely used – except when no other anaesthesia is suitable.

General Anaesthesia. Once the most popular pain relief for delivery, general anaesthesia – which puts the patient to sleep – is used today almost exclusively for surgical births, and occasionally for delivering the head in a vaginal breech. Because of ease of administration, it is most likely to be used in emergency caesareans, when there is no time for a regional anaesthetic to be administered.

Inhalants, such as those used for analgesic effect, are used to induce general anaesthesia – often in conjunction with other agents. This is done by an anaesthetist in an operating/delivery room. The mother is awake during the preparations and unconscious for only a few minutes as the baby is delivered (and in the case of a caesarean, while the incision is sutured). When she comes to she may be groggy, disoriented, and restless. She may experience nausea and vomiting, and her bowels and bladder may be sluggish. A temporary drop in blood pressure is another possible side effect.

The major problem with general anaesthesia is that as the mother is sedated, so is the foetus. Sedation of the foetus can be minimized, however, by administering the anaesthesia as close to the actual birth as possible. That way the baby can be delivered before the anaesthetic has reached him or her. Administering oxygen to the mother, and tilting her to the side (usually the left side), can also help reduce foetal sedation.

The other major risk of general anaesthesia is that the mother may vomit and aspirate (inhale) the vomited material, which can cause complications, such as aspiration pneumonia. That's why you are asked not to eat when in active labour and why, if you do have general anaesthesia, a tube will be inserted through your mouth into your throat to prevent aspiration. You may also be given oral antacids to neutralize the acids in your stomach.

Because it's important to keep doses of anaesthetics moderate to avoid foetal sedation, the effect of general anaesthesia is occasionally too weak to entirely block out the mother's awareness of the surgery. Supplementary use of potent inhalants can avoid this problem.

Hypnosis. Despite the somewhat disreputable image it's developed on the nightclub circuit, hypnosis, in qualified hands, provides a legitimate, medically acceptable route to pain relief. There's really nothing mysterious about hypnosis. Suggestion, and the power of mind over matter, are taught in every good childbirth preparation class. With hypnosis a very high level of suggestibility is achieved, which (depending on an individual's susceptibility and the type of hypnosis used) can do anything from making the patient more relaxed and comfortable to com-

pletely eliminating awareness of pain. Only about one in four adults is hypnotizable to some degree. (A very small percentage can even go through an unmedicated caesarean section without feeling any pain.)

Training of a subject in hypnosis for childbirth should start weeks or months in advance, under a physician certified in the subject or another practitioner recommended by your physician. You may use auto- or self-hypnosis, or you may depend upon the practitioner to make the suggestions. Either way, use caution.

Acupuncture. There is a relatively new alternative treatment now available in Britain that can be used during pregnancy and labour to help relax and relieve pain: traditional Chinese acupuncture.

Acupuncture works fundamentally by treating the whole person on physical, mental and spiritual levels. It is a system which has been used in China to restore and maintain health for 4,000 years, and it is now gaining some serious respect in the west.

It's place within childbirth is for use anaesthetically and supportively to restore and balance the energies that may have become depleted in the labouring woman, thus assisting her to relax and cope with the situation better. There are certain acupuncture points on the body that will help to relieve pain but they are better used together with over all treatment rather than in isolation. It is therefore essential that you are treated by a fully qualified practitioner with some years experience.

A register of qualified practitioners and hospitals that allow this system of

medicine to be used can be obtained from the.
Traditional Acupuncture Society,
11, Grange Park,
Stratford-upon-Avon,
Warwickshire,
CV37 6XH

If your hospital is not on the list it is always worth raising the subject with your midwife or doctor if you are interested.

Transcutaneous Electrical Nerve Stimulation (TENS). This is a form of drug-free pain relief which is gradually becoming more popular in the UK. Although many hospitals still do not have it available for use on the maternity ward, it has been in use for some time in pain clinics, to assist with severe cases of arthritis, low back pain or cancer. It is a small box about the size of a calculator, from which 4 electrodes protrude. These are attached to the woman's back, covering the area where the nerve roots, which make up the nerve supply to the womb, emerge from the spinal cord. The box also has a 'personal demand switch' attached.

The theory upon which TENS is based, is that the sensation of pain is a gateway which can be opened and closed by particular nerve fibres. The electrical current provided by TENS is carried by fast nerve fibres in our bodies to a gateway in the spinal cord. The current causes the gate to shut, blocking the pain impulses which are carried by slower nerve fibres. At the same time, it is thought to stimulate the production of the body's own natural painkiller, endorphin.

As the woman requires greater pain relief, she can turn the personal demand switch to increase the frequency of electrical current.

The sensation of TENS has been described initially as the feel of butterfly wings on the spine. As the contractions build up, and the frequency is increased, it changes to birds' wings tapping rhythmically on the back.

The effect that it has on the contractions is to break the pain up, leaving a sensation rather like dull toothache – not exactly comfortable, but certainly not painful.

It doesn't work for everyone, but it is certainly worth trying as a possible alternative to the use of drugs.

Making the Decision

Women have more options in childbirth today than ever before. And, with the exception of certain emergency situations, the decision of whether or not to have medication during your labour and delivery will be largely yours. Here's how to make the best decision possible, for you and your baby:

☆ Discuss pain relief and anaesthesia with your doctor long before labour begins. Your practitioner's expertise and experience make him or her an invaluable ally in your decision-making process. Well before your first contraction, find out: what kinds of drugs or procedures he or she uses most often; what side effects may be experienced by mother and/or child; when he or she considers medication absolutely necessary; when he or she considers the option to be yours.

☆ Recognize that childbirth isn't supposed to be a trial by ordeal. Nor is it a test of your bravery, strength, or endurance. Medical technology has given women who are in pain during childbirth the option of relief through medication. Not only is it an acceptable option, it is, in certain cases, the best option. The pain of childbirth has been described by some as the most intense in the human experience. Seeking relief from such pain doesn't mean you've failed yourself, your partner, or your baby.

☆ Don't make up and close your mind in advance. Investigate and familiarize yourself with the various options in analgesia and anaesthesia; think about what might be best for you; discuss it with your doctor and your partner. But don't try to make a final decision before the time comes. It's impossible to predict what kind of labour and delivery you'll have, and thus it would be foolhardy to decide in advance whether or not you'll want or need medication. Even if you're scheduled for a caesarean, you can plan only tentatively on an epidural or spinal; last-minute complications could necessitate general anaesthesia.

☆ If during labour you feel you need medication, discuss it with your partner and the midwife or doctor. But don't insist on it immediately. Try holding out 15 minutes or so, and putting that time to the best possible use – concentrating extra-hard on your relaxation or breathing techniques; taking in all the comfort your partner can give you. You may find that with a little more support you can handle the pain, or that the progress you make in those 15 minutes gives you the will to go on without help. (If your physician decides that you need medication immediately, for your sake or your baby's, waiting may not be advisable.) If after waiting you find that you need the relief as much or even more, ask for it – and don't feel guilty.

☆ Remember that, as with all aspects of pregnancy, labour, and delivery, the well-being of you and your baby is your priority, and not some pre-conceived, idealized childbirth scenario. All decisions should be made on that basis, and on no other.

12
The Eighth Month

WHAT YOU CAN EXPECT AT THIS MONTH'S CHECKUP

In this month you can expect the following to be checked, depending upon your particular needs and upon your doctor or midwife's style of practice:[1]

☆ Weight and blood pressure

☆ Urinalysis

☆ Foetal heartbeat

☆ Blood test for haemoglobin if indicated

☆ Height of fundus (top of uterus)

☆ Degree of engagement of foetal head in relation to pelvis

☆ Size (you may get a rough weight estimate) and position of foetus, by palpation

☆ Feet, hands and legs for oedema (swelling); legs and vulva for varicose veins

☆ Ultrasound scan if needed

☆ Symptoms you have been experiencing, especially unusual ones

☆ Questions or problems you want to discuss – have a list ready

WHAT YOU MAY BE FEELING

You may feel all of these symptoms at one time or another or only a few of them. Some may have continued from last month, others may be new or hardly noticeable. You may also have other, less common symptoms.

Physically:
☆ Strong, regular foetal activity

☆ Increasing heavy whitish vaginal discharge (leukorrhoea)

1. See appendix for an explanation of the procedures and tests performed

☆ Increased constipation

☆ Heartburn and indigestion, flatulence and bloating

☆ Occasional headaches, faintness or dizziness

☆ Nasal congestion and occasional nosebleeds; ear stuffiness

☆ Leg cramps

☆ Backache

☆ Mild oedema (swelling) of ankles and feet, and occasionally hands and face

☆ Varicose veins of legs and/or haemorrhoids

☆ Itchy abdomen

☆ Increasing shortness of breath as uterus crowds the lungs

☆ Difficulty sleeping

☆ Increasing Braxton Hicks contractions, abdominal achiness

☆ Increasing clumsiness

☆ Colostrum, either leaking or expressed, from breasts (though this premilk substance may not appear until after delivery)

Emotionally:

☆ Increasing anxiousness to be over with the pregnancy

What You May Look Like

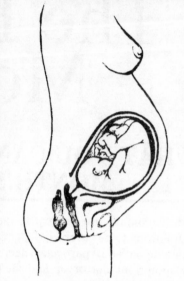

By the end of the eighth month, the baby is about 18 inches long and weighs 5 pounds. Growth, especially of the brain, is great in this period. Calcium, protein, and iron are more important than ever in the last weeks. Most systems are well developed, but the lungs may still be immature. Baby has an excellent chance of survival if born now.

☆ Apprehension about the baby's health, labour, and delivery

☆ Increasing absentmindedness

☆ Excitement at the realization that *it* won't be long now

WHAT YOU MAY BE CONCERNED ABOUT

Shortness of Breath

'Sometimes I have trouble breathing. Could this mean that my baby isn't getting enough oxygen?'

Shortness of breath doesn't mean you – or your baby – are short of oxygen. Changes in the respiratory system during pregnancy actually allow women to take in *more* air, and to use it more efficiently. Still, most women experience varying degrees of difficulty breathing (some describe it as feeling a conscious need to breathe more deeply) – particularly in the last trimester, when the expanding uterus presses against the diaphragm, crowding the lungs. Relief usually arrives when lightening occurs (when the foetus settles back down into the pelvis, generally two to three weeks before delivery). In the meantime, you may find it easier to breathe if you sit straight up instead of slumped over, sleep in a semi-propped-up position, and avoid over-exertion.

Your Weight Gain and the Baby's Size

'I've gained so much weight that I'm afraid the baby will be very big and difficult to deliver.'

Just because you've gained a lot of weight doesn't necessarily mean your baby has. Even a 35- to 40-pound weight gain can yield a 6- or 7-pound baby. On the average, however, a larger weight gain will produce a larger baby. Your baby's size may also be influenced by your own birth weight (if you were born large, your baby will tend to be) and by your pre-pregnancy weight (in general, heavier women have heavier babies). By palpating your abdomen and measuring the height of your fundus (the top of your uterus), your practitioner will be able to give you some idea of your baby's size, though such 'guesstimates' can be off by a pound or more. An ultrasound scan may more accurately gauge size but it may be off, too.

Even if your baby is large, that doesn't automatically portend a difficult delivery. Though a 6- or 7-pound baby often slithers out faster than an 8- or 9-pounder, many women are able to deliver a bigger baby naturally and normally. The vital factor is whether the baby's head (its largest part) can fit through the mother's pelvis. If it can, delivery should be no problem. At one time, an x-ray was routinely ordered to try to determine whether or not a foetopelvic disproportion existed. But experience and research have shown that the x-ray is not an accurate predictor of whether or not the baby can actually fit through the birth canal, partly because it can't forsee to what extent the foetal head will mould in order to squeeze through. Though the risk of the x-ray is slight, it is not recommended except in very unusual circumstances, when the benefits outweigh that risk.

More commonly today, when there is some suspicion of foetopelvic disproportion, the midwife or doctor will allow a trial labour. If you progress, the labour will continue. If you don't, labour may get a boost with the administration of oxytocin. If labour still doesn't progress, a caesarean will usually be performed.

How You're Carrying

'Everyone says I seem to be carrying small and low for the eighth month. Could it be that my baby isn't growing properly?'

It would be a good idea to make

earplugs and an eye mask a part of every pregnant woman's maternity wardrobe. Wearing them for nine months would enable her to avoid the worry generated by the misguided commentary and advice of relatives, friends – even strangers – and prevent invidious comparisons of her belly to those of other pregnant women, who are larger, smaller, lower, or higher.

Just as no two prepregnant figures are proportioned in precisely the same fashion, no two pregnant silhouettes are identical. How you carry, both in size and shape, is dependent on whether you started out tall or short, thin or not-so-thin, petite or voluptuous. And it is seldom an indication of *what* you're carrying. A petite woman carrying low and small may give birth to a larger infant than a bigger-boned woman carrying high and wide.

The only accurate assessments of your baby's progress and well-being are likely to come from your practitioner. When you're not in his or her office, keep your earplugs in and your eye mask on – and you'll have a lot less to worry about.

Carrying Baby, Eighth Month

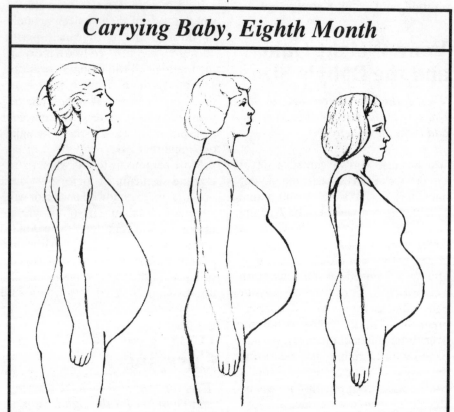

These are just three of the very different ways that a woman may carry near the end of her eighth month. The variations are even greater than before. Depending on the size and position of your baby, as well as your own size and weight gain, you may be carrying higher, lower, bigger, smaller, wider, or more compactly.

Presentation and Position of the Baby

'My doctor says the baby is in a breech position. How will this affect my labour and delivery?'

It's never too early to prepare yourself for the possibility of a breech birth, but it's definitely too early now to resign yourself to one. Most babies turn and settle into a head-down position between the 32nd and 34th weeks, but a few keep their parents and doctors guessing until only a few days before delivery.

Some midwives recommend doing exercises in the last eight weeks, designed to encourage a breech baby to turn. There's no medical proof that these exercises work, but there's none to suggest that they hurt, either. When the foetus is still in a breech position near term, some physicians advocate foetal version – a turning of the breech foetus to the vertex, or head-down, position. The doctor, applying his or her hands to the mother's abdomen, gently, and often with ultrasound guidance, gradually shifts the position of the foetus. The foetal condition is monitored continuously to be sure that the umbilical cord isn't accidentally compressed or the placenta disturbed. Version is best done in very late pregnancy or very early labour, when the uterus is still relatively relaxed. Some doctors claim a successful turning rate of 75%, but other physicians hesitate to use this procedure for fear of complications. Certainly, only an experienced obstetrician – who is ready to do an emergency caesarean if trouble arises – should attempt version.

Breeches are more common when the foetus is smaller than average and not cradled snugly in the uterus, when the uterus is unusually shaped, when there is an excess of amniotic fluid, when there is more than one foetus, and in women who have had babies before and whose uteri are more relaxed. If your baby is one of the 3% or 4% in breech position at term, you should discuss the delivery possibilities with your physician (nurse-midwives do not usually handle breech births). You may be able to have a normal vaginal delivery, or, depending on various conditions, you may indeed have to undergo a caesarean. (Which is *not* the end of the world, and for which eventuality every pregnant woman should be prepared anyway. See page 216.)

If your obstetrician routinely performs caesarean sections for breech presentations, don't ask for a vaginal delivery. Vaginal deliveries are perfectly safe in about one third to one half of breech births, but *only* if the doctor is experienced in the proper protocol. Some studies of vaginal breech deliveries show the potential risk is not always from the delivery itself, but from the reason for the breech: for example, the baby is premature or undersize, there are multiple foetuses, or there is some other congenital problem.

Experienced doctors and midwives will usually permit vaginal deliveries when all the following conditions are met:

☆ The baby is a frank breech (with the legs folded flat up against the face), the most common breech position.

☆ The baby is determined to be small enough (usually under 8½ pounds) for easy passage through the pelvis.

☆ The mother has no obstetrical or medical problem that would complicate a vaginal delivery.

☆ The presenting part is engaged, or descended into, the pelvis as labour begins.

☆ The foetal head is not hyperextended, but is tucked down toward the chest.

Breech labour is begun on a trial basis in a surgically equipped delivery room. If all goes well, it continues. If not, or if the cervix dilates too slowly, the doctor and surgical team are ready to perform a caesarean section in a matter of minutes. Continuous electronic foetal monitoring is absolutely essential. Often a pudendal nerve block (see page 204) is administered to prevent the mother from bearing down too hard before she is fully dilated (which might lead to the cord being compressed between the baby and the pelvis). Forceps may be used to keep the head properly flexed, and to help deliver the head without pulling too much on the body or neck. A wide episiotomy is sometimes made to facilitate the birthing process.

'How can I tell if my baby is lying the right way for delivery?'

Playing 'name that bump' (trying to figure out which are shoulders, elbows, and bottom) may be better evening entertainment than TV, but it's not the most accurate way of determining your baby's position. Your doctor or midwife can probably

How Does Your Baby Lie?

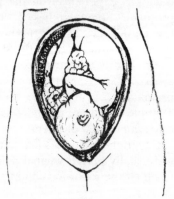

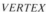
VERTEX

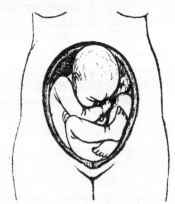
BREECH

About 96 out of every 100 babies present head first (vertex). The rest are usually in one or another breech position (buttocks first). The complete breech is illustrated here. The frank breech, in which the baby's legs are folded straight up, is the easiest breech to deliver vaginally.

get a better idea than you, by palpating your abdomen with the flat of his or her trained hands, for recognizable baby parts. The baby's back, for instance, is usually a smooth, convex contour opposite a bunch of little irregularities which are the 'small parts' – hands, feet, elbows. In the eighth month, the head has usually settled near your pelvis; it is round, firm, and – when pushed down – bounces back without moving the rest of the body. The baby's bottom is a less regular shape, and softer, than the head. The location of the baby's heartbeat is another clue to its position – if the presentation is head first, the heartbeat will usually be heard in the lower half of your abdomen; it will be loudest if the baby's back is toward your front. If there's any doubt, an ultrasound scan will be used for verification.

Adequacy For Delivery

'I'm 5 feet tall and very petite. I'm afraid I'll have trouble delivering a baby normally.'

Fortunately, when it comes to giving birth, it's what's inside, not what's outside, that counts. The size and shape of your pelvis is what determines whether your delivery will be easy and normal. And you can't always tell a pelvis by its cover. A short, slight woman can have a roomier pelvis than a tall, stocky woman. Only your practitioner can make an educated guess about its size – usually by measurements taken at your first prenatal exam. If there's some doubt whether your pelvis is

adequate while you're in labour an ultrasound scan will be taken. (See Foetopelvic Disproportion, page 218.)

Of course, in general the overall size of the pelvis, as of all bony structures, is smaller in people of smaller stature. For example, Oriental women usually have smaller pelvises than Nordic women. Luckily nature, in its wisdom, rarely presents an Oriental woman with a Nordic-size baby – even if the father is a 6-foot fullback. Instead, all things being equal, babies are generally fairly well matched to the size of their mothers.

Your Safety During Childbirth

'I know medical science has taken most of the risk out of giving birth, but I'm still afraid of dying during delivery.'

There was a time when mothers routinely risked their lives to have children; they still do in some areas of the world. In the West today, the risk to maternal life in labour and delivery is virtually nonexistent. Just 1 in 10,000 women dies in childbirth. And this number include not only women with chronic heart conditions and other serious illnesses, but those who give birth in backwoods shacks and dingy tenements, without medical assistance.

In short, even if your pregnancy falls into the highest-risk category – and certainly if it doesn't – you stand a lot better chance of surviving labour and delivery than you do a trip to the supermarket in your car, or a stroll across a busy street.

Having A Caesarean Section

'My doctor just told me I will have to have a caesarean. But I'm afraid the surgery will be dangerous.'

Though popular lore has it that the caesarean section got its name because Julius Caesar was born via abdominal delivery, that's virtually impossible. Julius might have survived such an operation, but his mother wouldn't have – and it is known that Mrs. Caesar lived for many years after his birth.

Today, however, caesareans are nearly as safe as vaginal deliveries for mother, and in difficult deliveries or when there's foetal distress, they are often the safest route for baby. Even though it is technically considered major surgery, a caesarean carries relatively minor risks – much closer to those of a tonsillectomy than a gall bladder operation, for instance.

Learning all you can about caesarean sections before delivery – from your doctor, in your childbirth class (a special class on caesareans is ideal), and through reading – will help to prepare you and to ease your fears.

'The doctor says I may have to have a caesarean section. I'm worried that this may be dangerous for the baby.'

Chances are that if you have a caesarean, your baby will be at least as safe, and possibly safer, than if you had had a vaginal delivery. Every year thousands of babies who might not have survived the perilous journey through the birth canal (or might have survived impaired) are lifted from their mother's abdomen sound and unscathed.

Though there has been some speculation that caesareans are somehow harmful to babies, there's no hard evidence that this is so. Of course, a higher proportion of caesarean babies do have medical problems after birth – but most often because of the original distress that necessitated the operation, not because of the operation itself. Many of these infants would never have made it at all if left to a natural delivery.

In most ways, babies delivered via caesarean don't differ from those delivered vaginally – though caesarean babies do have the edge in appearance. Because they don't have to accommodate to the narrow confines of the pelvis, they usually have nicely unmoulded heads.

Apgar scores (the rating scale used to evaluate an infant's condition one and five minutes after birth) on babies from both types of delivery are comparable. Caesarean-born babies do have the slight disadvantage of not having some of the excess mucous squeezed out of their respiratory tracts in the birthing process, but the mucous can be easily suctioned after delivery. Very, very rarely is there any serious damage done to a baby during caesarean delivery – much more rarely than during vaginal deliveries.

The most likely kind of damage a baby delivered abdominally might suffer is psychological – not from the delivery itself, but because of the mother's attitude toward it. Occasionally a mother who has had a caesarean will subconsciously resent the baby who she feels deprived her of her finest hour and brought such insult to her body.[2] She may allow the jealousy she feels toward mothers who've delivered vaginally, and the guilt she feels about failing, to interfere with the establishment of a good relationship with her baby. Or she may incorrectly assume that the caesarean-born infant is unusually fragile (few are) and become over-protective. If such feelings develop, the mother should try to confront and deal with them and, if necessary, seek professional help in resolving them.

But often, destructive attitudes can be avoided right from the start. First, by recognizing that the method by which a baby is delivered in no way reflects on either the mother or the child. Second, by making sure that there is an opportunity for bonding with your baby at the earliest possible time (if this is important to you). Long before you go into labour, let your doctor know that if you have a caesarean you would like to be able to hold or even nurse the baby on the operating table, or if that's not possible, in the recovery room. If you wait until delivery day to state your case you may not have the strength or opportunity to make it. Planning ahead also gives you the opportunity to challenge contrary hospital rules, such as those requiring every caesarean-delivered newborn, even healthy ones, to spend some time in the Special Care Baby Unit (SCBU). If you present a strong argument in a

rational, non-hysterical way, you may be able to effect a change in the rules.

If, good intentions notwithstanding, you turn out to be too weak to participate in any serious mother-baby bonding (and many women are, whether they've had abdominal or vaginal deliveries), or if your baby needs to be observed or cared for in the Special Care Baby Unit (SCBU) for a while, don't panic. There is no evidence, despite the hoopla the concept has aroused, that bonding *must* take place immediately after birth. It can, of course, but it can also take place weeks, even months, later (see page 292).

'I so much want a natural birth; but it seems like everybody is having a caesarean these days and I'm terrified I'll have to have one too.'

Not quite 'everybody' is having a caesarean these days – but far more women are than ever before. In the early 1960s your chances of having a caesarean would have been 1 in 20. Today they are at least 1 in 9.

The major reason for the increase in caesareans is *good* medicine: Caesareans save the lives of babies who cannot be delivered safely via the vagina. Most doctors perform caesareans not for convenience or because they are afraid of malpractice, but because they believe that in certain circumstances this surgery is the best, sometimes the only, way to protect the baby they are about to deliver. (The dramatic decrease in newborn deaths that has corresponded with the increase in caesareans suggests they may be right.)

2. Women who deliver vaginally may have a similar resentment, almost always temporary, because of the pain of delivery.

Several changes in obstetrical practice have also contributed to the increase in caesareans. Caesarean delivery has become extremely quick and safe – and in most instances mothers can be awake to see their babies born. The foetal monitor, and a variety of foetal tests, can more accurately (though not infallibly) indicate when a foetus is in trouble and needs to be delivered in a hurry. Finally, thanks to better understanding and management of their problems, more women at high risk are able to have successful pregnancies, frequently aided by surgical deliveries.

Most women won't know whether or not they will have a caesarean until they are well into labour. There are, however, several advance indications that point to the possibility:

One or More Previous Caesarean Births.
Though repeat caesareans are routinely performed by some doctors, they are not always necessary.

Breech or Transverse (Crosswise) Presentation of the Foetus.
Or other difficult-to-deliver presentations (see pages 213, 279).

Foetopelvic Disproportion.
A mismatch between the baby's head and the mother's pelvic outlet, which will not permit vaginal delivery, is not usually apparent until labour fails to progress, but may be suggested in advance by ultrasound examination, or by previous difficult deliveries.

Pre-eclampsia or Eclampsia That Doesn't Respond to Treatment.
In such cases the only way to protect both mother and baby is prompt delivery. If induction does not bring on labour, or if the foetus is very immature or in distress, a caesarean will put less stress on the baby than a vaginal delivery.

Placenta Praevia
(abnormally low positioning of the placenta). If the placenta partly or completely covers the cervical opening, caesarean delivery is absolutely essential. This may be determined by an ultrasound examination prior to labour or by an internal exam once the cervix has begun to dilate. But vaginal delivery, with the help of foetal monitoring, can sometimes be attempted when the placenta is to the side and hasn't begun to separate from the uterus.

Abruptio Placenta
(premature separation of a normally located placenta from the wall of the uterus). The separation before labour begins causes bleeding, and threatens the lives of both mother and baby if prompt delivery is not effected – either through induced vaginal delivery, if the separation is not extensive and there is no foetal distress, or through surgical delivery.

Rh Complications.
When the baby has Rh disease, which is rare today (see page 46), he or she may not be strong enough to tolerate vaginal delivery.

Active Maternal Herpes
(within four weeks of delivery). Since a baby can contract herpes passing through the birth canal of a mother with an active infection, a caesarean is definitely indicated in such cases. (See page 47.)

A Dysmature Foetus (A foetus more than two weeks overdue, whose placental nourishment has begun to rapidly diminish).

Maternal Diabetes. Early delivery is often best for the babies of diabetic mothers, to prevent their becoming overly large and dysmature. Depending upon the condition of both foetus and mother, and on other factors, labour may be induced or caesarean performed.

Maternal Hypertension or Kidney Disease. Either of these may necessitate delivery by caesarean.

Preterm Foetal or Maternal Distress. When a mother or her foetus is suddenly in trouble and a speedy delivery seems necessary, a caesarean is usually the preferred route, both because it is faster than inducing labour and because it is less traumatic for the immature foetus.

It's during labour that most indications for a possible caesarean are first noted. They include:

Failure of Labour to Progress After 16 to 18 Hours. This may be due to ineffective or weak contractions;[3] a foetus that is too large for the mother's pelvis; an unusually shaped pelvis that won't allow for the passage of the foetus; lack of pelvic flexibility, particularly in women over 40 who are having their first babies; and a foetus

who is presenting face-first or 'sunny-side up.'

Foetal Distress. When the foetus is in trouble, prompt delivery is imperative. Foetal distress is most often diagnosed today through the use of an electronic foetal monitor. (Expert reading of the monitor print-out is important to avoid misdiagnosis.)

Prolapsed Cord (An umbilical cord that comes down into the cervix or the vagina). The cord becomes wedged between the cervix and the baby, impairing blood flow to the foetus. An emergency caesarean is a necessary unless delivery is imminent.

If caesareans are so safe, and sometimes lifesaving, why do most of us dread the prospect of having one? Partly because major surgery even when it's routine and almost risk free, is still a little scary, but mostly because, although we spend months preparing ourselves for an idyllic natural childbirth, we usually enter the labour-room utterly unprepared for the fact that we may have a caesarean instead. For nine months, we block that unpleasant possibility out of our minds. We devour childbirth primers, but we bypass chapters on caesarean section. We ask dozens of questions about natural delivery in childbirth class, but not one about a surgical birth. We look forward to holding our partner's hand as we pant and push our baby into the world – not to lying passively, and possibly unconscious, as sterile instruments slice into our abdomen to extract him or her, like a hot appendix. When suddenly faced with a caesarean, we feel

---

3. The doctor may try to stimulate contractions with oxytocin, the drug used in the induction of labour, before resorting to caesarean in such cases.

Caesarean Questions to Discuss With Your Doctor

☆ Will it be possible to try some other alternatives before caesarean is resorted to (except in emergency situations)? For example, oxytocin to stimulate contractions, or squatting to make contractions more effective?

☆ What kinds of anaesthesia might be used? A general anaesthesia that puts you to sleep is usually necessary when time is of the essence, but spinal or epidural anaesthesia will allow you to be awake during a nonemergency abdominal delivery. (See All About Childbirth Medication, page 201.)

☆ Does he or she routinely use the low-segment, or 'bikini,' incision whenever possible, so that vaginal delivery can be considered next time around?

☆ Can your partner be present if you are awake? If you are asleep?

☆ Will you and your partner be able to hold the baby immediately after birth (if you are awake and all is well), and will you be able to nurse in the recovery room? Will your partner be able to hold the baby if you're asleep?

☆ If the baby doesn't need special care, can he or she still room-in with you, possibly along with your husband, to help you out?

☆ After an uncomplicated caesarean birth, how much recovery time will you need both in and out of the hospital? What physical discomforts and limitations can you expect to experience?

☆ If the foetal monitor indicates the baby may be in distress, will other methods (such as checking the scalp pH) be used to verify the monitor readings before a caesarean is decided upon?

deprived of control over the birth of our baby. As we see it, medical technology has taken over, ushering in frustration, disappointment, anger, and guilt.

But that's not how it has to be. Not if you are as prepared for an abdominal delivery as for a vaginal one, if you start looking forward to the birth of your baby instead of to an idealized childbirth experience, and if you recognize that a caesarean birth can be beautiful, too.

Several steps taken now can make the prospect of caesarean less ominous and the reality more fulfilling. Even if you have no suspicion that you might need a caesarean, be sure at least one session on the subject is included in your childbirth preparation course. If you do have some reason to believe a caesarean section might be necessary, try to take a full preparatory course. Do some reading on your own, too.

Discuss the topic of a caesarean section with your doctor or midwife. Don't be put off by assurances that you aren't likely to need one; explain that you want to be prepared, just in case. Let the doctor know that you would like to be part of the decision-making team if a caesarean seems to be necessary.

If your obstetrician decides in advance that a caesarean will be necessary, be sure to ask for a detailed explanation of why. Ask if there are any alternatives, such as a trial labour. Once in labour, you would be permitted to continue without a caesarean on the condition that the labour progresses normally.

Whether you're preparing for a scheduled caesarean or just for the possibility of one, there are a number of issues you should talk over with your doctor (see Caesarean Questions to Discuss With Your Doctor, page 220).

Of course, few pregnant women would select caesarean as their delivery of choice; and almost 90% will have the vaginal delivery they've hoped for. But for those who don't, there's no reason for disappointment, or feelings of guilt or failure. Any delivery (vaginal or abdominal, medicated or unmedicated, with an episiotomy or without) that yields a healthy baby is an unqualified success.

Pets and the Baby

'We have a dog who's been like an only child. He's never been exposed to children, and we are very worried that there will be problems when we bring the baby home.'

There's no bigger baby than the kind with four legs and a wagging tail – particularly when the affections and attentions of his 'parents' (and possibly his place in their bed) are suddenly usurped by a noisy, red-faced, demanding, unfamiliar, and thoroughly unwelcome newcomer. To minimize the jealousy your pooch may feel when baby makes four, start his transition from 'only child' to secondary sibling well in advance of delivery:

☆ If your dog isn't obedience-trained already, get him trained now. It's vitally important that his behaviour be controllable and predictable (especially since the baby's won't be). Dogs who are obedience-trained feel more secure and stable, and are less likely to get out of hand.

☆ Expose your dog to babies and children now if he's never been around them before. It's good for him to be familiar with the sounds and erratic movements babies make.

☆ Bring a baby-sized doll home, and treat it like a baby. Put it in the baby's crib, cuddle it, sing to it, carry it around, take it into bed with you. If your dog's going to vent his jealous feelings, now is the time.

☆ If your dog has always slept with you but won't be allowed to once the baby comes home, get him used to a solitary sleeping arrangement now. Make up a comfortable doggie bed – perhaps with a favourite blanket or pillow for solace.

☆ Before you bring the baby home from the hospital, acquaint your dog with the baby's scent by sending home a piece of clothing that the baby has worn.

☆ Once the baby is home, don't make the mistake of being over protective – which will only make the dog more jealous. Try to help the dog make friends with the baby, and make him feel that he's still part of the family. Pet him while you nurse the baby, walk him while you walk the baby, welcome him into the baby's room while you are there.

☆ If, despite all you've done, your dog shows hostility toward the baby, you may have to keep him tied up (inside or outside) until you are certain he has adjusted. It's dangerous to assume that a dog who's never bitten before isn't capable of causing harm.

Travel Safety

'I've got an important business trip scheduled this month. Is it safe for me to travel, or should I cancel?'

If you can possibly avoid travelling in the last trimester, do. Not only is travelling in late pregnancy uncomfortable, it can be hazardous – since you could suddenly go into labour (premature labour can't always be predicted) hundreds or thousands of miles from your doctor. The threat of labour occurring at thousands of feet in the air (and hours away from landing) is enough to keep airlines from allowing pregnant women in their ninth month to fly without a doctor's letter of permission. That letter may prove difficult to obtain, since most doctors don't recommend travel in the last trimester, particularly in the eighth and ninth months. If you must travel, refer to the tips on page 161. It's particularly important to secure the name of a local obstetrician.

Driving

'Should I still drive?'

Long car trips are too exhausting late in pregnancy, no matter who's driving. but as long as you're not experiencing any dizzy spells, and as long as you can still fit behind the wheel, you can safely drive short distances up to delivery day. Don't, however, try to drive yourself to the hospital while in labour.

Braxton Hicks Contractions

'Every once in a while my uterus seems to bunch up and harden. What's going on?'

These are Braxton Hicks contractions, which usually begin to rehearse the pregnant uterus for labour sometime during the latter half of pregnancy. Your uterus is flexing its muscles, practicing and preparing itself for the contractions which will soon push your baby out. You'll feel these contractions as a painless (but possibly uncomfortable) tightening of your uterus, beginning at the top and gradually spreading downward before relaxing. These contractions usually last about 30 seconds (ample time to practice your breathing exercises), but may last as long as 2 minutes or more.

As pregnancy draws to a close in the ninth month, Braxton Hicks contractions begin to get more frequent, intense – sometimes even painful – and thus more difficult to distinguish from true labour contractions (see Prelabour, False Labour, Real Labour, page 238). Though they're not efficient enough to deliver your baby, Braxton Hicks contractions may get the prebirth processes of effacement and dilation started, thereby giving you a leg up on labour before it ever begins.

Bathing

'My mother says she wasn't permitted to bath after the 34th week. My doctor says it's okay. Why?'

This is one case where mother doesn't know best. Though well intentioned, she is misinformed. Her doctor, like most 20 or 30 years ago, believed that foreign substances, such as dirty bath water, could travel up the vagina to the cervix in pregnancy and cause an infection. But while further research remains to be done, doctors today believe that water does not enter the vagina unless it is forced, as in a douche; thus, worry about infection is not justified. Even if water does enter the vagina, the cervical mucous plug that seals the entrance to the uterus effectively protects the membranes that surround the foetus, the amniotic fluid, and the foetus itself from invading infectious organisms. Therefore, unless membranes have ruptured or the plug has been discharged, most doctors permit bathing in normal pregnancies.

Baths, however, aren't totally risk-free, particularly in the last trimester when ungainliness can lead to slips and falls. Bath with care – and preferably with someone to help you in and out of the tub.

Making Love Now

'I'm confused. I hear a lot of conflicting information about sexual intercourse in the last weeks of pregnancy.'

The problem is that existing medical evidence on the subject is confusing and conflicting. It is widely believed that neither intercourse nor orgasm alone precipitate labour unless conditions are ripe (though many impatient-to-deliver couples have enjoyed trying). For that reason, many doctors and midwives allow patients with normal pregnancies to make love – assuming they're still interested – right up until delivery day. And most couples apparently can do so without complication.

There does, however, seem to be some risk of sexual intercourse triggering premature labour, at least in women at high risk for preterm delivery (such as those carrying multiple foetuses, those who start effacing and dilating early, and those with a history of premature labour). Premature rupture of the membranes (PROM), at term or preterm, may also be related to intercourse, particularly when there is also inflammation of the membranes. Some cases of chorion amnionitis (infection of the amniotic sac) and postpartum infection have been tentatively linked to late pregnancy intercourse, and may be prevented by the use of condoms in the last eight weeks.

Ease your confusion by checking with your practitioner to see what the latest medical consensus is. If you get a green light, then by all means make love – if you want to and feel comfortable about it. If the light is red (and it will be if you are at high risk for premature delivery, have placenta praevia or abruptio, are experiencing unexplained bleeding, or if your membranes have ruptured), then find your intimacy in other ways. Try a romantic rendezvous at a candlelit restaurant, or walking hand-in-hand under the stars. Or try an evening at home snuggling in bed or under a rug in front of the TV, hugging and kissing on the sofa, soaping each other in the shower, or using massage – of the neck, back, feet, and of course, belly – as the medium.

WHAT IT'S IMPORTANT TO KNOW: FACTS ABOUT BREASTFEEDING

Thirty years ago, when the eldest of the authors had her first baby, she was the only woman in the maternity wing to breastfeed. Just recently, when the youngest had her first baby, there was only one woman in maternity who *wasn't* planning to nurse.

Today there is clearly a back-to-breast trend. At the turn of the century, nearly every baby was fed at the breast; there was no other choice. But in the early 1900s, women began to demand rights they'd never had – to vote, to work, to smoke cigarettes, to let down or bob their hair, to peel off confining undergarments, and to set their sights outside the kitchen and the nursery. Breastfeeding was old-fashioned, it was restricting, and it represented all that women sought freedom from. To be a modern woman was to bottle-feed. And by the 1950s, the only remaining breastfeeders (besides our senior author and an assortment of bohemian stragglers) were those with whom emancipation hadn't caught up.

Ironically, it was the revitalised women's movement of the 1960s and 1970s that brought breastfeeding back into vogue. Women wanted not only freedom, but control – control of their lives, control of their bodies. They knew that control came with knowledge, and knowledge told them that breastfeeding was best – for their babies and, on the whole for themselves.

Why Breast Is Best

There is no question but that given normal circumstances, breastfeeding provides your newborn with the most perfect food for human infants:

☆ Human breast milk contains at least a hundred ingredients that are not found in cow's milk and that cannot be perfectly duplicated in formulas. Breast milk is individualised for each infant; raw materials are selected from the mother's bloodstream as needed, altering from day to day, feeding to feeding, as the baby grows and changes. The nutrients are matched to infant needs. Variations from breast milk in cow's milk formulas can lead to nutritional deficiencies.

☆ Breast milk is more digestible than cow's milk. The proportion of protein in mother's milk is lower (1.5%) than in cow's milk (3.5%), making it easier for the infant to handle. The protein itself is mostly lactalbumin, which is more nutritious and digestible than the major protein component of cow's milk, caseinogen. The fat content of both milks are similar, but the fat in mother's milk is more easily digested by the baby.

☆ Breast milk is less likely to cause overweight in infants.

☆ No baby is allergic to breast milk (though some can have allergic reactions to a certain food or foods in their mothers' diets). Beta-lactoglobulin, a substance contained in cow's milk, can trigger an allergic response and, following the formation of antibodies, can even cause anaphylactic shock (a life-threatening allergic reaction) in infants – which some suspect could be a contributing factor in the sudden infant death syndrome (or crib death). The soy milk formulas, which are often substituted when an infant is allergic to cow's milk, stray even farther in composition from what nature intended.

☆ Nursed babies are never constipated, because of the easier digestibility of breast milk. They also rarely have diarrhoea – since breast milk seems both to destroy some diarrhoea-causing organisms and to encourage the growth of beneficial flora in the digestive tract, which further discourage digestive upset. On a purely aesthetic note, the bowel movements of a breastfed baby are sweeter-smelling (at least until solids are introduced) and less apt to cause nappy rash.

☆ Breast milk contains one third the mineral salts of cow's milk. The extra sodium is difficult for immature kidneys to handle.

☆ Breast milk contains less phosphorus. The higher phosphorus content of cow's milk is linked to a decreased calcium level in the formula-fed infant's blood.

☆ Breastfed babies are less subject to illness in the first year of life. Protection is provided by the transfer of immune factors in breast milk and in the premilk substance, colostrum.

☆ Nursing at the breast, because it requires more effort than sucking on a bottle, encourages optimum development of jaws, teeth, and palate.

☆ Breast milk is safe. There is no risk of contamination or spoilage.

☆ Breastfeeding is convenient. It requires no advance planning or packing, no equipment; it is always available (in the car, on an aeroplane, in the middle of the night), and at just the right temperature. When mother and baby aren't together (if the mother works,for instance), milk may be expressed in advance and stored in the freezer for bottle feedings as needed. (Breast milk is so vital to the well-being of a premature infant that, if his mother can't nurse, human milk is often supplied by a donor – preferably a woman who delivered prematurely.

☆ Breastfeeding is economical. There is no investment in bottles, sterilizers, or formula; there are no half-emptied bottles or opened cans of formula to waste. And a nutritious diet (such as the Best-Odds Nursing Diet, page 82), which enables a nursing mother to feed her infant well, probably costs less than a typical western diet – unsaturated with empty but expensive fast-food calories.

☆ There is evidence that breastfeeding decreases a woman's risk of developing breast cancer later in life.

☆ Nursing helps speed the shrinking of the uterus back to its prepregnant size and decreases the flow of lochia (the postpartum vaginal discharge).

☆ Lactation suppresses ovulation and menstruation, at least to some degree. Though it shouldn't be relied on for birth control, it may postpone resumption of a woman's periods for months, or at least for as long as she nurses.

☆ Nursing can help burn off the fat accumulated during pregnancy. If a woman is careful to consume an adequate number of only quality calories, she can fill all of her infant's nutritional needs while losing weight.

☆ Breastfeeding enforces rest periods for the new mother – particularly important during the first six postpartum weeks.

☆ Nursing in public is becoming more acceptable. With a little discretion and a big napkin, both mother and baby can dine at the same restaurant table.

☆ Breastfeeding brings mother and baby together, skin to skin, at least six to eight times a day. The emotional gratification, the intimacy, the sharing of love and pleasure, can be very special and very fulfilling.

(A special note to mothers of twins: All the advantages of breastfeeding a single child are doubled for you. See page 303 for tips that make breastfeeding for two easier.)

Why Some Prefer The Bottle

Just as there were hold-outs against bottle-feeding 30 years ago, however, there are women today who choose not to breastfeed. And though the advantages of bottle-feeding seem to be dwarfed by those of breastfeeding, they can be real and convincing for some women.

☆ Bottle-feeding doesn't tie the mother down. She's able to work, shop, go out in the evening, even sleep through the night – letting someone else feed the baby.

☆ Bottle-feeding allows the father to share the feeding responsibilities and the bonding benefits more easily. (Although he can also give baby a bottle of expressed mother's milk.)

☆ Bottle-feeding doesn't interfere with a couple's sex life (unless baby wakes up for a feeding at the wrong time). Breastfeeding, on the other hand, can. First, because lactation hormones can keep the vagina dry;

and second, because leaky breasts are a turnoff to some couples during lovemaking. For bottle-feeding couples, the breasts can remain sensual instead of utilitarian.

☆ Bottle-feeding doesn't dictate your diet, cramp your eating style. You can eat all the garlic, spicy foods, and cabbage you want, and you don't have to drink even one glass of milk.

☆ Bottle-feeding may be preferable for a woman who is inhibited about her body, squeamish about having such intimate contact with her infant, and uncomfortable about the possibility of nursing in public. Or for a woman who feels she is too high-strung or impatient to breastfeed.

Making the Choice

For more and more women today, no choice need be made. They know they will opt for breast over bottle long before they even decide to become pregnant. Others, who've never given it much thought before pregnancy, choose breastfeeding once they've read up on its many benefits. Some women teeter on the brink of indecision right through pregnancy, uncertain about their own feelings, uncertain about their partner's. A few women, though convinced that nursing isn't for them, can't shake the nagging feeling that they ought to do it anyway.

For all of these women, we have one suggestion: Try it – you may like it. You can always quit if you don't, but at least you will have eased those nagging doubts. Best of all, you and your baby will have reaped the benefits of breastfeeding, if just for a brief time.

Give breastfeeding a fair trial, though. The first few weeks are always difficult, even for the most ardent breastfeeders. Some experts suggest that a full month of nursing is needed to establish a successful feeding relationship.

When You Can't Or Shouldn't Breastfeed

Unfortunately, the choice of whether or not to breastfeed isn't open to every new mother. Some women can't or shouldn't nurse their newborns. The reasons may be emotional or physical, due to mother's health or the baby's, temporary or long-term – and the following are factors:

☆ Serious debilitating illness (such as cardiac or kidney impairment, or severe anaemia) or extreme underweight.

☆ Serious infection, such as tuberculosis.

☆ Conditions that require medications which pass into the breast milk and might be harmful to the baby such as: antithyroid, anticancer, or antihypertensive drugs, lithium, tranquillizers, sedatives. If you take any kind of medication, check with your doctor before beginning breastfeeding.[4]

4. A temporary need for medication, such as penicillin, even at the time you begin nursing, need not necessarily eliminate the chances of breastfeeding. It may be possible to start the baby on formula temporarily, express milk to get your milk supply going, and, as soon as medication is halted, switch to breastfeeding.

☆ Breast cancer or a family history of breast cancer before menopause, particularly on your mother's side. If you have such a history, discuss the advisability of breastfeeding with your doctor. (Some recent research has suggested that a virus for breast cancer might be transmitted through breast milk.)

☆ Drug abuse – including the use of tranquillizers, heroin, methadone, marijuana, cigarettes, and heavy use of caffeine or alcohol.

☆ A deep-seated aversion to the idea of breastfeeding.

Conditions in the newborn that interfere with breastfeeding include:

☆ A disorder such as lactose intolerance or phenylketonuria (PKU), in which neither human *nor* cow's milk can be digested.

☆ Cleft lip and/or cleft palate, or other mouth deformities that make sucking at the breast difficult.

Making Bottle-Feeding Work

Though breastfeeding is a good experience for both mother and child, there is no reason why bottle-feeding can't be, too. Millions of happy, healthy babies have been raised on the bottle. When you can't, or don't wish to, breastfeed, the danger lies not in the bottle, but in the possibility that you might communicate any guilt or frustration you feel to your baby. Know that, with a little extra effort, love can be passed from mother to child through the bottle as well as through the breast. Make every feeding a time to cuddle your baby, just as you would if you were nursing: Never feed baby in the crib with a propped bottle; make skin-to-skin contact by opening your shirt, when practical, and letting the baby rest against your bare breast while feeding.

13
The Ninth Month

WHAT YOU CAN EXPECT AT THIS MONTH'S CHECKUP

After about the 36th week, you will see your doctor or midwife weekly. Both the tenor and content of these examinations will be reminders that you are getting closer to D-day. In general, you can expect your doctor to check the following, though there may be variations depending upon your particular needs and upon your doctor or midwife's style of practice:[1]

☆ Weight (gain will probably slow down or cease) and blood pressure (it may be up slightly over what it was at mid-pregnancy)

☆ Urinalysis

☆ Foetal heartbeat

☆ Height of fundus

☆ Blood test for haemoglobin

☆ Inquiry into any unusual vaginal discharge or bleeding, or any urinary symptoms

☆ Feet, hands, and legs for oedema (swelling); legs and vulva for varicose veins

☆ Your cervix, for effacement and dilatation, usually some time after the 38th week (by internal examination) but not always routine

☆ Symptoms you have been experiencing, especially unusual ones

☆ Inquiry into whether or not the baby is moving well

☆ Frequency and duration of Braxton Hicks contractions you may be having and which you may be noticing

☆ X-ray for pelvimetry or assessment of foetus if indicated

☆ Instructions from your doctor as to when to call if you think you are in labour

1. See appendix for an explanation of the procedures and tests performed

☆ Questions and problems you want to discuss, particularly those related to labour and delivery – have a list ready, especially when to come into hospital or summon the midwife

WHAT YOU MAY BE FEELING

You may feel all of these symptoms at one time or another or only a few of them. Some may have continued from last month, others may be new. Still others may hardly be noticed because you are used to them and/or because they are eclipsed by new and more exciting signs indicating that labour may not be far off.

Physically:

☆ Changes in foetal activity (more squirming and less kicking, as the uterus becomes a more cramped home)

☆ Vaginal discharge (leukorrhoea) becomes heavier and contains more mucous, which may be streaked red with blood or tinged brown or pink after intercourse or a pelvic exam

☆ Constipation

☆ Heartburn and indigestion, flatulence and bloating

☆ Occasional headaches, faintness, dizziness

☆ Nasal congestion and occasional nosebleeds; ear stuffiness

☆ Leg cramps during sleep

☆ Increased backache and heaviness

☆ Buttock and pelvic discomfort and achiness

What You May Look Like

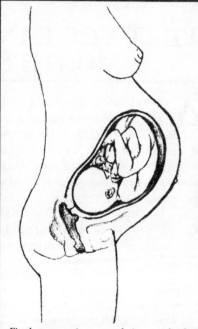

Final preparations are being made for birth, which can safely take place any time now. Lungs are mature. About 2 inches and 2½ pounds are added to baby's length and weight (the average baby will be 20 inches, 7½ pounds at term). More confined, and possibly engaged in the pelvis, the foetus may seem less active.

☆ Increased oedema (swelling) of ankles and feet, occasionally hands and face

☆ Varicose veins of legs and/or haemorrhoids

☆ Itchy abdomen

☆ Easier breathing after the baby 'drops'

☆ More frequent urination after the baby drops

☆ Increased difficulty sleeping

☆ Increasing and intensifying Braxton Hicks contractions (some may be painful)

☆ Increasing clumsiness and difficulty getting around

☆ Colostrum, either leaking or expressed, from breasts (though this premilk substance may not appear until after delivery)

☆ Fatigue or extra energy, or alternate periods of each

☆ Increase in appetite, or loss of appetite

Emotionally:

☆ More excitement, more anxiety more apprehension, more absent-mindedness

☆ Relief that you're almost there

☆ Irritability and oversensitivity (especially with people who keep saying: 'Are *you* still around?')

☆ Impatience and restlessness

☆ Dreaming and fantasizing about the baby

WHAT YOU MAY BE CONCERNED ABOUT

Changes In Foetal Movements

'My baby, who used to kick so vigorously, isn't kicking at all now – just squirming.'

When you first heard from your baby, way back in the fifth month, there was ample room in the uterus for acrobatics – and lots of kicking and punching. Now that conditions are getting a little cramped, gymnastics are curtailed. In this uterine straightjacket, there is room for little more than turning, twisting, and wiggling. And once the head is firmly engaged in the pelvis, baby will be even less mobile.

It's not important what kind of foetal movement you feel at this stage – as long as you're conscious of activity every day. Should the rate of activity suddenly decrease dramatically, or movements cease altogether or become very weak, a call to your doctor or midwife is warranted. He or she may ask you to try this test: Lie down and relax. Then over a period of half an hour or an hour, count the movements. Repeat, possibly two or three times during the day. Ten or more movements per hour during each test period will assure everyone that everything is okay. Fewer might suggest that further evaluation is needed, although even then there is no cause for alarm. Many babies who are relatively inactive in the womb turn out to be perfectly healthy. But if inactivity indicates foetal distress, prompt medical action is vital to the well-being of your baby.

'I've read that foetal movements are supposed to slow down as delivery approaches. My baby seems more active than ever. Could that mean he's going to be hyperactive?'

Before birth is too soon to start worrying about hyperactivity. Studies show that foetuses who are very active in the womb are no more likely than quiet foetuses to become hyperactive in childhood.

Recent reserach also contradicts the notion that the average foetus becomes lazy just before delivery. In late pregnancy, there is generally a gradual decline in movement (from about 25 to 39 movements an hour at 30 weeks to 18 to 28 at term), probably related to tighter quarters, a decrease, in amniotic fluid, and improved foetal coordination. But unless they're counting, many women never notice a significant difference.

Bleeding or Spotting

'Right after my partner and I made love this morning, I began to bleed. Does this mean that labour is beginning – or is the baby in some kind of danger?'

Any new symptom in the ninth month immediately raises one of two questions – or both: Is it time? Is something wrong? Bleeding and spotting are two such anxiety-provoking events. What they indicate depends on the type of bleeding you experience and the circumstances that surround it:

☆ Pinkish-stained or red-streaked mucus appearing soon after, or

brownish-tinged mucus or brownish spotting appearing about 48 hours after, intercourse or vaginal examination is probably just a result of the sensitive cervix being bruised or manipulated. This is normal and not a danger sign – although it should be reported to your practitioner. He or she may advise abstinence from intercourse until delivery.

☆ Bright red bleeding or persistent spotting could be originating at the placenta and requires immediate medical evaluation. Call your practitioner at once. If he or she can't be reached, have someone take you to the hospital.

☆ Pinkish- or brownish-tinged or bloody mucus accompanied by contractions or other signs of oncoming labour (see Prelabour, False Labour, Real Labour, page 238) could be signalling the start of labour. The fact that this blood-streaked mucus appeared just after intercourse could be a coincidence. Put in a call to your doctor.

Lightening and Engagement

'If I'm past my 38th week and haven't dropped, does it mean I'm going to be late?'

'Dropping,' also called 'lightening,' is the descent of the foetus into the pelvic cavity. In first pregnancies, lightening generally takes place two to four weeks before delivery. In women who have had children previously, it rarely occurs until they go into labour. But as with almost every aspect of pregnancy, exceptions to the rules are the rule. A first-time mother can drop four weeks before her due date and deliver two weeks 'late,' or she can go into labour without having dropped at all.

Often, lightening is quite apparent. The pregnant woman notes that her bulging belly seems to have dropped and tilted forward. As the uterus moves away from the diaphragm, she may find breathing less of an effort; with the stomach less crowded, she may be able to eat more at a sitting. These added comforts are offset by the discomfort of pressure on the bladder, the pelvic joints, and the perineal area – which results in increased frequency of urination, difficult mobility, the sensation of increased perineal pressure, and, sometimes, pain. Sharp little shocks or twinges may occur when the foetal head presses on the pelvic floor. Some women sense a rolling in their pelvis when the head turns. And often, because her centre of gravity has again shifted, a pregnant woman feels off balance once lightening has occurred.

It is very possible, however, for lightening to occur without your ever realising it. If, for instance, you carried low to begin with, the shape of your abdomen might not be altered significantly. Or if you never experienced difficulty breathing or urinated frequently throughout pregnancy, you might not notice any obvious change.

When the broadest diameter of the foetal head has reached the upper boundary of the bony pelvis, it is said to be "engaged." Only your practitioner knows for sure whether or not your baby's head is snugly engaged in your pelvis. He or she relies on two basic indicators: on internal examination, the presenting part (the part of the foetus closest to the exit, most commonly the head) is felt in the pelvis; on palpating the head externally, it is found to be fixed, no longer 'floating.'

How far the presenting part has progressed through the pelvis is measured in 'stations,' each a centimetre long. A fully engaged baby is at 'zero (or 0) station' – that is, the foetal head has descended to the level of the ischial spines (prominent bony landmarks on either side of the midpelvis). A baby who has just begun to descend may be at -4 or -5 station. Once delivery begins, the head continues on through the pelvis past 0 to $+1$, $+2$, and so on, until it begins to 'crown' at the external vaginal opening at $+5$. Though a woman who goes into labour at 0 station probably has less pushing ahead than the woman at -3, this isn't invariably true, since station isn't the only factor affecting the progression of labour.

Though the engagement of the foetal head suggests that the baby can probably get through the pelvis without difficult, a foetus that is still floating going into labour is not necessarily going to have trouble. And in fact, a majority of them come through the pelvis smoothly.

When You Will Deliver

'Can the doctor or midwife tell exactly how close I am to going into labour?'

No. And don't believe it if he or she tells you otherwise. There are clues that labour may soon begin, which your practitioner begins to look for in the ninth month. Has lightening or engagement taken place? What station (level in the pelvis) has the baby's presenting part reached? Have effacement (thinning of the cervix) and dilatation (opening of the cervix) begun?

But 'soon' can mean anywhere from an hour to three weeks or more. Ask the woman whose euphoria at being told by her practitioner, 'You'll be in labour by this evening,' dissolves into depression as weeks of pregnancy proceed to pass with nary a contraction.

A practitioner's prognostication that, since effacement and dilatation haven't yet begun, labour is weeks away can be equally unreliable. As women will testify who, upon hearing such a prediction, have sagged home from the doctor's office resigned to another long month of pregnancy, only to give birth by the following morning.

The fact is that engagement, effacement, and dilatation can occur gradually over a period of weeks or even a month or more in some women. In others they can occur in a matter of hours. No one, no matter how well trained, can accurately predict the onset of labour – because no one knows exactly what triggers it. (That's why some doctors are as loath to venture guesses on when you will deliver as on whether it's going to be a girl or a boy.)

So like every pregnant woman before you, you'll just have to play a waiting game, knowing for certain only that your day, or night, will come – sometime.

Labour and Delivery Rooms

'I'm very uneasy about going into the hospital and having my baby in unfamiliar surroundings.'

The labour and delivery floor is by far the happiest in the hospital. Still, if you don't know what to expect, you can be filled with trepidation. Most hospitals allow – in fact, encourage – tours of the labour and delivery suite by expectant couples. Inquire when you make your booking. You can also stop in during visiting hours, and though you won't see the actual labour and delivery area, you can see what patient rooms look like in the postpartum section, and also take a good look at the nursery. Besides making you feel more comfortable, this will give you the opportunity to see what a newborn looks like before you hold your own in your arms.

Labour and delivery rooms vary from hospital to hospital. Some are very sterile and businesslike; others are more homey. Birthing rooms are becoming more and more common and boast the at-home look, with rocking chairs, bright pictures on the walls, curtains on the windows, and birthing beds that look more as if they came out of a home furnishing showroom than a hospital supply catalogue.

Though it's nice to be in pleasant surroundings, in the long run it won't be the talent of the hospital's interior designer but the skill and caring of the medical staff that will be important to your well-being and that of your baby.

The Overdue Baby

'I'm a week overdue and my doctor's arranged to give me a non-stress test. Is it possible that I might never go into labour on my own?'

The magic date is circled in red on the calendar; every day of the 40 weeks that precede it is crossed off with great anticipation. Then, at long last, the big day arrives. And, as in the majority of pregnancies, the baby doesn't. Anticipation dissolves into discouragement. The baby carriage and crib sit empty for another day. And then a week. And then, in 10% of pregnancies, two weeks. Will this pregnancy never end?

Though women who have reached the 42nd week might find it hard to believe, no pregnancy on record ever went on forever – even before the advent of labour induction. (It's true an occasional pregnancy progresses to the 44th week or beyond, but today most are induced before they go past the 42nd.)

When a pregnant woman appears to be post-term (technically 42 weeks or more, though most doctors will take action 10 days after the expected delivery date) the practitioner evaluates the situation, considering two major factors: One, is the estimated due date accurate? He or she can be reasonably sure that it is if the date corresponded throughout pregnancy with the fundal height and the size of the uterus, and if the timing of both the first foetal movements felt by the mother and the first foetal heartbeats detected by the examiner also correlated with it. Sometimes ultrasonography and urine and blood tests are used to verify the gestational age. It is estimated that about 70% of apparent post-term pregnancies are due to a miscalculation of the time of conception.

Two, is the foetus continuing to thrive? Many babies continue to grow and flourish well into the tenth month (although this can be a problem if the baby becomes too large to pass easily through the mother's pelvis). Occasionally, however, the aging placenta begins to deteriorate, and the foetus ceases to thrive. These 'dysmature' babies may lose weight in the uterus and be born with long, thin limbs and dry, parchment-like skin that hangs loosely because of the depleted fat layers. Though the risk of distress during labour is greater for dysmature babies than for normal-term infants, they usually develop normally following birth.

There are several procedures which can determine the condition of the post-term foetus and its placenta. Such tests are performed at the discretion of the practitioner – either routinely, when the delivery is overdue by a week or more, or occasionally, because there is some sign of foetal or maternal difficulty.

The Non-Stress Test (NST) is simple and safe. The mother is hooked up to a foetal monitor so that the response of the foetal heart to foetal movemens can be observed. Normally, the heart rate will accelerate immediately following each foetal movement. Two such accelerations in a 20-minute period indicate a reactive, and thus healthy, foetus.

The Stress Test, or Oxytocin Challenge Test (OCT), also evaluates the reactivity of the foetal heart, but to uterine contractions that stimulate labour rather than to foetal movements. In this somewhat more complex and time-consuming test (it may take up to 3 hours), the mother is hooked up to a foetal monitor, just as she would be in labour. If contractions are not occurring frequently enough on their own, they are initiated via the intravenous administration of oxytocin, or by stimulation of the mother's nipples (with hot towels and, if necessary, manually by the mother). Foetal response indicates the probable condition of foetus and placenta, as well as whether or not they can safely meet the strenuous demands of labour.

Levels of Oestriol (an oestrogenic hormone produced by the foetal-placental unit) in the blood or urine of the mother may also be evaluated, sometimes in conjunction with a stress or non-stress test, or both. Normally, oestriol levels rise from the 28th week of pregnancy until term. A series of oestriol determinations that show a trend that is either stationary or decreasing is an indication that living conditions in the uterus are no longer optimal and prompt delivery is advisable. Several maternal factors are known to affect oestriol levels (e.g., chronic disease, change in level in activity, medications), and results are interpreted accordingly. Low levels of HPL (human placental lactogen) may also indicate placental dysfunction.

If the foetus passes all its tests, the doctor will probably allow the pregnancy to follow nature's course for a while longer. Tests will be repeated at least weekly. If at any point results indicate placental insufficiency (a foetal scalp pH may be taken to verify this), a decision will be made to remove the foetus from the deteriorating environment, by either induction of labour or caesarean.

Membranes Rupturing in Public

'I live in fear of my membranes rupturing in public.'

You're not alone in your fear. The idea of the 'bag of waters' rupturing on a bus or in a crowded department store is as mortifying to most pregnant women as that of losing bladder control in public. One woman reportedly became so obsessed with her worry that she carried a jar of pickles in her handbag, ready to be dropped at the first tell-tale trickle of amniotic fluid.

But before you start rummaging through your cupboards for a jar of onions, there are two things you should know. First, the rupture of membranes before labour begins is uncommon – occurring in less than 15% of pregnancies. And once they do break, the flow of amniotic fluid is unlikely to be heavy except when you are lying down (something you aren't likely to do in public). When you are walking or sitting, the foetal head tends to block the opening of the uterus as a cork does in a wine bottle.

And second, should your membranes rupture and the amniotic fluid gush suddenly, you can be sure that those around you will not point, shake disapproving heads, or – worse – chuckle. Instead they will (as you would if you were a bystander) either offer you assistance or discreetly ignore you. Keep in mind, after all, that no one is likely to overlook the fact that you're pregnant or to mistake amniotic fluid for anything else.

Wearing a panty liner in the last weeks may give you a sense of security, as well as keeping you fresher as leukorrhoea increases.

Breastfeeding

'My breasts are very small and my nipples are flat. Will I be able to breastfeed?'

As far as hungry babies are concerned, satisfaction comes in all kinds of packages. Breasts don't have to be centrefold-shaped or sized, and they can come equipped with almost any kind of nipple – small and flat, large and pointy, even inverted. All combinations of breasts and nipples have the capacity to produce and dispense milk – the quantity or quality of which is not in the least dependent on outward appearance. Unfortunately, because so many fallacies and old wives' tales exist about what kinds of breasts can and cannot satisfy a baby, many women are unnecessarily discouraged from breastfeeding.

Inverted nipples that don't become erect with sexual stimulation generally need some special priming prior to childbirth. The use of a breast shield is the best way to 'pull out' an inverted nipple. Worn for as many hours as possible during the day in the last few months of pregnancy, the mild suction of the shield gently draws the nipple out. A manual breast pump used several times a day can also help to correct inverted nipples.

Some experts recommend that all women who expect to nurse try to prepare their breasts in advance by expressing a small amount of colostrum from the nipples daily from the eighth month on (though not every woman will be able to do this) and by pulling, twisting, or rolling the nipples between forefinger and thumb to toughen them. Others say that nursing comes naturally to nipples, without special preparation.

'My mother says she had milk leaking from her breasts by this time; I don't. Does this mean I won't have any milk?'

The thin, yellowish discharge that some pregnant women can express, or may notice leaking from their breasts, is not milk. It is a premilk fluid called colostrum. Richer in protein and lower in fat and milk sugar than the breast milk that comes in two or three days after delivery, it contains antibodies that may be important in protecting the baby against disease.

Many women, however, don't have any noticeable colostrum until after delivery. Even then, they may not be aware of it. This in no way predicts difficulty in breastfeeding.

Mothering

'Now that the baby's arrival is so close, I'm beginning to worry about taking care of it. I've never even held a newborn before.'

Women are not born mothers, instinctively knowing how to rock a crying baby to sleep, change a nappy, or give a bath. Motherhood – or parenthood, for that matter – is a learned art, one that requires plenty of practice to make perfect (or even near-perfect). A hundred years ago, that practice commonly took place at an early age, when female children learned to care for younger siblings – much as they learned to bake bread and mend socks.

Today, a high percentage of fully grown women have never kneaded bread dough, taken a needle to a worn sock, or held – let alone taken care of – an infant. Their training for motherhood comes on the job, with some reading on the side. Which means that for the first week or two, the baby may do more crying than sleeping, the nappies may leak, and many a tear may be shed over the 'no-more-tears' lather. Slowly but surely, however, the new mother begins to feel like an old pro. Her trepidation turns to assurance. The baby she was afraid to hold (won't it break?) is now cradled casually in her left arm while her right sets the table or pushes the vacuum cleaner. Dispensing vitamin drops, giving baths, slipping squirming arms and legs into sleepers, have ceased to be dreaded ordeals. They, like all the daily tasks of parenting, have become second nature. She's a mother, and – difficult though it may be to imagine – you will be one, too.

WHAT IT'S IMPORTANT TO KNOW: PRELABOUR, FALSE LABOUR, REAL LABOUR

It always seems so simple on TV. Somewhere around 3 A.M., the pregnant woman sits up in bed, puts a knowing hand on her belly, and reaches over to rouse her sleeping husband with a calm, almost serene, 'It's time, honey.'

But how, we wonder, does this woman know it's time? How does she recognise labour with such cool, clinical confidence when she's never *been* in labour before? What makes her so sure she's not going to get to the hospital, be examined by the midwife, and be found to be uneffaced, undilated, and nowhere near her time? That she won't be sent home – amidst snickers from the night shift – just as pregnant as when she arrived?

On our side of the TV, we're more likely to awaken at 3 A.M. with complete uncertainty. Are those really labour pains, or just some more Braxton Hicks? Should I turn on the light and start timing? Should I bother to wake my husband? Do I call the doctor in the middle of the night to report what might really be false labour? If I do, and it isn't time, will I turn out to be the pregnant woman who cried 'labour' once too often, and will anybody take me seriously when it's for real? Or will I be the only woman in my class not to recognise labour? Will I leave for the hospital too late, maybe giving birth in a taxi cab? The questions multiply faster than the contractions.

The fact is that most women, worry though they might, *don't* end up misjudging the onset of their labour. The vast majority, thanks to instinct, luck, or no-doubt-about-it killer contractions, show up at the hospital neither too early nor too late, but at just about the right time. Still, there's no reason to leave your deliberations up to chance. Becoming completely familiar with the signs of prelabour, false labour, and real labour will help to allay the concerns and clear up the confusion.

No one knows exactly what triggers labour. Several theories have been suggested – none of which, in isolation, holds up under scientific scrutiny. Probably a combination of foetal, placental, and maternal factors are responsible for setting into motion the events of labour.

Prelabour Symptoms

The process of prelabour can precede real labour by a full month or more – or by only an hour or so. Prelabour is characterized by the beginning of cervical effacement and dilatation, which only your practitioner can confirm, as well as by a wide variety of related signs which you may notice yourself.

Lightening and Engagement. Usually somewhere between two and four weeks before labour begins in first-time mothers, the foetus begins to descend into the pelvis. This milestone is rarely reached in second or later births until labour has actually commenced.

Increasing Pressure Sensations in the Pelvis and Rectum. Crampiness and groin pain are particularly common in second and later pregnancies. Persistent low backache may also be present.

Loss of Weight or Cessation in Weight Gain. As labour approaches, some women lose up to 2 or 3 pounds; in general, weight gain slows in the ninth month.

Changes in Energy Levels. Some ninth-monthers find that they are increasingly fatigued. Others experience energy spurts. An uncontrollable urge to scrub floors and wash woodwork has been related to the 'nesting instinct' – mother preparing the nest.

Changes in Vaginal Discharge. You may find that your discharge increases and thickens.

Loss of Mucous Plug. As the cervix begins to thin and dilate, the 'cork' of mucous that seals the opening of the uterus becomes dislodged. This can happen a week or two before the first real contractions, or just as labour begins.

Pink, or Bloody, Show. As the cervix effaces and dilates, capillaries frequently rupture, tinting the mucous pink or streaking it with blood. This 'show' usually means labour will start within 24 hours – but it could be as much as several days away.

Intensification of Braxton Hicks Contractions. These practice contractions may become more frequent and stronger, even painful.

Diarrhoea. Some women experience loose bowel movements just prior to the onset of labour.

False Labour Symptoms

Real labour probably has not begun if:

☆ Contractions are not regular and don't increase in frequency or severity.

☆ Pain is in the lower abdomen rather than the lower back.

☆ Contractions subside if you walk around or change your position.

☆ The uterus relaxes and contractions ease if you have an alcoholic drink.

☆ Show, if any, is brownish.[2] (This is usually a result of an internal exam

---

2. Bright red blood requires immediate consultation with your doctor.

or intercourse within the past 48 hours.)

☆ Foetal movements intensify briefly with contractions.

Real Labour Symptoms

When contractions of prelabour are replaced by stronger, more painful, and more frequent ones, the question arises: 'Is this the real thing or false labour?' It is probably real if:

☆ The contractions intensify, rather than ease up, with activity and aren't relieved by a change in position or by an alcoholic drink.

☆ Pain begins in the lower back and spreads to the lower abdomen; it may also radiate to the legs. Contractions may feel like a gastrointestinal upset and be accompanied by diarrhoea.

☆ Contractions become progressively more frequent and painful, and generally (but not always) more regular. (This progression isn't absolute – not every contraction is more painful or longer than the previous one, but their general intensity does build up as real labour progresses. Nor does frequency always increase in regular, perfectly even intervals but it does increase.)

☆ Show is present and pinkish or blood-streaked.

☆ Membranes rupture. In 15% of labours the membranes rupture – either as a gush of waters or a trickle – before labour begins.

What to Take to the Hospital

For the Labour or Birthing Room

☆ This book.

☆ A watch or clock with a second hand for timing contractions.

☆ A radio or a cassette player equipped with your favourite tapes, if music soothes and relaxes you.

☆ A camera, tape recorder, and/or video equipment, if you don't trust your memory to capture the moment completely (and if the hospital rules allow media coverage of births).

☆ Powder, lotions, or anything else you'd like to be massaged with.

☆ A small paper bag, to breathe into in case you begin to hyperventilate from breathing exercises.

☆ A tennis ball or plastic rolling pin, for firm counter-massage should backache be a problem.

☆ Sugarless lollipops to keep your mouth moist (though sugar-full candies are usually recommended, they will only make you thirstier and more dehydrated).

☆ Heavy socks, in case your feet become cold.

☆ A hairbrush, if having someone brush your hair is comforting.

☆ A washcloth for sponging down with, though the hospital may provide this (don't bring a white one which might accidentally end up in the hospital laundry).

☆ A sandwich or other snack for Dad (a partner who faints from hunger can't be effective).

☆ A bottle of champagne, wrapped and labelled with your name, for celebrating (your partner can ask the nurse to keep it in the fridge), though depending on the hour you deliver, you may be more in the mood for an orange juice toast.

For the Hospital Room

☆ A robe and/or nightgowns, if you'd rather wear your own than the hospital's. Be forewarned, however, that though pretty nightgowns can boost your spirits, they may get bled on and permanently stained. Ditto bathrobes. A good compromise might be a favourite bedjacket to wear over the hospital gown.

☆ Perfume, powder, or whatever else makes you feel fresh.

☆ Toiletries, including shampoo, toothbrush, toothpaste, lotion (your skin may be dry from a loss of fluids), a bar of soap in a carrying case, deodorant, hairbrush, hand mirror, makeup, and any other essentials of beauty and hygiene.

☆ Sanitary pads, preferably the adhesive variety, though pads and a belt are usually provided by the hospital.

☆ Playing cards, books (including what-to-name-your-baby books if you're leaving that decision for the last minute), and other distractions.

☆ Packs of raisins, nuts, wholewheat crackers, and other healthy snacks to keep you regular in spite of a hospital diet.

☆ A going-home outfit for you, keeping in mind that you'll still be sporting a sizable abdomen.

☆ A going-home outfit for baby – a kimono or stretch suit, T-shirt, booties, a shawl, and a heavy blanket if it's cold; nappies will probably be provided by the hospital, but take along an extra, just in case.

When to Call the Doctor or Midwife

When in doubt, call. Even if you've checked and rechecked the above lists, you may still be unsure of whether you're really in labour. Don't wait to find out for sure – unless you'd prefer an unplanned home birth. Call the doctor or midwife. He or she will probably be able to tell from the sound of your voice, as you talk through a contraction, whether it's the real thing. (But only if you don't try to cover up the pain in the name of good manners.) Fear of being embarrassed if it doesn't turnout to be labour shouldn't prevent your calling the doctor or midwife. If it does turn out to be a false alarm, nobody's going to snicker. You wouldn't be the first patient to misjudge her labour signs – and you certainly won't be the last.

☆ Call anytime, night or day, if all signs indicate that you're ready to go to the hospital. Don't let an overdeveloped sense of guilt or politeness keep you from waking your doctor or midwife up in the middle of the night, or disturbing his or her weekend at home. People who deliver babies for a living don't expect to work a 9-to-5 shift.

☆ Your doctor or midwife has probably specified that you should call when your contractions have reached a particular frequency – say, 5, 8, or 10 minutes apart. Call when at least some of your contractions are that frequent. Don't wait for perfectly even intervals; they may never come.

☆ Your doctor or midwife has probably also intructed you about when to call if your membranes rupture, or if you think they have ruptured, but labour has not begun. Some say: 'If they break at 3 A.M., wait until morning.' Others say to call immediately. Follow your doctor or midwife's instructions, unless: your due date is still several weeks away; you know your baby is small or is not engaged in the pelvis; or the amniotic fluid is not clear, but is stained greenish brown. In these cases, call immediately since there is a risk of foetal distress, and go straight to hospital.

☆ Don't assume that if you're not sure it's real labour, it necessarily isn't. Err on the side of caution and call your doctor or midwife.

14
Labour and Delivery

WHAT YOU MAY BE CONCERNED ABOUT

Bloody Show

'I have a pink mucous discharge. Does it mean labour's about to start?'

Don't send your husband out for the cigars yet. Passage of 'bloody show,' a mucous discharge tinged pink or brown with blood, is a sign that your cervix is dilating and that the process that leads to delivery is beginning. But it's a process with an erratic timetable that will keep you in suspense until the first contractions. Labour could be one, two, or even three weeks away, with your cervix continuing to dilate gradually over that time. Or it could be less than an hour away.

If your discharge should suddenly become red or bloody, contact your practitioner immediately. Fresh-bleeding could indicate a premature separation of the placenta, which requires you to get prompt medical attention.

Rupture of Membranes

'I woke up in the middle of the night with a wet bed. Did I lose control of my bladder, or did my membranes rupture?'

A sniff of your sheets will probably clue you in. If the wet spot smells sort of sweet and not like ammonia, it's likely to be amniotic fluid. Another clue: You'll probably still be leaking the pale, straw-coloured amniotic fluid (which won't run dry because it continues to be produced until delivery, replacing itself every three hours). If you stand up or sit down, however, the baby's head may act like a cork and slow down the leak.

Some women never experience a gushing of amniotic fluid when their membranes rupture – partly because of the cork effect, partly because there are no contractions to force the fluid out. All they notice is a constant trickle. (A leak that starts and then stops, particularly several weeks before term, probably indicates a tear in the membranes that healed itself.)

'My water just broke, but I haven't had any contractions. When is labour going to start, and what should I do in the meantime?'

If you're like the majority of pregnant women whose membranes rupture prior to labour, your labour will begin within the next 12 hours. If you're not, you'll probably be feeling the first contractions within 24 hours. About 1 in 10 women take even longer to go into labour. Because of the increasing risk of infection to baby and/or mother through the ruptured amniotic sac, most doctors or midwives will induce labour after 24 hours, though a few wait as little as 6 hours. When the membranes rupture before the 34th week, or if there is another reason to suspect foetal immaturity, some doctors or midwives recommend a carefully controlled delay of 48 to 72 hours, during which drugs are administered to accelerate the maturation of the foetal lungs. This approach, however, is still a matter of controversy.

If you think your membranes have ruptured, call your doctor or midwife. In the meantime, keep the vaginal area as clean as possible to avoid infection. Don't take a bath or have sexual relations; use sanitary napkins to absorb the flow of amniotic fluid; don't try to do your own internal exam; and wipe front to back at the toilet.

Rarely, in premature rupture of the membranes (more often in breech and premature births), when the presenting part is not engaged in the pelvis, the umbilical cord becomes 'prolapsed' – swept into the neck of the uterus (the cervix) or even the vagina, with the gush of amniotic fluid. Because pressure on the cord can cut off the baby's oxygen supply, prolapse requires immediate medical attention. If a loop of cord appears at your vagina, get onto your hands and knees; this will reduce the pressure on the cord. If the cord still protrudes in this position, support it gently (do not compress it) with warm, wet gauze pads or a clean cloth. Have someone rush you to the hospital, or call an ambulance.

Darkened Amniotic Fluid (Meconium Staining)

'My membranes ruptured, and the fluid is greenish-brown. What does this mean?'

Your amniotic fluid is stained with meconium, a greenish-brown substance that comes from your baby's digestive tract. Ordinarily, meconium is passed after birth as the baby's first stool. But sometimes – particularly when there is some kind of foetal stress, and very often when the baby is postmature – it is passed prior to birth into the amniotic fluid.

Meconium staining alone is not a sure sign of foetal distress, but because it hints at the possibility, notify your practitioner immediately.

Induction of Labour

'My doctor wants to induce labour. I'm upset because I had wanted a natural delivery.'

Though some doctors 20 years ago believed it was safe to routinely induce labour in their patients so that birth would come at a convenient time, doctors today rarely induce without good cause, because they recognize that, when possible, it's best to let nature take its time taking its course.

In certain circumstances, however, when labour hasn't begun on its own, or is weak or erratic, nature needs a little prodding. For example, when there is:

☆ Foetal distress – and there is time for a vaginal delivery.

☆ Premature rupture of membranes – to reduce the risk of getting an infection if labour has not begun spontaneously within 24 hours. (Some practitioners will wait longer, some not as long; some will suggest first trying to stimulate contractions 'naturally' with mineral oil and/or nipple stimulation, under medical supervision in the hospital. See below.)

☆ Postmaturity – when the pregnancy has gone two or more weeks past a due date that is considered accurate, or when a stress or non-stress test shows that the placenta is no longer functioning optimally because of age.

☆ Arrested or inefficient labour – which could put both mother and child in jeopardy if delivery is delayed indefinitely.

☆ Maternal diabetes. Induced delivery of babies of diabetic mothers before the due date is often indicated because their placentas tend to deteriorate prematurely, and because, if carried to term, the babies are often oversized.

☆ Other maternal illness – such as high blood pressure or kidney disease, in which carrying a baby to term may present increased hazard.

☆ Severe Rh disease – when the foetus may not survive unless delivered early.

Though artificial rupture of the membranes (if they haven't already ruptured naturally) is sometimes indicated to try to bring on labour, oxytocin is much more commonly used for uterine stimulation.

Oxytocin is a hormone produced naturally by the maternal pituitary gland throughout pregnancy. As pregnancy progresses, the uterus becomes more and more sensitive to the hormone, although it isn't clear whether it plays a significant role in the triggering of labour. It is known that the hormone may be released by the pregnant woman when her nipples are stimulated, causing the uterus to contract. Some practitioners may in fact advise nipple self-stimulation to bring on, or speed up contractions before resorting to less natural methods. The artificial administration of oxytocin, however, is a more reliable method of induction. When conditions are ripe, it is capable of initiating labour that mimics the naturally occurring variety, with contractions that may be a little more regular, and slightly different in quality.

The hormone (trade name syntocinon) can be administered intramuscularly (injected into a muscle), sublingually (placed under the tongue), or intranasally (sniffed) – but the intravenous (IV) oxytocin drip, utilizing an infusion pump, is the safest and easiest route to control. The IV is introduced via a needle in the arm or the back of the hand, and connected by tubing to two bottles of neutral (unmedicated) IV solution. The pump releases oxytocin into the primary bottle, one drop at a time. (The second bottle remains on standby.) Usually the induction begins slowly with very little oxytocin being released, and the reaction of the uterus and the foetus are carefully monitored. (A doctor or midwife must be in attendance at all times during induction.) The rate of infusion is increased gradually until effective contractions are established. Should the woman's uterus prove extremely sensitive to the drug, and be overstimulated into either too long or too powerful contractions, this method allows the infusion to be immediately reduced or halted entirely, with the IV being switched to the standby bottle.

If, after six to eight hours of oxytocin administration, labour hasn't begun or progressed, the procedure will probably be terminated in favour of an alternative. Treatment may also be terminated if contractions are well established and continue on their own.

Induction of labour is not considered appropriate when there is serious foetal distress; if there is any doubt the foetus can fit through the mother's pelvis; when a woman is judged to be in false labour; and, generally, in women who have had five or more previous births.

Some women find the sudden onset of hard labour that usually occurs with induction unpleasant; some even feel cheated by the short duration of their labouring experience. Others enjoy such down-to-business births. With their partners at their side, they go through their induced labours otherwise naturally, using all the breathing exercises and other coping mechanisms learned in childbirth classes. And so can anyone who keeps in mind that labour (no matter how it started) is labour. There's no reason why a labour that doesn't begin 'naturally' can't turn out to be a fully satisfying, memorable birth experience.

Short Labour

'Can a short labour actually be harmful to the baby?'

Short labour isn't always as short as it seems. Often the expectant mother has been having painless contractions for hours, days, even weeks, which have been dilating her cervix gradually. By the time she feels the first contraction, she is often well into the transition stage of labour (see the stages of childbirth on page 259). This kind of slow-buildup, quick-resolution labour certainly places no extra strain on the foetus, and may be even less stressful than the average 12-hour labour.

Occasionally a cervix dilates very

rapidly, accomplishing in a matter of minutes what most cervixes (particularly those of first-time mothers) take hours to do. But even with this abrupt, or precipitous, labour (one that takes three hours or less from start to finish), there is rarely any threat to the baby. There is no evidence to support the notion that an infant must go through a minimum amount of labour in order to arrive in good condition.

Calling Your Doctor or Midwife During Labour

'I just started getting contractions and they're coming every three or four minutes. I feel silly calling the doctor, who said we should spend the first several hours of labour at home.'

Most first-time mothers-to-be (whose labours often begin slowly, with a gradual buildup of contractions) *can* safely count on spending the first several hours at home. But if your contractions start off strong – lasting at least 45 seconds and coming more often than every five minutes – your first several hours of labour may very well be your last. Chances are that much of the first stage of labour has passed painlessly, and that your cervix has dilated significantly during that time. This means that not calling your doctor – and chancing a dramatic dash to the hospital at the last minute – would be considerably sillier than picking up the phone now.

Before you do, however, it is best to have timed several consecutive contractions. Be clear and specific about their frequency, duration, and strength when you report them. Don't try to minimize your discomfort when you describe it by trying to maintain a calm voice. (Your practitioner is used to judging the stage of labour in part by the sound of a woman's voice as she talks through a contraction.)

If you feel you're ready, but your practitioner doesn't seem to think so, don't take 'wait' for an answer. Ask if you can go to the hospital and have your progress checked. (See Calling the Doctor, in Prelabour, False Labour, Real Labour, page 238.) You can take the suitcase along 'just in case,' but be ready to turn around and go home if you've only just begun to dilate.

Back Labour

'The pain in my back since my labour began is so bad I don't see how I'll be able to make it through delivery.'

Technically, 'back labour' occurs when the foetus is in a posterior (or occipitoposterior) position, with the back of its head pressing against the mother's sacrum – the rear boundary of the pelvis. It's possible, however, to experience back labour when the baby is not in this position, or after the baby has turned from a posterior to an anterior position – possibly because the area has become a focus of tension.

When you're having that kind of pain – which often doesn't let up between contractions and becomes excruciating during them – the cause is not really a crucial consideration. How to relieve it, even slightly, is. There are several measures that may help; all are at least worth trying:

☆ Stay off your back. Try to take the pressure off by changing your position – walk around (though this may not be humanly possible once contractions are coming fast and furiously), crouch or squat, get down on all fours, or do whatever is most comfortable and least painful for you. If you feel you can't move, and would prefer to be lying down, do it on your side, with your back well rounded.

☆ Your partner can apply heat (a hot water bottle wrapped in a towel, warm compresses, a heating pad) or cold (ice packs, cold compresses) – whichever soothes best.

☆ Apply counterpressure. Have your partner experiment with different ways of applying pressure to the area of greatest pain, or to adjacent areas, to find one or more that seem to help. He can try his knuckles, or the heel of one hand reinforced by pressure from the other hand on top of it, using direct pressure or a firm circular motion. Pressure can be applied while you are sitting or, to allow greater force, while you are lying on your side. The relief you may get from really intense counterpressure will be well worth any black-and-blue marks you find the morning after.

☆ Use acupressure. This is probably the oldest form of pain relief – and you don't have to be Chinese to try it. In the case of back labour, it involves applying strong finger pressure just below the centre of the ball of the foot.

☆ Aggressively massage the area. This may spell relief either in place of counterpressure or alternated with it. A rolling pin or a tennis ball can be used for especially firm massage (although it will probably leave you aching afterwards). Oil or powder can be rubbed on periodically to avoid irritation.

Irregular Contractions

'In class we were told not to go to the hospital until the contractions were regular and five minutes apart. Mine are less than five minutes apart, but they aren't at all regular. I don't know what to do.'

No two women have exactly the same fingerprints. And no two women have exactly the same labours. The labour described in books, in childbirth education classes, or by your practitioner is what is typical – close to what many women can expect. But far from every labour is true-to-textbook, with contractions regularly spaced and predictably progressive.

If you are having strong, long, frequent (five minutes apart or less) contractions, even if they vary considerably in length and time elapsed between them, do not wait for them to become 'regular' before calling your doctor or midwife or heading for the hospital – no matter what you've heard or read. It's possible that your contractions are about as regular as they are going to get, and

Emergency Home (or Office) Delivery

1. Call 999 for an ambulance (all ambulancemen are trained to deliver babies in an emergency), or the hospital or surgery, who will send out a midwife or doctor.

2. The mother should start panting to keep from bearing down.

3. During all the preparations and during the delivery, comfort and reassure the mother.

4. If there's time, wash the vaginal area and your hands with detergent or soap and water.

5. If there's no time to get to a bed or table, place newspapers or clean towels or folded clothing under the buttocks, to give some height for delivering the baby's shoulders.

6. If there is time, place the woman onto the bed (or a desk or a table) sideways, with her buttocks slightly hanging off, her hands under her thighs to keep them elevated. A couple of chairs can serve as supports for her feet.

7. Protect delivery surfaces, if possible, with shower curtains, newspapers, plastic tablecloths, towels, and so on. A dish pan or basin can be used to catch the amniotic fluid and blood.

8. As the top of the baby's head begins to appear, instruct the mother to pant or blow (not push), and apply gentle counterpressure to keep the head from popping out suddenly. Let the head emerge gradually – *never* pull it out. If there is a loop of the cord around the baby's neck, hook a finger under it and gently work it over the baby's head.

9. When the head has been delivered, gently stroke the nose downward, the neck and under the chin upward, to help expel mucous and amniotic fluid.

10. Now take the head gently in two hands and press it very slightly downward, asking the mother to push at the same time, to deliver the frontward shoulder. As the upper arm appears, lift the head carefully, watching for the rearward shoulder to deliver.

11. Quickly wrap the baby in blankets, towels, or anything else that is available (preferably something clean; something recently ironed is relatively sterile). Place it on the mother's abdomen, or if the cord is long enough (don't tug at it), at her breast.

12. Don't try to pull the placenta out. But if it arrives on its own before the ambulance comes, wrap it in towels or newspaper, and keep it elevated above the level of the baby, if possible. Don't try to cut the cord.

13. Keep both mother and baby warm and comfortable until help arrives.

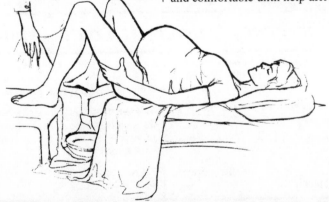

that you are well into the 'active' phase of your labour. Waste no time in calling your doctor or midwife and getting to the hospital; she who hesitates in a case like this could end up with an unscheduled home birth.

Not Getting to the Hospital in Time

'I'm afraid that I won't get to the hospital in time.'

Fortunately, most surprise deliveries take place in the movies and on television. In real life, deliveries rarely occur without ample warning. But once in a great while, a woman who has had no labour pains, or just erratic ones, suddenly feels an overwhelming urge to bear down; often she mistakes it for a need to go to the bathroom. If it happens to you, don't panic. Even if you don't know the first thing about delivering a baby, your lack of experience won't stop the baby from arriving. It is a good idea, however, for you and your husband to be familiar with a few basics (see boxes).

Enemas

'I've heard that enemas early in labour aren't really necessary, and that they interfere with natural birth.'

Enemas were until fairly recently, administered in early labour, as part of the hospital admissions procedure. The theory was, and still is in many hospitals, that emptying the bowels before delivery prevents compression of the birth canal by hard faecal matter in the rectum (which would hinder the baby's descent) and contamination of the sterile birthing setup by involuntary evacuation during the pushing stage of labour.

These theories are less in favour today. It is recognized that compression of the birth canal is not likely to be a problem if a woman has had a bowel movement in the past 24 hours, or if no hard faecal mass is felt in her rectum on internal examination. And the use during delivery of disposable sterile gauze pads to whisk away faecal matter virtually eliminates the threat of faecal contamination to mother and baby. (According to some

---

Emergency Delivery If You're Alone

1. Call 999 for an ambulance, or the hospital or surgery who will send out a midwife or doctor.

2. Find a neighbour or someone to help, if possible.

3. Start panting to keep from bearing down.

4. Wash your hands and the perineal area, if you can.

5. Spread some clean towels, newspapers, or sheets on a bed, sofa, or the floor, and lie down to await help.

6. If the baby starts to arrive before help does, gently ease it out by pushing each time you feel the urge, catching it with your hands.

7. Proceed with steps 9 to 13 on page 249, as best you can.

Emergency Delivery En Route to the Hospital

1. If you're in your own car and delivery is imminent, pull over. If you have a CB, call for help. If not, put your hazard warning lights or signal on. If someone stops to help, ask them to get to a phone and call 999. If you're in a cab, ask the driver to radio for help.

2. If possible, help the mother into the back of the car. Place a coat, jacket, or blanket under her. Then proceed as on page 249. As soon as delivery is completed, continue to the nearest hospital in a hurry.

studies, the possibility of neonatal infection from bowel organisms is highly remote to begin with.) For these reasons, most hospitals have abandoned the routine enema.

Shaving the Pubic Area

'The idea of having my pubic hair shaved is unpleasant to me. Is it ever necessary?'

It is very unlikely you will have to have your pubic area shaved. It was once believed that pubic hair harboured bacteria which would infect the baby as it passed through the vaginal outlet. But since the entire area around the vagina is swabbed with an antiseptic solution prior to delivery, infection of this type is not likely. And in fact, some studies have shown a *higher* rate of infection among women who are shaved prior to delivery than those who aren't, probably because the small – sometimes microscopic – nicks which even very careful shaving can produce may serve as excellent breeding grounds for bacteria. From the woman's point of view, the humiliation of the shaving itself and the postpartum burning and itching as the hair grows back are

additional reasons to object to the procedure. In the UK now, shaving the area is almost never done.

Routine IVs

'When we had our visit to the hospital, I saw a woman being wheeled from the delivery room with an IV attached. Is that necessary with a normal labour and delivery?'

In some consultant units, it is routine to set up an IV (intravenous drip) containing a simple solution of nutrients and fluid for a woman in labour. This is done partly to be certain that the woman does not become dehydrated from lack of fluids or weak from lack of food during labour, partly to allow ready access for medication should the need arise (it's injected right into the IV bottle or line, instead of into the patient). In these instances, the IV is precautionary.

Some doctors and midwives, on the other hand, prefer to wait until there is a clear need for the IV – for instance, because the labour is lengthy and the labouring woman is weakening. Ask your doctor or midwife in advance what his or her policy is. If you strongly object to a routine IV, say so. It may be possible to hold off until the need for one arises.

If, however, it's your doctor's policy to give IVs routinely, or if you end up needing one, don't despair. The IV is only slightly uncomfortable as it's inserted and thereafter should barely be noticed. When it's hung on a movable stand, you can take it with you to the bathroom or on a brief constitutional.

Though you can't always make the decision about whether or not you should have an IV, you do have a right to know what the IV is pumping into your veins. Ask the nurse or doctor who inserts it. Or have your partner check the label on the bottle.

Foetal Monitoring

'My doctor believes in foetal monitoring at all births. I've heard that monitoring can lead to unnecessary caesareans and also makes labour more uncomfortable.'

For someone who's spent the first nine months of his or her life swimming peacefully in a warm and comforting amniotic bath, the trip through the narrow confines of the maternal pelvis will be no joy ride. Your baby will be squeezed, moulded, compressed, and pushed with every contraction.

It is because there is an element of risk in this stressful journey (and not to promote maternal discomfort or unnecessary caesareans) that foetal monitors have come into such common use. In some hospitals, all labour and delivery patients are electronically monitored. In virtually every hospital, at least half of the patients – particularly those in high-risk categories, who have meconium staining of the amniotic fluid, who are receiving oxytocin, or who are having a difficult labour – are monitored electronically.

A foetal monitor gauges the baby's response, via its heart rate, to the contractions of the uterus. The reader of the monitor printout may be able to pick up signs of foetal stress and distress through variations from the normal reactions to labour. Sometimes an alarm is preset to go off if such variations occur. Foetal monitoring can be external or internal:

External Monitoring. In this type of monitoring, used most frequently, two devices are strapped to the abdomen. One, an ultrasound transducer, picks up the foetal heartbeat. The other, a pressure-sensitive gauge, measures the intensity and duration of uterine contractions. Both are connected to a monitor which displays or prints out the readings. This doesn't mean the labouring woman must be confined to bed, hooked up to a machine, like Frankenstein's monster, for hours on end. In most cases, monitoring will be required only intermittently, and you will be able to walk around between readings.

During the second (pushing) stage of labour, when contractions may come so fast and furiously that some women aren't sure when to push and when to hold back, the monitor may accurately signal the beginning of each contraction, so that pushing can be most effective. Or the use of the monitor may be all but abandoned during this stage, so as not to interfere with the mother's concentration. In this case, the foetal heart rate will be checked periodically.

Internal Monitoring. When more accurate results are required – often when foetal distress is suspected – an internal monitor may be used. Since the electrode that reads the foetal heartbeat is clipped, or otherwise attached, to its scalp through the cervix, internal monitoring is possible only once the cervix is dilated to at least 1 or 2 centimetres and the membranes have ruptured. Contractions can be measured either with the pressure gauge strapped to the maternal abdomen or with a fluid-filled catheter (tube) inserted into the uterus. Because an internal monitor can't be periodically disconnected and reconnected, mobility is somewhat limited – but changes in position are possible.

Sometimes internal monitoring employs telemetry, which reads and transmits vital signs via radio waves. This technique, pioneered in the space programme, allows the patient to be monitored without being confined by equipment. With telemetry, the labouring woman is totally mobile – able to strike any position she finds comfortable, to go to the bathroom, or even to take strolls.

Like any invasive medical procedure (one that enters or intrudes upon the body), internal foetal monitoring entails some risk – mostly of infection. In some instances the foetus may later develop a rash, or occasionally an abscess, on the site where the electrode was placed, or, very rarely, may even have a permanent bald spot. It may also be possible that the insertion of the electrode causes momentary pain or discomfort to the baby. Because of the risks, though they are slight, internal foetal monitoring is best used when its benefits are significant.

If your foetal monitor signals trouble, don't panic. The technology is far from perfect and the machine often produces false readings. Sometimes it just isn't working right; sometimes it is misread. Frequently the mother's position causes an undesirable change in the foetal heart rate, because pressure on the baby's cord or her vena cava is interfering with blood flow to the foetus. A change in position often rectifies the problem. If administration of oxytocin is causing the problem, reducing the dosage or terminating the infusion completely will generally eliminate it. Oxygen to the mother may also do the trick.

If the abnormal readings continue, several possible steps can be taken. If the danger to the foetus seems great, the physician may opt for an immediate abdominal delivery. If the reading is inconclusive, there will be a speedy check for other indications of distress, such as meconium in the amniotic fluid or an abnormal foetal blood pH (taken from a scalp sample). In order to make these determinations, the membranes must be ruptured, which will probably be accomplished artificially at this point, if it hasn't already occurred spontaneously. A check of the mother's medical and obstetrical history may be made to see if the foetal heartbeat abnormalities might be related to maternal medication, infection, or chronic disease. An experienced and knowledgeable obstetrician will take all factors into account before concluding that the baby is actually in trouble. If foetal distress is diagnosed, then an immediate caesarean is usually called for. If, in the doctor or midwife's judgment, the baby is not threatened by labour, vaginal delivery will be allowed to continue.

It is estimated that foetal monitoring saves thousands of babies each year whose life-threatening difficulties in the birth canal would otherwise have gone unnoticed until it was too late. Yet because electronic monitoring has led to an increase in unnecessary caesareans in some hospitals (largely through misreadings), and because some view it as just another technological intrusion into the natural birthing process, its use remains controversial.

How expectant parents respond to the monitoring depends a great deal on their own attitudes. If they come into the labour or birthing room resentful and fearful of all that isn't 'natural,' they will probably find the foetal monitor objectionable. If they want the best of both worlds – the natural and the scientific – they will feel reassured and more in control at seeing their baby's heartbeats registering rhythmically on the bedside monitor.

The Sight of Blood

'The sight of blood makes me feel faint. What if I pass out while I'm watching my delivery?'

The sight of blood makes many people feel weak-kneed. But remarkably, though they might faint while watching a film of someone else's delivery, even the most squeamish women manage to get through their own without smelling salts.

First of all, there isn't all that much

blood – not much more than you see when you're menstruating (though there can be some additional bleeding with an episiotomy or a tear). Second, you won't be a spectator at your delivery – you'll be a very active participant, putting every ounce of your concentration and energy into pushing your baby those last few inches. Caught up in the excitement and anticipation, (and, let's face it, the pain and fatigue), you are very unlikely to notice, much less be unsettled by, any bleeeding. Few new mothers would be able to tell you just how much blood, if any, there was at their deliveries.

If you feel strongly that you don't want to see any blood, simply avert your eyes from the mirror (if one has been provided for you) during the episiotomy and at the moment of birth. Instead, just look down past your belly for a good view of the real thing as it emerges. From this vantage point, virtually no blood will be visible.

Episiotomy

'My childbirth teacher says we shouldn't have episiotomies – they aren't natural. My doctor says that's ridiculous. I don't know whether to have one or not.'

To have or not to have an episiotomy? That is the question that has many obstetricians shooting it out with some childbirth educators and feminists – catching pregnant women in the crossfire.

The minor surgical procedure which is the centre of this heated controversy was originated in Ireland in

1742 to help facilitate difficult births, but it wasn't commonly performed until the middle part of this century. Today, the episiotomy (a surgical incision made in the perineum to enlarge the vaginal opening just before the birth of the baby's head) is performed in 80% to 90% of first births, and in about 50% of subsequent deliveries.

There are two basic types of episiotomies: the midline and the mediolateral. The midline incision is made directly back toward the rectum. In spite of its advantages (it provides more space per inch of incision, heals well and is easier to repair, causes less blood loss, and results in less postpartum discomfort), it is far less frequently used because it has a greater risk of tearing completely through to the rectum. To avoid this tearing, most physicians prefer the medio-lateral incision, which slants toward the side, away from the rectum.

Traditional medical wisdom supports the use of episiotomy for several reasons. Its straight edges are easier to repair than a ragged tear; timed well, it can prevent injury to the muscles of the perineum and vagina; it spares the foetal head from battering against the perineum; and it can shorten the pushing stage of labour by 15 to 30 minutes – especially useful when there may be foetal distress and/or maternal exhaustion.

Opponents (including many antenatal teachers, midwives, and women) counter that episiotomies are an unnatural, largely unnecessary, technological intrusion into the birth process. They claim that the cuts made are often more extensive than tearing would be, and that they result in excessive bleeding, immediate postpartum discomfort, painful intercourse for months to come, and possible infection. Instead, they support the use of Kegel exercises and local massage to prepare and strengthen the perineum before delivery, and massage to gradually stretch the perineum during delivery, so that birth can take place without episiotomy and hopefully, without tearing.

What hard-liners (those who routinely perform episiotomies, even when they're not needed, and those who routinely refrain from performing them, even when they are needed) fail to recognize is that 'to have or not to have an episiotomy' is a question that shouldn't be answered in the classroom or the office – but in the delivery or birthing room, as the baby's head crowns. It is only then that an unbiased birthing attendant can make a realistic judgment as to whether or not the perineum can stretch sufficiently to accommodate the baby's head without tearing and without jeopardizing foetal or maternal well-being by prolonging labour. The prudent doctor or midwife who has some doubt will generally opt for the controlled episiotomy rather than risk an uncontrolled tear.

What decision should the expectant mother make on episiotomies? None. She can form an opinion and can discuss this opinion with her doctor or midwife so that it can be taken into account at the time of childbirth. But the decision is going to be made, and should be made, by the birthing attendant, with the speedy and safe delivery of the baby and the well-being of the mother the prime considerations.

Being Stretched by Childbirth

'The thing that frightens me most is my vagina stretching and tearing. Will I ever be the same again?'

The vagina is a remarkably elastic organ that is composed of accordion folds that open for childbirth. It is normally so narrow that inserting a tampon may be difficult, yet it can expand to allow the passage of a 7- or 8-pound baby without tearing. After birth, it returns to almost its original size – though some women report a slight increase in roominess. For those who were unusually small before conception, this is a plus, because intercourse becomes more pleasurable. For most others, the widening is slight, even imperceptible, and does not interfere with sexual enjoyment.

The perineum, the area between the vagina and the rectum, is also elastic, but less so than the vagina. In some women, the perineum will stretch enough without tearing to allow the birth of a baby. But in others, it will tear unless an episiotomy is performed by the birth attendant. Stretching may leave the muscles a little slacker than will a carefully timed episiotomy, one in which the perineum wasn't allowed to stretch excessively before the incision was made.

But exercising the muscles of childbirth long before you get to the delivery room may enhance elasticity and certainly will hasten their return to normal tone. Kegel exercises, which strengthen the perineal area (see page 323), should be done regularly during pregnancy and for at least six months following childbirth.

Many couples report that sex after delivery is even more satisfying than it was before, thanks to the increased muscular awareness and control a woman may develop as a result of prepared childbirth training.

In other words, you may not be the same after childbirth you may be even better!

The Use of Forceps

'I've heard all kinds of horror stories about forceps. What if my doctor wants to use them?'

It was in 1598 that British surgeon Peter Chamberlen the Elder designed the first pair of forceps, using the tong-shaped instrument to ease babies out of the birth canal when a difficult delivery might otherwise cost both mother and infant their lives. Instead of writing himself up in the latest obstetrical journal, however, Dr Chamberlen kept his discovery a secret – privy only to four generations of Chamberlen medical men and their patients, many of them royalty. Indeed, the use of forceps might have ended forever with the career of the last Chamberlen doctor had a hidden box of instruments not been uncovered beneath a floorboard in the family's ancestral home in the 1800s.

Today, forceps deliveries are used if the second stage needs to be speeded up. The reasons they are used include foetal distress; the failure of the baby to turn sufficiently to come through the birth canal; or a delay in second stage, when the head ceases to descend. This delay can be caused by a number of factors, including the baby's position, Pethidine or an epidural preventing full cooperation with contractions; exhaustion after a long labour; or the woman lying too flat on her back. In some cases, changing position to squatting and/or on all fours could help to start the head descending again, before forceps are used.

There are two types of forceps:–
1. 'High' Keillands or Neville-Barnes, to turn the baby's head from a difficult position, and then end the delivery.
2. 'Low' Wrigleys for lift out deliveries, to assist the woman to deliver her own baby.

For a forceps delivery, your legs will be put up in stirrups, then a local anaesthetic or pudendal block will be given, if you have not already had an epidural. An episiotomy will be made, then the two separate, curved blades (shaped rather like salad servers), will be slipped in on either side of the baby's head, then locked into position.

Vacuum extraction (ventouse) is sometimes used instead of forceps, for turning and delivering the baby, usually if it is necessary to speed up the delivery before the cervix is fully dilated. Your legs will be put up in stirrups, and a suction cap will be placed on the baby's head, and suction applied by a machine to help with the delivery.

In both forceps and ventouse deliveries, it is possible for you to help your baby to be born, by relaxing and pushing, whether or not you have had an epidural.

The Baby's Condition

'The doctor said the baby is okay, but her Apgar score was only 7. Is she really all right?'

Your doctor is right. Any Apgar score of 7 or over indicates the baby is in good condition. A score of under 4 indicates severe distress – but even most of these babies turn out to be normal and healthy.

The Apgar test was developed by the late Dr Virginia Apgar, a renowned paediatrician, to enable medical personnel to evaluate quickly the condition of a newborn. At 60 seconds after birth, the midwife or doctor checks the infant's *A*ppearance (colour), *P*ulse (heartbeat), *G*rimace (reflex), *A*ctivity (muscle tone), and *R*espiration. Hence the acronym, APGAR. (See Apgar Table, page 259.) Those who score between 4 and 6 often need resuscitation – which generally includes suctioning their airways and administering oxygen. Those who score under 4 require more dramatic lifesaving techniques.

The Apgar test is administered once again at five minutes after birth. If the score is 7 or better at this point, the outlook for the infant is very good. Though it has long been believed that a low score at five minutes often indicates future neurological trouble, more recent studies show little correlation between a low Apgar and later problems.

'The baby was distressed during childbirth. Then she was taken away from me immediately. Why?'

If the baby is in distress during childbirth, what will happen? In most cases of distress, the foetus is getting inadequate oxygen – because of compression of the cord, separation of the placenta, or for some other reason. At birth it is crucial to establish a good breathing pattern immediately. If the baby is breathing poorly or not at all, the midwife will first of all suck out any mucous that is in the lung. If necessary oxygen will then be administered through a face mask. If breathing problems persist, the baby will be taken to the special care baby unit (SCBU). It is usual for fathers to be able to visit the baby in the SCBU, and mothers are encouraged to spend as much time as possible with their babies.

What happens if my baby dies before she is born?

Unless a baby dies during labour, it is usual for parents to learn that their baby is no longer alive before the end of the pregnancy. The baby usually stops moving in the womb, and many women instinctively feel that there has been a change in their pregnancy.

The couple will come into hospital, often after being given some time at home to talk about the death, and to prepare themselves for labour. Labour may be induced, and allowed to progress as normal, or may start naturally, within a few days of the death of the baby.

Many midwives and doctors encourage parents to hold their baby, and give her a name, but this is a decision that must be made by both parents.

The woman will receive her postnatal care either on the postnatal ward, in a side room if at all possible or at home, according to her individual needs. Parents will be able to arrange their own funeral, or leave the arrangements to the hospital.

It is natural that you will both grieve about the loss of your baby. Allow yourself time to recover from the birth, and ask for support from your family and friends. Some useful organisations to contact are:–

Stillbirth and Perinatal Death Association.
37 Christchurch Hill, London NW3 1JY (01–794 4601).

Compassionate Friends.
5 Lower Clifton Hill, Clifton, Bristol. BS8 1BT (0272 292778 – office hours).

Foundation for the Study of Infant Deaths.
5th Floor, 4/5 Grosvenor Place, London SW1X 7HD (01–235 1721/01–245 9421).

What happens if my baby is handicapped?

This is a natural concern that all parents have at some stage of their pregnancy.

If your baby is born handicapped, it may be necessary for her to be taken to the SCBU (special care baby unit) soon after she or he is born. If at all possible you will be given a chance to cuddle and greet him or her in the delivery room, unless immediate medical attention is necessary.

Both of you will be given every opportunity to visit and care for your baby in SCBU. A hospital paediatrician will be available for you to discuss your baby's illness, and the likely course of treatment.

Apgar Table

SIGN	POINTS		
	0	1	2
Appearance (colour)*	Pale or blue	Body pink, extremities blue	Pink
Pulse (heartbeat)	Not detectable	Below 100	Over 100
Grimace (reflex irritability)	No response to stimulation	Grimace	Lusty cry
Activity (muscle tone)	Flaccid (no or weak activity)	Some movement of extremities	A lot of activity
Respiration (breathing)	None	Slow, irregular	Good (crying)

* In non-white children, colour of mucous membranes of mouth, of the whites of the eyes, of lips, palms, hands, and soles of feet will be examined.

You will be linked up with any support groups that exist, either locally or nationally, and given the opportunity to talk to other parents in a similar situation. When you return home, your community midwife and health visitor will be able to advise you about any further help that is available.

The baby is distressed when she is born. Why have they taken her away without showing her to us?

If your baby is not breathing strongly when he or she is born, it is necessary to make sure that she or he does so as soon as possible.

The midwife will take the baby and suck out any mucous that is in the lungs. If necessary, she or he will be given oxygen through a face mask. If there is still difficulty with breathing, he or she may be taken to the special care baby unit (SCBU). It is usual for fathers to be able to visit the baby in SCBU, and mothers are encouraged to spend as much time as possible with their babies, although they usually need to be escorted from the ward.

WHAT IT'S IMPORTANT TO KNOW
THE STAGES OF CHILDBIRTH

Few pregnancies seem as though they could have been lifted right from the pages of an obstetrical manual – with morning sickness that vanishes at the end of the first trimester, first foetal movements felt at precisely 20 weeks, and lightening that occurs exactly two weeks before the onset of labour. Likewise, few childbirth experiences mirror the textbook – commencing with mild regular contractions, widely spaced, and progressing at a predictable pace to delivery. Yet just as it's useful to have a general idea of what a typical woman can expect when she's expecting, it's valuable to know what an average childbirth is like – as long as you allow for the likelihood of variations that will make your experience yours alone.

Childbirth is divided (more loosely by nature, more rigidly by obstetrical science) into three stages. The first stage is labour, with its early, active, and transitional phases; the second stage is delivery, culminating in the birth of the baby; and the third is delivery of the placenta, or afterbirth. The whole process averages about 14 hours or less for first-time mothers, about 8 hours for women who have already had children.

All women who carry to term go through all three phases of labour, dilating from 0 to 10 centimetres in the process. Some, however, may not recognize that they are in labour until the second, or even the third, phase because their initial contractions were mild or painless. For a very few women, all of dilatation passes unnoticed; they don't realize they're in labour until they feel the urge to push that signals the second stage.

The timing and intensity of your contractions can help pinpoint where you are at any particular time. An internal exam, to check on the progress of dilatation, will confirm your progress.

THE FIRST STAGE OF CHILDBIRTH: LABOUR

The First Phase: Early or Latent Labour

This is usually the longest and, fortunately, the least intense phase of labour. The dilatation (or opening) of the cervix to 3 centimetres and the accompanying effacement (thinning out) which characterize this phase can be reached over a period of days or weeks with no noticeable or bothersome contractions, or over a period of two to six hours (and, less commonly, up to 24 hours) of unmistakable labour.

Contractions in this phase (if they are felt) usually last 30 to 45 seconds. They are mild to moderately strong, may be regular or irregular (between 5 and 20 minutes apart), and become progressively closer together, but not necessarily in a consistent pattern.

You will probably go to the hospital at the end of this phase or the beginning of the next.

What You May Be Feeling or Noticing. The most common signs and symptoms in this phase include backache (either with each contraction or constant), menstrual-like cramps, indigestion, diarrhoea, a sensation of warmth in the abdomen, bloody show (a blood-tinged mucus

Labour Positions

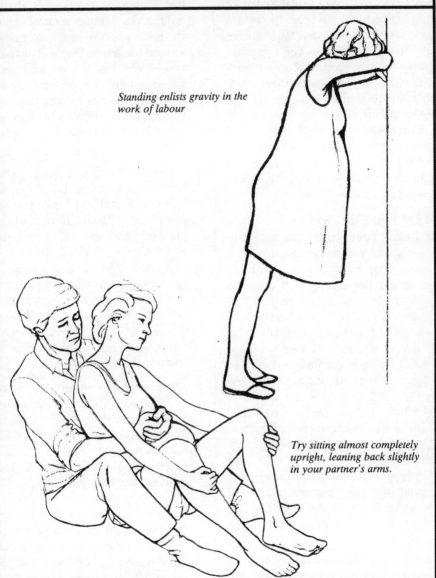

Standing enlists gravity in the work of labour

Try sitting almost completely upright, leaning back slightly in your partner's arms.

Talk to your doctor or midwife in advance about the possibility of remaining at least partially upright during labour: perhaps standing, walking, or sitting (in a rocking or beanbag chair, or in your partner's arms). Studies show that upright positions can shorten labour by speeding dilatation and descent – though the position that works best and is most comfortable varies from woman to woman. Lying flat on your back cannot only slow down labour, but can also compress important blood vessels (especially if you are on a firm surface), possibly interfering with blood flow to the foetus. If you are more comfortable lying down, lie on your side, switching sides and doing pelvic tilts periodically.

discharge). You may experience all of these, or just one or two. Membranes may have ruptured before the onset of contractions, but it is more likely that they will rupture sometime during labour itself. (If they don't rupture spontaneously, your doctor or midwife may elect to rupture them artificially anytime after you've gone into active labour.)

Emotionally, you may feel excitement, relief, anticipation, uncertainty, anxiety, fear; some women are relaxed and chatty, others tense and apprehensive.

What You Can Do:

☆ Relax. Your practitioner has probably told you not to call until you are in more active labour. Or he or she may have suggested that you call early on if labour begins during the day or if your membranes have ruptured. Definitely call, however, if your membranes have ruptured and the amniotic fluid is murky or greenish, if you have any bright red bleeding, or if you feel no foetal activity (it may be hard to notice because you are distracted by contractions, so you might want to try the test on page 231). Although you may not feel like it, it's best if you, not your partner, make the call and talk to the doctor. A lot can be lost in third-party translations.

☆ If it's the middle of the night, try to sleep (but not on your back; see page 157 for the recommended sleeping position). It's important to rest now, because you probably won't be able to later. And you needn't fear that you'll sleep through the next phase – the contractions will be too insistent. If sleep eludes you, don't just lie in bed timing contractions – that'll only make labour seem longer. Instead, get up and do things around the house that will distract you. Clean out a cupboard; put sheets on the baby's bed; finish packing your bag for the hospital (see page 241); make your partner a sandwich to take along; play solitaire.

☆ If you're labouring during daylight hours, go about your usual routine – as long as it doesn't take you far from home. If you have nothing planned, find something to keep you occupied. Try the distractions suggested above, take a walk (gravity aids the work of labour), watch TV, make and freeze a casserole or two for easy postpartum dining. Put your partner on alert, but it's not necessary for him to come running home – yet.

☆ Make yourself comfortable. Take a warm bath (only if your membranes haven't ruptured) or a shower; use a heating pad if your back is hurting – but *do not* take aspirin or lie on your back. A glass of wine may help you relax.

☆ Eat a light snack if you're hungry (broth, toast with apple butter, or fruit juice). Don't eat heavily, and avoid hard-to-digest foods, such as meats, dairy products, and fats. Not only will digesting a heavy meal compete with the birthing process for body resources, but a full stomach could cause problems if you should need anaesthesia later on.

On to the Hospital

Getting to the Hospital. Sometime near the end of the early phase or the beginning of the active phase (probably when your contractions are five minutes apart or less, sooner if you live far from the hospital or if this isn't your first baby), your doctor or midwife will have told you to pick up your bag and get going. Getting to the hospital will be easier if you've planned your route in advance, are familiar with parking regulations, and know which entrance will get you to the obstetrical floor more quickly. (If parking will be a problem, taking a cab may be more sensible.) You may be more comfortable if you stretch out in the rear seat with a blanket, if you've got chills, and a pillow for your head. Always phone the hospital to tell them you are coming.

Hospital Admission. Procedures will vary, but you can probably expect something like the following:

☆ On admission, brief details will be taken.

☆ Once in the labour and delivery suite, you will be taken to a labour or birthing room by your midwife for this shift. Depending on hospital regulations, your partner and family members may, rarely, be asked to wait outside while you are being admitted and 'prepped'. (Note to your partner: This is a good time to make a few priority phone calls, to get a snack, and to arrange for stowing your partner's luggage in her room and for chilling the celebratory champagne. If you aren't called to join your partner within 20 minutes or so, remind someone at the ward office. You may be asked to change into a sterile outfit.)

☆ Your midwife will take a brief history, asking, among other things, when the contractions started, how far apart they are, whether your waters have broken, when it was that you last ate.

☆ Your midwife will ask you for your signature on routine hospital consent forms.

☆ Your midwife will give you a hospital gown to change into and will request a urine sample. She will check your pulse, blood pressure, respiration, and temperature; inspect your perineum for leaking amniotic fluid, bleeding, or bloody show; listen to the foetal heartbeat with a stethoscope, or hook you up to a foetal monitor, and, possibly, evaluate the position of the foetus and take a blood sample.

☆ A midwife will examine you internally to see how far dilated and effaced your cervix is. If your membranes haven't ruptured spontaneously and you are at least 3 or 4 centimetres dilated (many practitioners prefer to wait until at least 5 centimetres of dilatation), your membranes may be artificially ruptured – unless it is decided to leave them intact until later in labour. The procedure is painless; all you will feel is a warm gush of fluid. The intensity of contractions may increase; for this reason, artificial rupture of the membranes is often useful in stimulating sluggish labour.

If you have any questions that haven't been answered before, now is the time to speak your mind. Have your partner speak it for you, if you don't feel up to it.

☆ Time contractions for a half-hour span if they seem to be getting closer than 10 minutes apart, and periodically even if they don't. But don't be a clock watcher.

☆ Urinate frequently to avoid bladder distention, which could inhibit the progress of labour.

☆ Use your relaxation techniques if they help, but don't start your breathing exercises yet, or you will be exhausted and bored long before you really need them.

What Your Partner Can Do.

☆ Practice timing contractions. The interval between contractions is timed from the beginning of one to the beginning of the next. Time them periodically, and keep a record. When they are coming less than 10 minutes apart, time them more frequently.

☆ Be a calming influence. During this early phase of labour, your most important function is to keep the expectant mother relaxed. And the best way to do this is to keep yourself relaxed, both inside and out. Your own anxiety and tension can be transferred to her unwittingly, communicated not just through words but through touch. Relaxation techniques, a gentle, unhurried massage, or a glass of wine may be helpful. It's too soon, however, to begin using breathing exercises.

☆ Keep your sense of humour, and help her keep hers; time flies, after all, when you're having fun. It'll be easier to laugh now than when contractions are coming fast and hard.

☆ Help distract the expectant mother. Suggest activities that will help keep both your minds off her labour; reading aloud, playing board games or cards, viewing engrossing (and preferably light) television fare, taking short walks.

☆ Offer comfort, reassurance, and support. She'll need them all from now on.

☆ Keep up your own strength, so you'll be able to reinforce hers. Eat periodically, even though she can't. Prepare a sandwich to bring along to the hospital (but nothing with an overpowering odour that might make you, or your partner, feel queasy – such as salami or tuna).

The Second Phase: Active Labour

The second, or active, phase of labour is usually shorter than the first, lasting an average of two to three-and-a-half hours (though variations on this average are great). The uterus's efforts are more concentrated now, accomplishing more in less time. With contractions becoming stronger and more frequent (generally three to four minutes apart and lasting 40 to 60 seconds), the cervix dilates to 7 centimetres. The pattern of contractions may still not be regular. Each contraction probably has a distinct peak (acme or apex) now, which constitutes from 40% to 50% of its total duration. There is less resting time between contractions.

You will probably be in the hospital by early in this phase.

What You May Be Feeling or Noticing. The most common signs and symptoms in this phase include increasing discomfort with contractions (you may be unable to talk through them now), increasing backache, leg discomfort, fatigue, increasing bloody show. You may experience all of these, or just one or two. Rupture of membranes may occur now if it hasn't earlier. (If they don't rupture spontaneously, your doctor or midwife may elect to rupture them artificially sometime during this phase.)

Emotionally, you may feel restless and find it more difficult to relax; or your concentration may become more intense, and you may become completely absorbed in the work at hand. Your confidence may begin to waver, and you may feel it's never going to end; or you may feel that things are really starting to happen.

What You Can Do:

☆ Start your breathing exercises, if you plan to use them, as soon as contractions become too strong to talk through. (If you have never practiced exercises, some simple breathing suggestions from the midwife may help make you more comfortable.) If the exercises seem to make you less comfortable, or more tense, however, you don't have to use them. Women have given birth without them for centuries.

☆ Don't eat or drink anything, but suck on ice chips to replace the fluids you're losing and to keep your mouth moist.

☆ Make a concerted effort to relax between contractions. This will be increasingly difficult as they come more frequently, but it is also increasingly important as your energy begins to wane.

☆ Walk around, if possible, or at least change position frequently, experimenting to see which provides the most comfort. (See page 261 for useful labour positions.)

☆ Remember to urinate periodically; because of tremendous pelvic pressure, you may not notice the urge to empty your bladder.

☆ If you feel you need some pain relief, don't be afraid to discuss it with your attendant. He or she may suggest waiting for 20 minutes or half an hour before actual administration – at which point you may have made so much progress that you won't need it, or you may have renewed strength and no longer want it.

What Your Partner Can Do:

☆ If possible, keep the door of the labour or birthing room closed, the lights low, and the room quiet to promote a restful atmosphere. Soft music, if permitted, may also help. Continue relaxation techniques between contractions. And stay as calm as possible yourself.

☆ Time the contractions. If your partner is on a foetal monitor, ask the doctor or the midwife to show you how to read it so that later, when contractions are coming one on top of the other, you can warn your partner as each new contraction begins. (The monitor may detect them before she can feel them.) You can also encourage her by telling her when each peak is ending. If there is no monitor, learn to recognize the arrival and departure of contractions by placing your hand on your partner's abdomen. This will give both of you some sense of control over the labour.

☆ Breathe with her through difficult contractions, if that helps her. Don't pressure her to do the exercises if she is uncomfortable with them, they make her tense, or they annoy her.

☆ If she shows any symptoms of hyperventilation (dizziness or lightheadedness, blurred vision, tingling and numbness of fingers and toes), have her exhale into a paper bag (the midwife will be able to supply one if you haven't brought one along) or into cupped hands. She should then inhale the exhaled air. After repeating this several times, she should feel better.

☆ Reassure your partner of her progress; praise, never criticize. Remind her to take her labour one contraction at a time, and that each pain brings her closer to seeing the baby.

☆ Massage her abdomen or back, or use counterpressure or any other techniques you've learned, to make her more comfortable. Take your cues from her; let her tell you what kind of stroking or touching or massage helps. If she prefers not to be touched at all (some women find it annoying), then it might be best to comfort her verbally.

☆ Don't pretend the pain doesn't exist; even if she doesn't verbalize it, tell her you know how uncomfortable she must feel. She needs your sympathy, not to have you avoid the subject.

☆ Remind her to relax between contractions.

☆ Remind her to urinate at least once an hour.

☆ Don't take it personally if she doesn't respond to – or even seems irritated by – your verbal comfort. A woman's moods during labour are mercurial. Stand by to offer support as she needs and wants it. Remember that your role is important, even if you sometimes feel superfluous.

☆ Be sure she has an ample supply of ice chips to suck on. From time to time ask her if she would like some.

☆ Use a damp washcloth to help cool her body and face; rechill it frequently.

☆ If her feet are cold, offer to get her a pair of socks and help her to put them on.

☆ Continue with distractions she finds useful (card games, conversation between contractions, reading aloud), encouragement, and support.

☆ Suggest a change of position; walk around with her, if that's possible.

☆ Serve as her go-between with medical personnel as much as possible. Intercept questions that you can answer, ask for explanations of procedures, equipment, any medication, so you'll be able to tell her what's happening. Be her advocate when necessary, but try to fight her battles quietly, perhaps outside the room, so that she won't be disturbed. (One thing you might want to check on now is if a mirror will be provided so that she can view the delivery.)

☆ If she requests medication, transmit her request to the midwife or doctor, but suggest a waiting period before the administration. During that time, the doctor will probably want to discuss the need for medication and to do an internal exam to check on the progress of labour. It's possible that a good progress report (or even just a brief period to think it over) may give your partner renewed strength to continue unmedicated. Don't be disappointed if she and the doctor or midwife decide that medication is needed. This isn't a test of endurance, and your partner hasn't failed if she needs some pain relief.

What Hospital Personnel Will Do:

☆ Provide a relaxed, comfortable, supportive environment, and answers to your questions and concerns.

☆ Continue monitoring the baby's condition with a stethoscope or electronic foetal monitor, and through observation of the amniotic fluid (greenish-brown staining is a sign of possible foetal distress). Foetal position may be assessed with external palpation.

☆ Continue checking your blood pressure.

☆ Periodically evaluate timing and strength of contractions and quantity and quality of bloody discharge. (Pads beneath your buttocks will be replaced as needed.) When there is an obvious change in the pattern or intensity of contractions, or the show becomes more bloody, an internal exam will be done to check the progress of your labour.

☆ Stimulate labour, if it is progressing very slowly, by the use of oxytocin, nipple self-stimulation, or artificial rupture of the membranes (if this wasn't done earlier).

☆ Possibly rupture your membranes, if they haven't ruptured spontaneously by the time you've reached the end of this phase.

☆ Administer sedatives and/or analgesics as needed and desired.

The Third Phase: Advanced Active or Transitional Labour

Transition is the most exhausting and demanding phase of labour. Suddenly, the intensity of the contractions picks up. They become very strong, two to three minutes apart, and 60 to 90 seconds long – with very intense peaks that last for most of the contraction. Some women, particularly women who have given birth before, experience multiple peaks. You may feel as though the contractions never completely disappear, and

If You Aren't Making Progress

Progress in labour is measured by the dilatation of the cervix and the descent of the foetus through the pelvis. Good progress is believed to require three main components: strong uterine contractions that effectively dilate the cervix; a baby that is small enough and in a position for easy exit, and a pelvis that is sufficiently roomy to permit the passage of the baby.

If one or more of these factors is not present, abnormal (or dysfunctional) labour, in which the progress is slow or nonexistent, generally occurs. There are several types of abnormal labour:

Prolonged Latent Phase – when little or no dilatation occurs after 20 hours of labour in a first-time mother, or after 14 hours in one who has delivered previously. Sometimes progress is slow because labour hasn't really begun, and the contractions felt are those of false – not real – labour. Sometimes the reason is overmedication before labour is well established. Sometimes, it is theorized, the cause may be psychological: a woman (almost always a first-time mother) panics when labour begins, triggering the release of chemicals in the brain that interfere with uterine contractions.

In general, the practitioner may suggest stimulating a slow first phase of labour with activity (such as walking) or the opposite (sleep and rest, possibly aided by the use of relaxation techniques or an alcoholic drink and, if the labouring woman is too agitated to relax naturally, the administration of a sedative). Such treatment will also help rule out false labour (the contractions of false labour will usually subside with activity, an alcoholic drink, or a nap). Once true latent phase labour is established, it may be speeded up with an enema or mineral oil, with nipple self-stimulation, or with the administration of oxytocin. (It is also a good idea to urinate periodically, as a full bladder could interfere with descent.) If these tactics are unsuccessful, the practitioner may explore the possibility of a disproportion in size between the foetus's head and the mother's pelvis (foetopelvic disproportion). A caesarean will usually be performed after 24 or 25 hours (sometimes sooner) if insufficient progress has been made by that time.

Primary Dysfunction of Active Phase – when the second, or active, phase of labour progresses very slowly (less than 1 to 1.2 centimetres per hour in women having their first babies, and 1.5 centimetres per hour in those with previous deliveries). When any progress, albeit slow progress, is being made, many practitioners will let the uterus set its own pace – on the theory that the

---

that you can't completely relax between them. The final 3 centimetres of dilatation, to 10 centimetres, will probably take place in a very short time: on average, 15 minutes to an hour.

What You May Be Feeling or Noticing. In transition, you are likely to feel strong pressure on the lower back and/or perineum. Rectal pressure, with or without an urge to push or move bowels, may cause you to grunt involuntarily. Body temperature may be erratic. You may feel either very warm and sweaty or chilled and shaky, or alternate between the two. Your bloody vaginal show will increase as capillaries in the cervix rupture; your legs may be crampy and cold and may tremble uncontrollably. You may

woman will eventually deliver naturally, as two thirds of those who experience primary dysfunction do. (Most of the remaining one third will end up being delivered surgically because of a foetopelvic disproportion. Such a mismatch is frequently suspected when progress of labour ceases completely, and can often be confirmed by ultrasound and other examinations.) A labouring woman may be able to speed up the work of her uterus by walking, if possible, staying off her back, and keeping her bladder empty. Intravenous fluids will probably be administered during a lengthy labour.

Secondary Arrest of Dilatation – when, during active labour, there is no progress for two hours or more. In about half of these cases, it is estimated, foetopelvic disproportion exists, necessitating a caesarean delivery. This is a situation where the size and shape of the baby does not match that of the pelvis, which is likely to lead to complications during birth, i.e. the baby becomes stuck and unable to move down the birth canal, so it cannot be delivered vaginally. In most other cases, oxytocin (sometimes along with artificial rupture of the membranes) will reestablish labour, particularly when a uterus is only suffering from exhaustion. Again, the woman may be able to make some contribution to the battle against sluggish labour by utilizing gravity (sitting upright, squatting, standing, when possible) and keeping her bladder empty.

Abnormal Descent of the Foetus – when the baby moves down the birth canal at a rate of less than 1 centimetre per hour in women having their first babies, or 2 centimetres per hour in others. In most such cases delivery will be slow, but otherwise uneventful. Stimulation with oxytocin and/or artificial rupture of the membranes are the usual methods – once foetopelvic disproportion and a foetal position which would make vaginal delivery difficult have been ruled out.

Prolonged Second Stage – one that lasts longer than two hours in a first delivery, or slightly less in subsequent deliveries. Many doctors routinely use outlet forceps or perform a caesarean when a second stage goes beyond two hours; others allow the spontaneous vaginal delivery to continue if progress is being made and both mother and foetus (whose conditions are carefully monitored) are doing well. Sometimes the baby's head will be gently eased out those last few inches with outlet forceps. Rotation of the head (so that it faces front, providing for a better fit through the pelvis) may also be attempted, either manually or with outlet forceps. Gravity, again, can help; a semi-sitting or semi-squatting position is most effective for delivery.

experience nausea and/or vomiting; and sleepiness may overcome you between contractions as oxygen flow is shifted from your brain to the site of the delivery. Not surprisingly, you may feel exhausted.

Emotionally, you may feel vulnerable and overwhelmed, as though you're reaching the end of your rope. In addition to frustration over not being able to push yet, you may feel irritable, disoriented, discouraged, restless, and have difficulty concentrating and relaxing (it may seem impossible).

What You Can Do:

☆ Hang in there. By the end of this phase, your cervix will be fully dilated, and it will be time to push your baby out.

☆ Instead of thinking about the work

ahead, try to think about how far you've come.

☆ If you feel the urge to push, pant or blow instead, unless you've been instructed otherwise. Pushing against a cervix that isn't completely dilated can cause the cervix to swell, which can delay delivery.

☆ If you don't want anybody to touch you unnecessarily, if your partner's once comforting hands now irritate you, don't hesitate to let him know.

☆ If you find them useful, use breathing techniques you have learned (or ask the midwife for suggestions), adjusting them to the intensity of your contractions.

☆ Try to relax between contractions (if you find it humanly possible) with slow, rhythmic chest breathing.

What Your Partner Can Do:

☆ Be specific and direct in your instructions, without wasting words. She may find small talk annoying. If she doesn't want your help at any point and wants to be left alone, take her cue without feeling helpless or rejected.

☆ Offer lots of encouragement and praise, unless she would prefer you to keep quiet. At this moment, eye contact may communicate more expressively than words.

☆ Touch her only if she finds it comforting. Abdominal massage may be offensive now, though counterpressure may be helpful if her back hurts.

☆ Breathe with her through every contraction, if it helps her through them.

☆ Remind her to take one contraction at a time. She may need you to warn her when each begins, and to tell her as it declines.

☆ Help her relax between contractions, touching her abdomen lightly to show her when a contraction is over. Remind her to use slow, rhythmic breathing.

☆ If her contractions seem to be getting closer and/or she feels the urge to push – and she hasn't been examined recently – tell the doctor or midwife. She may be fully dilated.

☆ Offer her ice chips frequently, and mop her brow with a cool damp cloth often.

What Hospital Personnel May Do:

☆ Continue comfort and support.

☆ Continue monitoring your condition and that of the foetus.

☆ Continue checking duration and intensity of contractions, and the progress you are making.

☆ Prepare for delivery, ultimately moving you to a delivery room, if you are not delivering in a birthing or labour room.

☆ Administer anaesthesia if planned or needed.

THE SECOND STAGE OF CHILDBIRTH: PUSHING AND DELIVERY

Your active participation in the birth of your child has been, up to this point, negligible. Though you've undeniably taken the brunt of the proceedings, your cervix and uterus (and baby) have done most of the work. But now that the task of dilatation has been completed, your help is needed to push the baby down, through the birth canal, and out. This generally takes between half an hour and an hour, but can be accomplished in 10 short minutes or in two to three very long hours.

The contractions of the second stage are more regular than the contractions of transition. They are still about 60 to 90 seconds long, but sometimes farther apart (usually about two to five minutes) and possibly less painful – though sometimes they are more intense. There now should be a well-defined rest period, although you may still have trouble recognizing the onset of each new contraction.

What You May Be Feeling or Noticing. Common in the second stage is an overwhelming urge to push (although not every woman has it). You may experience a burst of renewed energy (a kind of second wind) or fatigue; tremendous rectal pressure; very visible contractions, with the uterus rising noticeably with each; a possible increase in bloody show; a tingling, stretching, burning, or stinging sensation at the vagina as the head crowns; and a slippery wet feeling as the baby emerges.

Emotionally, you may feel relieved that you can now start pushing (though some women feel embarrassed or inhibited); you may also feel exhilarated and excited or, if the pushing stretches on for much more than an hour, frustrated or overwhelmed. In prolonged second stages, the woman's preoccupation is often less with seeing the baby than with getting the ordeal over with; this is a natural, and temporary, reaction, which in no way reflects on her capacity for motherly love.

What You Can Do:

☆ Get into a pushing position (which one will depend upon hospital policy, your practitioner's predilection, the bed or chair you are in, and hopefully, what is most comfortable and effective for you). A semi-sitting or semi-squatting position is probably the best because it enlists the aid of gravity in the birthing process and affords you more pushing power.

☆ Give it all you've got. The more efficiently you push, and the more energy you pack into the effort, the more quickly your baby will make that trip through the birth canal. But keep your work coordinated and rhythmical. Listen carefully to instructions. Frantic, disorganized pushing wastes energy and accomplishes little.

A Baby Is Born

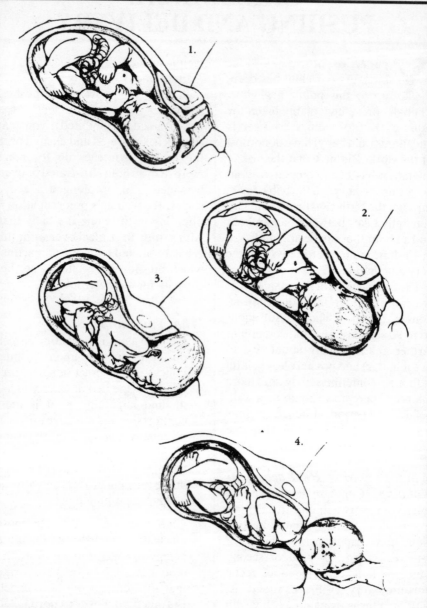

1. *The cervix has thinned (effaced) somewhat, but has not begun to dilate.* **2.** *The cervix has fully dilated and the baby's head has begun to press into the birth canal (vagina).* **3.** *To allow the narrowest diameter of the baby's head to fit through the mother's pelvis, the baby usually turns sometime during labour. Here the slightly moulded head has crowned.* **4.** *The head, the baby's broadest part, is out. The rest of the delivery should proceed quickly and smoothly.*

☆ Don't let inhibition or embarrassment break the pushing rhythm. Since you're bearing down on the whole perineal area, anything that's in your bowels may be pushed out, too; trying to control your bowels while you're pushing will impede your progress. A little involuntary evacuation is experienced by nearly everyone in delivery – even by some women who've had enemas. No one else in the room will think twice about it, and neither should you. Sterile pads will be used to whisk away any excretion immediately.

☆ Do what comes naturally. Push when you feel the urge, unless otherwise instructed. Take a few deep breaths while the contraction is building; take another and hold it. Then, as the contraction peaks, push with all your might until you can no longer comfortably hold your breath. You may feel as many as five urges to bear down with each contraction. Follow each urge, rather than trying to hold your breath and push through an entire contraction; breath-holding for long periods of time can exhaust you and may deprive the foetus of oxygen. Several deep breaths as the contraction wanes will help restore your respiratory balance. If nothing seems to be coming naturally – and it doesn't for every woman – your doctor or midwife will help direct your efforts, and redirect them if you lose your concentration.

☆ Be sure your thighs and perineum are relaxed as you push. Tenseness works against your pushing efforts.

☆ Stop pushing when you're instructed to (as you may be, to keep the baby's head from being born too rapidly). Pant or blow instead.

☆ Rest between contractions, with the help of your partner and the attendants. If you are very exhausted, especially when the second stage drags on, your practitioner may suggest that you don't push for several contractions so you can rebuild your strength.

☆ Don't become frustrated if you see the baby's head crown, then disappear again. Birthing is a two-steps-forward, one-step-backward proposition.

☆ Remember to keep an eye on the mirror (if one is available). Seeing your baby's head crown (and reaching down and touching it, if your practitioner approves) will give you the inspiration to push when the pushing gets tough. Besides, unless your partner is video-taping, there won't be any replays.

What Your Partner Can Do:

☆ Continue giving comfort and support, but don't feel hurt if your partner doesn't seem to notice you're there. Her energies are necessarily focused elsewhere.

☆ Guide her pushing and breathing, using the cues that you have both become familiar with during childbirth preparation; or relay instructions from the midwife or doctor.

☆ Don't feel intimidated by the

Pain Risk Factors

Your Perception of pain may be increased by:	It may be decreased by:
Being alone.	Having the company and support of those you love, and/or experienced medical personnel.
Fatigue.	Being well rested (try not to overdo things during the ninth month); trying to rest and relax between contractions.
Hunger and thirst.	Having light snacks during early labour; sucking ice chips throughout.
Thinking about and expecting pain.	Turning your mind to other thoughts and distractions; thinking of contractions in terms of how much they accomplish, rather than how much they hurt; and remembering that no matter how intense the discomfort, it will be of relatively brief duration.
Anxiety and stress; tensing up during contractions.	Using relaxation techniques between contractions; concentrating on your efforts during them.
Fear of the unknown.	Learning as much as you can about childbirth in advance; taking childbirth one contraction at a time; and not worrying about what's to come.
Self-pity.	Thinking about how lucky you are and about the wonderful reward to come.
Feeling out of control and helpless.	Having good childbirth preparation; knowing enough to feel some measure of control and confidence.

finesse and expertise of the professional medical team around you. Your presence is important, too. And in fact, your whispered 'I love you' may be more valuable to her at this stage than anything their experience can offer.

☆ Help her to relax between contractions, with soothing words, a cool cloth applied to forehead, neck, and shoulders, and, if feasible, back massage or counterpressure to help ease backache.

☆ Continue to supply ice chips to moisten her parched mouth, as needed.

☆ Support her back while she's pushing, if necessary; hold her hand, wipe her brow, stroke her arm – or do whatever seems to help her. If she slips out of position, help her back up.

☆ Periodically point out her progress. As the baby begins to crown, remind her to keep an eye on the mirror so she can have visual confirmation of what she is accomplishing; when she's not looking, or if there's no mirror, give her inch-by-inch descriptions. Take her hand and touch the head together for renewed inspiration (with the doctor or midwife's okay).

☆ If you're offered the opportunity to 'catch' your baby as it emerges or, later, to cut the cord, don't panic. Both are easy – and you'll get step-by-step directions, support, and backup from the attendants.

What Hospital Personnel May Do:

☆ Move you to the room in which you will deliver, if you aren't already there.

☆ Give support and direction to you as the delivery progresses.

☆ Continue to check the condition of the foetus, usually by foetal monitor.

☆ About the time the head crowns, prepare for the delivery – spreading sterile drapes and arranging instruments, donning surgical garments and gloves, dousing the perineal area with antiseptic.

☆ Perform an episiotomy just before the head is delivered, if necessary. (This will be painless if done at the height of a contraction, when the pressure of the baby's head naturally numbs the perineum, though the midwife may administer a local anaesthetic.)

☆ Elect to use outlet forceps to ease the baby's head out if the second stage lasts more than two hours (some doctors will wait longer if mother and baby are doing well), if the baby shows signs of difficulty tolerating the stresses of labour, if your medical condition prohibits further pushing, or if progress is impeded because of a slightly irregular foetal presentation or a slight disproportion between foetus and pelvis. (See Forceps Delivery, page 256.) A regional anaesthetic will be administered if an epidural or other block hasn't already been given, because forceps delivery can be painful. If forceps aren't feasible or don't work, a caesarean may be the safest route to delivery for baby and you.

☆ Once the head emerges, quickly suction the baby's nose and mouth to remove mucus, then assist the shoulders and torso out.

☆ Clamp and cut the umbilical cord, possibly with the newborn lying across your abdomen. Your partner may be asked to do the snipping. (Some practitioners prefer to wait until the placenta is delivered or the cord has stopped pulsating before cutting the cord.)

☆ Provide initial protective care for the newborn: evaluate his or her condition, and rate it on the Apgar scale at one minute and five minutes after birth (see page 259); give a brisk, stimulating, and drying rubdown; attach a bracelet with your name on it to the baby's wrist; weigh the baby, and wrap him or her for warmth. (In some hospitals additional procedures

A First Look at Baby

Those who expect their babies to arrive as round and smooth and pink as a Botticelli cherub may be in for a shock. Nine months of soaking in an amniotic bath and a dozen or so hours of sausage-like compression in a contracting uterus and cramped birth canal take their toll on a newborn's appearance.

Fortunately, most of the less-lovely newborn characteristics which follow are temporary. One morning, a couple of months after you've brought your wrinkled, slightly scrawny, puffy-eyed bundle home from the hospital, you'll wake to find that the Botticelli cherub has taken its place in the crib.

An Oddly Shaped Head. At birth, the infant's head is, proportionately, the largest part of the body, as wide around as the chest. As the baby grows, the rest of the body will catch up. Often, the head has moulded to fit through the mother's pelvis, giving it an odd, possibly pointed shape; pressing against an inadequately dilated cervix can further distort the head by raising a lump (called caput succedaneum). The caput will disappear in a day or two; the moulded look within two weeks – at which point your baby's head will begin to take on a Botticelli roundness.

Newborn Hair. The hair that covers the head at birth may have little relationship to the hair the baby will have later. Some newborns are virtually bald; others have thick thatches. Either way, the newborn hair will eventually fall out and be replaced by new growth.

Vernix Caseosa Coating. The cheesy substance that coats the foetus in the uterus is believed to protect the skin from the long exposure to the amniotic fluid. Premature babies have quite a bit of this coating at birth, postmature babies have almost none, except in the folds of their skin and under their fingernails.

---

may be performed in the delivery room; in others they will be attended to later, in the nursery.)

☆ Show your now cleaned-up baby to you and your partner. Depending on the situation and hospital policy, you may be able to hold the baby briefly or for a longer period. If there's time, and if you wish to, you may be able to try breastfeeding (Don't worry if you or your baby don't catch on immediately – see Getting Started Breastfeeding, page 298).

THE THIRD STAGE OF CHILDBIRTH: DELIVERY OF THE PLACENTA, OR AFTERBIRTH

The worst is over, the best has already come. All that remains is the tying up of loose ends, so to speak. During this final stage of childbirth (which generally lasts anywhere from five minutes to half an

Swelling of the Genitals. This is common in both male and female newborns, and is particularly pronounced in boy babies delivered via caesarean. The breasts of newborns, male and female, may also be swollen (occasionally even engorged, secreting a white substance nicknamed 'witch''s milk') due to stimulation by maternal hormones. The hormones may also stimulate a milky-white, even blood-tinged, vaginal secretion in girls. These effects are not abnormal, and disappear in a week to 10 days.

Lanugo. Fine downy hair, called lanugo, may cover the shoulders, back, forehead, and temples of full-term babies. This will usually be shed by the end of the first week. Such hair can be more abundant, and will last longer, in a premature baby.

Eyes. Caucasian babies' eyes are almost always a slate blue, no matter what colour they will be later on. In darker-skinned races, the eyes are brown at birth.

Birthmarks and Skin Lesions. A reddish blotch at the base of the skull, on the eyelid, or on the forehead is very common, especially in Caucasians. Mongolian spots, bluish-grey pigmentation of the deep skin layer that can appear on the back, buttocks, and sometimes the arms and thighs, are more common in Asians, Southern Europeans, and blacks. These markings will eventually disappear, usually by the time a child is four years old. Hemangiomas, elevated bright strawberry-coloured marks, vary from tiny to about quarter-size. They will eventually fade to a mottled pearly grey, then disappear entirely. Coffee-with-cream-coloured spots can appear anywhere on the body; they are usually inconspicuous, and don't fade. A variety of rashes, tiny 'pimples,' and whiteheads may also mar the newborn complexion, but all are temporary.

hour or more) the placenta, which has been your baby's life support inside the womb, will be delivered. You will continue to have mild contractions of approximately one minute's duration, though you may not feel them. The pressure these contractions exert separates the placenta from the uterus and moves it down into the lower segment of the uterus or into the vagina so you can push it out. Once the placenta is delivered, any necessary stitching up of episiotomy or tears will be taken care of.

What You May Be Feeling or Noticing.
Now that your work is done, you may feel fatigue or, conversely, a burst of renewed energy. You are likely to be very thirsty and, especially if labour has been long, hungry. Some women experience chills in this stage; all experience a bloody vaginal discharge (called lochia) comparable to that of a heavy menstrual period.

For many women, the immediate emotional reaction is a sense of relief. There may also be exhilaration and talkativeness, elation tempered by a new sense of responsibility, impatience at having to push out the placenta or submit to the repair of the episiotomy or tear, though you may be too excited or tired to care. Some women feel a strong closeness to their husbands and an immediate bond with their new baby; others feel somewhat detached (who is this stranger at my breast?), even resentful (how he's made me suffer!), particularly after a difficult delivery. (See pages 165, 238, 292 for more on bonding and new mother love.)

What You Can Do:

☆ Help expel the placenta, by pushing as directed.

☆ Hold still and be patient while any repair of episiotomy or tears is being done.

☆ Nurse or hold the baby, though your husband may do the holding until the placenta is expelled. In some hospitals, and under some circumstances, the baby may be kept in a heated bassinette for a while.

☆ Take pride in your accomplishment, relax, and enjoy!

What Your Partner Can Do:

☆ Give the new mother some well-earned words of praise.

☆ Share in bonding with the new baby.

☆ Don't forget to do some bonding with your partner, too.

☆ Ask the midwife for some juice for your partner; she'll be very dry. After she's been rehydrated, and if both of you are in the mood, break out the bubbly you've had the hospital staff keep chilled.

☆ Take pictures, if you've brought your camera, or tape the baby's first cries, if you have your tape recorder along.

What Hospital Personnel May Do:

☆ Help extract the placenta. The exact procedure will vary depending upon the practitioner and the situation. Some will pull the cord gently with one hand while pressing and kneading the uterus with the other; others will exert downward pressure on the top of the uterus. Many physicians will use oxytocin, by injection or IV, to encourage uterine contractions, which will speed expulsion of the placenta and minimize bleeding.

☆ Examine the placenta to be sure it is intact. If it isn't, the practitioner will inspect the uterus manually for placental fragments and remove any that remain.

☆ Cut the cord, if it wasn't cut earlier.

☆ Stitch an episiotomy or tear, if any. A local anaesthetic (if none was previously given, or if it has worn off) will probably be used to numb the area.

☆ Check your vaginal bleeding.

☆ Sponge bath the lower part of your body, help you into a clean gown, and help you put on a perineal pad (sanitary pad held in place by a belt).

☆ Wheel you into the recovery room, or to your own room.

BREECH DELIVERY

As far as the mother and father are concerned, labour and vaginal delivery of a breech baby don't differ much from that of a vertex (head-down) baby; tips for coping and comforting are virtually identical. The activities of the hospital staff will be different, however, and will vary further depending on the type of breech position and the delivery procedure that the' practitioner elects to follow.

Up until the second stage, a vaginal breech delivery progresses about the same as a vertex delivery. But it is always considered a trial labour, allowed to proceed only as long as it progresses normally. Because of the ever-present possibility that a caesarean may become necessary, you will probably be transferred to a delivery/operating room at the end of the first stage. Depending upon your baby's exact breech position, your doctor will determine the safest and most effective way to proceed. (What is most advisable in such a case also depends on the practitioner's experience. Asking a doctor to perform a procedure for breech extraction that you've read or heard about, but with which he or she is not comfortable, is *never* in your or your baby's best interest.)

A common procedure is to allow the baby to deliver naturally until the legs and lower half of the torso are out. Then a local anaesthetic is administered and the shoulders and head are delivered by the practitioner, with or without the aid of forceps.

A vaginal delivery is not likely to be attempted if the baby is in the complete breech (see page 213) or footling breech (with one leg dangling down) position, if the foetus is estimated to be oversized or the mother's pelvis inadequate, if the delivery is premature, or if there are signs of foetal distress.

A large episiotomy is often necessary with a breech, but occasionally it can be avoided. The delivery position for the vaginal breech birth will vary, again depending on the situation and on your practitioner's experience. Some find they have more control if the woman is flat on her back, legs up in stirrups. Others suggest that a woman may be more comfortable if she is placed in a sitting position.

Once the baby is delivered, the proceedings continue as with a vertex birth.

CAESAREAN SECTION: SURGICAL DELIVERY

At a caesarean delivery, unlike a vaginal one, you won't be able to participate actively. And, in fact, your most important contribution to the comfort and success of your baby's caesarean birth can be made before you arrive at the hospital – possibly before you even know that you're having a caesarean. That contribution is preparation. Being prepared both intellectually and emotionally for a caesarean, in case it should become necessary, will minimize the disappointment many women feel and help make your surgical delivery experience a positive one.

Thanks to regional anaesthesia and the liberalization of hospital regulations, most women (and often their husbands) are able to be spectators at their caesarean deliveries. Because they aren't preoccupied with pushing or discomfort, they are often able to relax and appreciate the birth – something women delivering vaginally can rarely do.

This is what you can expect in a typical caesarean birth:

☆ Your pubic and/or abdominal hair may be shaved, and a catheter (a narrow tube) will be inserted into your bladder to keep it empty and out of the surgeon's way.

☆ In the operating room, sterile drapes will be arranged around your exposed abdomen, which will be washed down with an antiseptic solution. If you are to be awake for the delivery, a screen will be put up at about shoulder level, so that you won't see the incision being made.

☆ An IV infusion will be started to provide easy access if additional medication is needed.

☆ Either an epidural or a spinal block (which numb the lower part of your body but allow you to be awake) or a general anaesthetic (which puts you to sleep – sometimes necessary when the baby must be delivered immediately) will be administered.

☆ If your partner is going to attend the delivery, he will be suited up in sterile garb. He will sit near your head, giving you support, holding your hand, and has the option of viewing the actual surgery. (Whether or not you know in advance you are going to have a caesarean, it's a good idea to discuss with your doctor ahead of time the possibility of your spouse being with you in case you do need surgery.)

☆ If yours is an emergency caesarean, things may move very quickly. Don't be upset by the seeming storm of activity around you. In such a situation, hospital policy, expediency, and concern for the safety of you and your baby may dictate that your husband leave during the delivery, which will only take about 5 or 10 minutes. You should both be prepared for this possibility.

☆ Once the physician is certain that the anaesthetic has taken effect, an incision (a cut) is made in the lower abdomen. If you are awake, you may feel a sensation of being 'unzipped,' but no pain.

☆ A second incision is then made, this time in the lower segment of your uterus. The amniotic sac is ruptured and the fluid suctioned out; you may hear a sort of gurgling or swooshing sound.

☆ The baby is then eased out, either by hand or with forceps, usually with an assistant pressing on the upper end of the uterus. With an epidural (though not likely with a spinal block), you will probably feel some pulling and tugging sensations, as well as some pressure. If you're anxious to see your baby's arrival, ask the doctor if the screen can be lowered briefly, which will allow you to see the actual birth, but not the more graphic details.

☆ Your baby's nose and mouth are then suctioned; you'll hear the first cry, and if the cord is long enough, you will be allowed a quick glimpse.

☆ The cord will be quickly clamped and cut, and while the baby is getting the same routine attention as a vaginally delivered infant, the doctor manually removes the placenta.

☆ Now the doctor will check your reproductive organs quickly and stitch up the incisions that were made.

☆ An injection of oxytocin may be given intramuscularly or into your IV bottle, to help contract the uterus and control bleeding.

☆ Depending upon your condition and the baby's, as well as hospital rules, you may or may not be able to hold the baby right there in the delivery room. If you can't, perhaps your husband can. If the infant has to be whisked away to the ICU nursery, don't fret. This is standard in many hospitals and doesn't indicate a problem with the baby's condition. As far as bonding is concerned, later can be just as good as sooner.

Part 3

LAST BUT NOT LEAST:

Postpartum, Fathers, and the Next Baby

15
Postpartum: The First Week

WHAT YOU MAY BE FEELING

Physically:

☆ Bloody vaginal discharge (lochia), turning pinkish toward week's end

☆ Afterpain in abdomen after first 24 hours

☆ Exhaustion, particularly if labour was difficult

☆ Perineal discomfort and/or pain and numbness, if you had a vaginal delivery (especially if you had stitches)

☆ Incisional pain and, later, numbness in the area, if you had a caesarean delivery (especially if it was your first)

☆ Sitting and walking may be uncomfortable if you had an episiotomy or a caesarean

☆ Difficulty urinating for a day or two

☆ Difficulty and discomfort with bowel movements for the first few days after delivery; constipation

☆ Sweating, possibly profuse, after the first couple of days

☆ Breast discomfort and engorgement about the third or fourth postpartum day

☆ Sore or cracked nipples, if you are breastfeeding

Emotionally:

☆ Elation, depression, or swings between the two

☆ Feelings of inadequacy and trepidation about mothering, especially about breastfeeding if you're nursing

☆ Frustration, if you're still in the hospital and would like to leave

☆ Little interest in sex; or less commonly, increased desire (intercourse won't be okayed until at least three weeks postpartum)

WHAT YOU MAY BE CONCERNED ABOUT

Bleeding

'I'd been told to expect a bloody discharge after delivery, but when I got out of bed for the first time and saw the blood running down my legs, I was really frightened.'

Don't be alarmed. This discharge of leftover blood, mucus, and tissue from your uterus, known as lochia, is normally as heavy as (sometimes even heavier than) a menstrual period for the first three postpartum days. And though it'll probably seem more copious than it really is, it may total up to two cups before it begins to taper off. A sudden gush on getting out of bed in the first few days is common, and no cause for concern. And since blood and an occasional blood clot are the predominant ingredients of lochia during the immediate postpartum period, your discharge will be quite red for two or three days, gradually turning to a watery pink, then to brown, and finally to yellowish white over the next week or two. Sanitary napkins, not tampons, should be used to absorb the flow, which may continue on and off for as long as six weeks.

Breastfeeding and the intramuscular or intravenous administration of oxytocin (routinely ordered by some doctors following delivery) may both reduce the flow of lochia by encouraging uterine contractions and helping to shrink the uterus back to normal size more quickly. The contraction of the uterus after delivery is important because it pinches off exposed blood vessels at the site where the placenta separated from the uterus, thus preventing haemorrhage. If the uterus is too relaxed and doesn't contract, excessive bleeding occurs. This can happen for several reasons: a long, exhausting labour; a traumatic delivery; a uterus that was over-distended because of multiple births, a large baby, or excess amniotic fluid; an oddly placed placenta, or one that separated prematurely; fibroids that prevent symmetrical contraction of the uterus; or generally weakened condition of the mother at the time of delivery (due to, for example, anaemia, pre-eclampsia, or extreme fatigue).

Postpartum haemorrhage can also occur because of lacerations to the genital tract, or because fragments of the placenta have been retained in the uterus. (In the latter case, bleeding may not occur until a week or two after delivery.) Occasionally internal bleeding causes swelling and severe pain over the site. Rarely, haemorrhage is caused by a previously undetected bleeding disorder. Infection can also cause postpartum haemorrhage, right after delivery or weeks later.

Most postpartum haemorrhages occur about 7 to 14 days after delivery, without any warning. Since this relatively rare complication of childbirth can be life-threatening, prompt diagnosis and treatment are vital. Any of the following signs of abnormal bleeding (some of which are also signs of postpartum infection) should be reported immediately to your doctor.

☆ Bleeding that saturates more than one pad an hour for more than a few hours.

☆ Frank (bright red) bleeding any time after the fourth day; but don't worry about an occasional blood-tinged discharge.

☆ Lochia that has a foul odour (it should smell like a normal menstrual discharge).

☆ Large clots in the lochia.

☆ Pain or discomfort in the lower abdominal area, beyond the first few days after delivery.

☆ A temperature of over 100 degrees for more than a day.

Afterpains

'I've been having cramp-like pains in my abdomen, especially when I'm nursing.'

These are probably 'afterpains,' which are believed to be caused by the contractions of the uterus as it makes its normal descent back into the pelvis following birth. The contractions are more likely to be felt by, and be more intense in, women whose uterine musculature is flaccid (lacking in tone) because of previous births or excessive stretching (as with twins).

Afterpains can be more pronounced during nursing, when contraction-stimulating oxytocin is released. Mild analgesics may be prescribed if necessary, but the pain should subside naturally within four to seven days. If analgesics don't relieve the symptoms, or if they persist for more than a week, see your doctor to rule out postpartum infection.

Pain in the Perineal Area

'I didn't have an episiotomy, and I didn't tear. Why am I so sore?'

You can't expect some 7 pounds of baby to pass by the perineum unnoticed. Even if the perineum was left intact during the baby's arrival, the area has still been stretched, bruised, and generally traumatised; and discomfort, ranging from mild to not-so-mild, is the very normal result.

'My episiotomy site is so sore, I'm afraid my stitches are infected. But how can I tell?'

The perineal soreness experienced by all vaginal deliveries is likely to be compounded if the perineum was torn or surgically cut. Like any freshly repaired wound, the site of an episiotomy or laceration will take time to heal – usually 7 to 10 days. Pain alone during this time, unless it is very severe, is not an indication that an infection has developed.

Infection is possible, but very unlikely if good perineal care has been practiced. While you're in the hospital, a midwife will check the perineum at least once daily to be certain that there is no inflammation or other indication of infection. She will also instruct you in postpartum perineal hygiene, which is important in preventing infection not only of the repair site but of the genital tract as well (puerperal fever). For this reason, the same precautions apply for those who were neither torn not had an episiotomy. Follow this 10-day plan for the care of the perineum:

☆ Use a fresh sanitary pad at least every four to six hours. Secure snugly so that it doesn't slide back and forth.

☆ Remove the pad front to back to avoid dragging germs from the rectum to the vagina.

☆ Pour or squirt warm water (or an antiseptic solution, if one was recommended by your doctor) over the perineum after urinating or defecating. Pat dry with gauze pads, or with the paper wipes which may come with hospital-provided sanitary pads, always from front to back.

☆ Keep your hands off the area until healing is complete.

Though discomfort is likely to be greater if you've had a repair (with itchiness around the stitches possibly accompanying soreness), suggestions for relief are usually welcomed by all recently delivered mothers:

☆ Warm salt baths, hot compresses.[1]

☆ Chilled witch hazel on a sterile gauze pad or a glove filled with crushed ice applied to the site.

☆ Local anaesthetics in the form of sprays, creams, or pads; mild pain

---

1. Use a heat lamp only under supervision in the hospital, or at home with instructions from your doctor on how to avoid burns.

relievers may be prescribed by your physician.

☆ Lying on your side; avoiding long periods of standing or sitting, to decrease strain on the area. Sitting on a pillow or inflated tube may help, as may tightening your buttocks before sitting.

☆ Doing Kegel exercises (see pages 166, 323) as frequently as possible after delivery, and right through the postpartum period, to stimulate circulation to the area, which will promote healing and improve muscle tone. (Don't be alarmed if you can't feel yourself doing them; the area will be numb right after delivery. Feeling will return to the perineum gradually over the next few weeks.)

Difficulty With Urination

'It's been several hours since I gave birth, and I haven't been able to urinate yet.'

Difficulty in passing urine during the first 24 postpartum hours is common. Some women feel no urge at all; others feel the urge but are unable to fulfill it. Still others do urinate, but with accompanying pain and burning. There are a host of reasons why bladder function often becomes such an effort after delivery:

☆ The holding capacity of the bladder increases because it suddenly has more room to expand – thus the need for urination may be less frequent.

☆ The bladder may have been trau-matised or bruised during delivery due to pressure created by the foetus, and become temporarily paralysed. Even when it's full, it may not send the necessary signals of urgency.

☆ Drugs or anaesthesia may decrease the sensitivity of the bladder or the alertness of the mother to signals.

☆ Pain in the perineal area may cause reflex spasms in the urethra, making urination difficult. Oedema (swelling) of the perineum may also interfere with urination.

☆ Any number of psychological factors may inhibit urination – fear that voiding may prove painful, lack of privacy, embarrassment or discomfort over using a bedpan or needing assistance at the toilet.

☆ The sensitivity of the site of an epi-siotomy or laceration repair can cause burning and/or pain with uri-nation. (Burning may be alleviated somewhat by standing astride the toilet while urinating so that the flow comes straight down, without touching sore spots.)

As difficult as urination may be after delivery, it's essential that the bladder be emptied within six to eight hours – to avoid urinary tract infec-tion, loss of muscle tone in the bladder from overdistension, and bleeding due to the bladder hindering the proper descent of the uterus. You can expect, therefore, that the mid-wife will ask you frequently after delivery if you've urinated. She may request that you void for the first time

postpartum into a container, so that she can measure your output, and may palpate your bladder to make sure it's not distended.

If you haven't urinated within eight hours or so, your doctors may have you catheterised (a tube is inserted into the urethra) to empty the bladder of urine. You may be able to avoid this with the following:

☆ Take a walk. Getting up from bed and going for a stroll as soon after delivery as you're allowed will help get your bladder (and your bowels) moving.

☆ If you're uncomfortable with an audience, have the midwife wait outside the room while you urinate. She can come back in when you've finished, to give you a demon-stration of perineal hygiene.

☆ If you're too weak to walk to the bathroom and must use a bedpan, ask for privacy; have the midwife warm the pan (if it's metal) and give you warm water to pour over the perineal area (which may stim-ulate the urge); and sit on the pan instead of lying on it.

☆ Warm the area in a salt bath or chill it with ice packs, whichever seems to induce urgency for you.

☆ Turn the water on while you try. Running the water in the sink really does help encourage your own faucet to flow.

After 24 hours, the problem of too little becomes one of too much. Post-partum women begin urinating fre-quently and copiously as the excess body fluids of pregnancy are excret-ed.If urinating is still difficult, or if output is scant during the next few days, it's possible you have a urinary tract infection. The symptoms of simple cystitis (bladder infection) include: pain and/or burning with urination (which continues even after the sensitivity of the episiotomy or laceration repair has lessened); frequency and urgency with little urine passed; and, sometimes, a low-grade fever. Symptoms of a kidney infection are more severe, and may include a fever of 101 to 104 degrees, back pain on one or both sides – usually in addition to the symptoms of cystitis. Your doctor will want to begin antibiotic treatment specific to the infection-causing organism, if infection is confirmed. You can help speed recovery by drinking plenty of extra fluids. (Also see page 180.)

Having a Bowel Movement

'I delivered almost a week ago and I haven't had a bowel movement yet. Although I've felt the urge, I've been too afraid that straining would open my episiotomy.'

The passage of the first bowel movement after childbirth is a milestone in the postpartum period. Every day that precedes it is fraught with increasing emotional and physical discomfort.

Several physiological factors may interfere with the return of normal bowel function after delivery. For one thing, the abdominal muscles that assist in elimination have been stretched during childbirth, making them flaccid and ineffective. For another, the bowel itelf may have been traumatised by delivery, leaving it sluggish. And, of course, it may have been emptied before or during delivery, and probably remained empty because no solid food was taken for the duration of labour.

But perhaps the most potent inhibitors of postpartum bowel activity are psychological: the unfounded fear of splitting open the stitches; the natural embarrassment over the lack of privacy in the hospital; and the pressure to perform, which often makes performance all the more elusive.

Although reregulating your system is rarely effortless, it isn't necessary to suffer endlessly. There are several steps you can take to resolve the problem:

Don't Worry. Nothing keeps you from moving your bowels more effectively than worrying about moving your bowels. Don't worry about opening the stitches – you won't. And don't worry if it takes a few days to get things moving; that's okay, too.

Request Roughage. Select whole grains and fresh fruits and vegetables from the hospital menu, if possible. Supplement the hospital diet, which many patients find constipating, with bowel-stimulating food brought in from outside. Apples, raisins and other dried fruit, nuts, bran muffins, and small boxes of bran cereal will help. Chocolate – so often a gift to hospital patients – will only worsen constipation.

Keep the Liquids Coming. Not only must you compensate for fluids lost during labour and delivery, you must take in additional liquids – especially water and fruit juices – to help soften stool if you're constipated.

Get Off Your Bottom. You won't be running marathons the day after delivery, but you should be able to take short strolls through the corridors. An inactive body encourages inactive bowels. Kegel exercises, which can be practiced in your bed almost immediately after delivery will help tone up not only the perineum, but also the rectum.

Don't Strain. Straining won't break your stitches open, but it can lead to haemorrhoids. If you do have haemorrhoids, you may find relief with salt baths, topical anaesthetics, suppositories, hot or cold compresses.

The first few bowel movements may pass with great discomfort. But as stools soften and you become more regular, the discomfort will ease.

Excessive Perspiration

'I've been waking up at night soaked with perspiration. Is this normal?'

What your doctor probably calls diaphoresis (but is more commonly referred to as perspiration or sweating) is one of the ways your body rids itself of pregnancy-accumulated fluids during the week following delivery. Often perspiration continues to be a problem for several weeks, because of the postpartum hormonal adjustments. Don't worry about it; but do make sure essential fluids are replaced – particularly if you're breast-feeding – by taking extra liquids. An absorbent towel over your pillow may help make you more comfortable if you do most of your perspiring during the night.

As a precaution, it's a good idea to take your temperature, and to report it to your doctor or midwife if it's over 100 degrees.

Adequacy of Your Milk Supply

'It's been two days since I delivered, and nothing comes out of my breasts when I squeeze them, not even colostrum. I'm worried that my baby is starving.'

Not only is your baby not starving, he or she isn't even hungry yet. Babies aren't born with an appetite, or with immediate nutritional needs. And by the time your baby begins to hunger for a breast full of milk (on the third or fourth postpartum day), you will undoubtedly be able to oblige.

Which isn't to say that your breasts are empty now. Colostrum (which provides your baby with enough nourishment and with important antibodies his or her own body can't yet produce, while helping to empty the digestive system of excess mucus and the bowels of meconium) is definitely present in the tiny amounts necessary. (A teaspoon or so is all your baby needs at this point.) But until the third or fourth postpartum day, when your breasts begin to swell and feel full, it's not that easy to express manually.

Even a day-old baby, with no previous experience, is better equipped to extract this premilk than you are.

Engorged Breasts

'My milk finally came in, leaving my breasts swollen to three times their normal size – and so hard, engorged, and painful that I can't bear to put on a bra. Is this what I have to look forward to until I wean my baby?'

If painfully tender, granite-hard breasts, the size of an exotic dancer's, were indeed what mothers had to look forward to for the duration of the breastfeeding experience, most babies would be weaned before they entered their second week of life. The engorgement, caused by the milk's arrival, can make nursing agonising for the mother and, because the nipples are flattened by the swelling, frustrating for the baby. The condition can be aggravated when the initial feeding doesn't begin until 24 to 36 hours after birth, as is common in some hospitals.

Happily, the engorgement and its distressing effects gradually diminish once a well-coordinated milk supply-and-demand system is established – within a matter of days. Nipple soreness, too – which usually peaks at about the 20th feeding – generally disappears rapidly as the nipples toughen up from frequent nursing. Some women, particularly those with fair skin, may also experience nipple cracking and bleeding. This, with proper care, is also only temporary.

Until breastfeeding becomes as gratifying and fulfilling as you had hoped it would be – and, believe it or not, painless – there are some steps you can take to reduce the discomfort and speed the establishment of a good milk supply (see Getting Started Breastfeeding, page 298).

Engorgement if You're Not Breastfeeding

'I'm not nursing. I understand that drying up the milk can be painful.'

Whether you nurse or not, your breasts will become engorged (overfilled) with milk on the third or fourth postpartum day. This can be uncomfortable, even painful. However, it is blessedly temporary.

Some physicians rely on hormones to suppress lactation. But since the drugs sometimes fail to relieve engorgement (and, if they do, it often returns a week or two after the medication is discontinued), most doctors prefer the natural course, letting the body itself take care of suppressing milk production. The breasts are designed to produce milk only as needed. If the milk isn't used, production ceases. Though sporadic leaking may continue for several days, or even weeks, severe engorgement shouldn't last more than 12 to 24 hours. During this time, ice packs and mild pain relievers may be prescribed. Wearing a well fitting, supportive bra is important until your breasts return to normal.

Bonding

'My new son was premature and I won't get to hold him for at least two weeks. Will it be too late for good bonding?'

Bonding, the process of attachment between a mother and her newborn child, has in recent years become a *cause célebre* in childbirth circles. The term originated in the 1970s, when some studies began to show that the separation of an infant from its mother immediately after birth posed a threat both to their lifelong relationship and to the infant's future relationships with others. Some very positive changes in postchildbirth procedure have come about because of this work. Today, many hospitals permit new mothers to hold their babies moments after birth, and to cuddle and nurse them for anywhere from 10 minutes to an hour or more, instead of whisking the newborns off to the nursery the moment the cord is cut.

But as sometimes happens with the popularisation of a good idea, the concept of bonding became misunderstood and abused (one of the doctors who published the first book on the subject now says: 'I wish we'd never written the statement'), with some unfortunate results. Mothers who have surgical deliveries and are unable to see their babies at birth worry that their parent-child relationship will be forever tarnished. The same worry haunts parents whose babies must be in the SCBU for several days or weeks, giving them little bonding opportunity. So frantic have some parents become about the necessity for instant bonding that they are demanding it even at risk to their infants.

Of course, initial bonding in the delivery room is nice. This early meeting of mother and baby gives them a chance to make contact, skin to skin, eye to eye. It's the first step in the development of a lasting parent-child bond. But only the *first* step. And it doesn't have to take place at the moment of birth. It can take place later in a hospital bed, or through the portholes of an incubator, or even weeks later at home. When your parents were born, they probably saw little of their mothers and even less of their fathers until they went home – usually 10 days after birth – and the vast majority of this 'deprived' generation grew up with strong, loving family ties. Mothers who had the chance to bond at birth with one child and not with another usually report no difference in their feelings toward the children. And adoptive parents, who often don't meet their babies until hospital discharge (or even much later) manage to foster strong bonds. Some experts believe, in fact, that bonding doesn't really take place until somewhere in the second half of the baby's first year. Certainly it is a complex process that isn't accomplished in minutes.

It's never too late to tie the bonds that bind. So, instead of wasting energy regretting the time you've lost, prepare to make the most of the lifetime of mothering you have ahead.

'I've been told that bonding brings mother and child closer together, but every time I hold my baby, she seems like a stranger to me.'

Love at first sight is a concept that flourishes in romantic books and movies, but rarely materialises in real life. The kind of love that lasts a lifetime usually requires time, nurturing, and plenty of patience to develop and deepen. And that's as true for the love between a newborn and its parents as it is between a man and a woman.

Physical closeness between mother and child immediately after birth does not guarantee instant emotional closeness. Feelings of affection don't flow as quickly and surely as lochia; those first few postpartum seconds aren't automatically bathed in the glow of maternal love. In fact, the first sensation a woman experiences after birth is far more likely to be relief than love – relief that the baby is normal and, especially if her labour was difficult, that the ordeal is over. It's not at all unusual to see that squalling and unsociable infant as a stranger – with very little connection to the cosy, idealised little foetus you carried for nine months – and to feel little more than neutral toward him or her. One study found that it took an average of over two weeks (and often as long as nine weeks) for mothers to begin having positive feelings toward their newborns.

Just how a woman reacts to her newborn at their first meeting may depend on a variety of factors: the length and intensity of her labour; whether she received tranquillizers and/or anaesthetics during labour, her previous experience (or lack of it) with infants; her feelings about having a child; her relationship with her partner; extraneous worries that may preoccupy her; her general health; and, probably most important of all, her personality. *Your* reaction is normal for *you*.

And as long as you feel an increasing sense of comfort and attachment as the days go by, you can relax. Some of the best relationships get off to the slowest starts. Give yourself and your baby a chance to get to know and appreciate each other, and let the love grow unhurriedly.

If you don't feel a growing closeness after a few weeks, or if you feel anger or antipathy toward your baby, discuss these feelings with your doctor or midwife. It's important to work them out early on, to prevent lasting damage to your relationship.

Rooming-in

'In childbirth class, having the baby room-in with me sounded like heaven. Since I gave birth, it's been more like hell. I can't get the baby to stop crying – yet what kind of mother would I be if I asked the midwife to take her?'

You would be a very human mother. You've just completed the more-than-Herculean task (Hercules couldn't have done it) of giving birth, and are about to embark on an even greater challenge: child rearing. Needing a few days' rest in between is nothing to feel guilty about.

Of course, some women handle rooming-in with ease. They may have had easy deliveries that left them feeling exhilarated instead of exhausted. Or they may have had experience caring for newborns, their own or other people's. For these women, an inconsolable infant at 3 A.M. may not be a joy, but it's not a nightmare, either. For a woman who's been without sleep for 48 hours, however, whose body has been left limp from an enervating labour, and who's never been closer to a baby than a nappy ad, such predawn bouts can leave her wondering tearfully: 'Why did I ever decide to become a mother?'

Playing the martyr can raise motherly resentments against the baby, feelings the baby will be likely to sense. If, instead, the baby is sent back to the nursery between feedings at night, mother and child, both well rested, may have a better chance to get acquainted when morning comes.

Full-time rooming-in is a wonderful new option in family-centred maternity care – but it's not for everyone. You are *not* a failure or a bad mother if you don't enjoy, or feel too tired for, rooming-in. Don't be pushed into it if you don't think you want it; and once you've committed yourself, don't feel you can't change your mind. Partial rooming-in (during the day but not at night) may be a good solution for you. Or you might prefer to get a good night's sleep the first night and start rooming-in on the second.

Be flexible. Be more concerned with the quality of the time you spend with your baby in the hospital than the quantity. Round-the-clock rooming-in will begin soon enough at home. And by then, if you are sensible now, you should be emotionally and physically ready to deal with it.

Going Home

'My labour was almost effortless, and I feel great. Why should I have to stay in the hospital if I have nothing to recover from?'

Chances are *you* don't have to stay in the hospital. Though 10-day hospital stays were once considered a necessary precaution after giving birth, it's now recognised that a woman who's had an uncomplicated delivery really doesn't need any hospitalisation. Your baby, on the other hand, sometimes does. Two or three days of observation is fairly standard, although that standard may be adjusted at the discretion of your doctor or midwife – and often now a doctor or midwife will allow for discharge within 24 hours after birth. The major reason for a delay in discharge is to watch for jaundice (a yellowing of the skin), which develops in more than 50% of newborns within the first 24 to 36 hours after birth. Though jaundice is rarely a major complication, many doctors and midwives prefer to keep the newborn in the hospital an extra day or two, or until it clears up. Others allow for early discharge in mild cases, assuming the infant is otherwise in good health, and providing that the doctor or midwife will be able to see him or her within a few days.

Of course, no one can hold you or your baby hostage in the hospital against your will. You have the right to sign yourself and your baby out of the hospital A.M.A. (against medical advice) at any time – if you take full legal, written responsibility for the consequences. But unless you have a degree in medicine, it would be extremely unwise to play doctor. If either your midwife or obstetrician recommends a prolonged stay, ask for an explanation – but do follow their professional advice. And try to make the best of your longer sojourn, getting as much rest as you can while you still have the chance.

Don't forget it's important to rest postpartum – in the hospital or at home.

Recovery from a Caesarean Section

'How different will my recuperation be from that of a woman with a vaginal delivery?'

Recovery from a caesarean section is similar to recovery from any major abdominal surgery – with a delightful difference: Instead of losing an old gall bladder or appendix, you've gained a brand new baby.

Of course, there's another difference, slightly less delightful. In addition to recovering from surgery, you'll also be recovering from childbirth. Except for a neatly intact perineum, you'll experience all the same postpartum discomforts you would have had if you'd delivered vaginally – afterpains, lochia, breast engorgement, fatigue, hormonal changes, hair loss, excessive perspiration, and the baby blues. (See this chapter and the next for tips on how to deal with all of these.)

As for your surgical recovery, you can expect the following in the recovery room:

A Wearing Off of Anaesthesia.
Until your general anaesthesia wears off, you will be observed carefully in the recovery room. Your memory of this time may later be fuzzy or totally absent. Since everyone responds differently to drugs – and each drug is

different – whether you are clear-headed and alert in a few hours or not for a day or two will depend upon you and upon the medications you were given. If you feel disoriented, or have hallucinations or bad dreams when you awaken, your partner or an understanding midwife can help you get back to reality quickly. You will also stay in the recovery room if you've had a spinal or epidural block. It will take longer for these to wear off – which they usually do from the toes up. You will be encouraged to wiggle your toes and move your feet as soon as you can. If you've had a spinal block, you will have to stay flat on your back for about 8 to 12 hours. You may be allowed to have both your husband and your baby visit with you in the recovery room.

Pain Around Your Incision.
Once the anaesthesia wears off, your wound, like any wound, is going to hurt – though just how much depends on many factors, including your personal pain threshold and how many caesareans you've had. (The first is usually the most uncomfortable.) You will probably be given pain relief medication as needed, which may give you a woozy or drugged feeling. It will also allow you to get some needed sleep. You needn't be concerned if you're nursing; the medication won't get into your colostrum, and by the time your milk comes in, you probably won't need any medication.

Possible Nausea, and Maybe Vomiting.
This doesn't always happen, but if it does, you may be given an anti-emetic preparation to

prevent vomiting. (If you vomit easily, you might want to talk to your doctor about giving you such a medication before the symptoms appear.)

Breathing and Coughing Exercises. These help rid your system of any leftover general anaesthetic, and help to expand your lungs and keep them clear to prevent pneumonia. Such necessary lung calisthenics may be very uncomfortable if you do them correctly. You may be able to minimize this discomfort by 'splinting' your incision with a pillow.

Regular Evaluations of Your Condition. A midwife will check your vital signs (temperature, blood pressure, pulse, respiration), your urinary output and vaginal flow, the dressing on your incision, and the firmness and level of your uterus (as it shrinks in size and makes its way back into the pelvis). She will also check your IV and urinary catheter.

Once you have been moved to your hospital room, you can expect:

Continuing Evaluation of Your Condition. Your vital signs, your urinary output and vaginal flow, your dressing, and your uterus, as well as your IV and catheter (as long as they remain in place) will be checked regularly.

Removal of the Catheter After 24 Hours. Urination may be difficult, so try the tips on page 288. If they don't work, the catheter may be reinserted until you can urinate by yourself.

Afterpains. These start about 12 to 24 hours after delivery. See page 286 for more about these occasional contractions.

Removal of the IV. About 24 hours after surgery, or when your bowels begin to show signs of activity (by producing gas), your IV will be discontinued and you will be allowed some fluids by mouth. Over the next few days, you will probably progress to soft foods, and then to a normal diet. Even if you feel as though you are starving, don't try to circumvent doctor's orders by having someone sneak in a Big Mac. Take it easy getting back to your normal diet. If you are breastfeeding, be sure to get plenty of fluids.

Referred Shoulder Pain. Irritation of the diaphragm following surgery can cause a few hours of sharp shoulder pain. An analgesic may help.

Possible Constipation. It may be a few days until you have a bowel movement, and that's all right. A stool softener may be prescribed to help move things along. Try some of the tips on page 289, but exclude the roughage for the first few days. If you haven't had a movement by the fifth or sixth day, you may be given a laxative, an enema, or a suppository.

Encouragement to Exercise. Before you are out of bed, you will be encouraged to wiggle your toes, flex your calves, bend your feet up at the ankles, push against the end of the bed with your feet, and turn from side to side. You can also try these; (1) Lie flat on your back, bend one knee, then extend the other leg, while tightening your abdomen slightly. Slide the bent leg slowly back down; repeat with the other leg. (2) Lie on your back, knees pulled up, feet flat on the bed, and raise your head for about 30 seconds. (3) On your back, knees bent, tighten your abdomen, and reach with one arm across your body to the other side of the bed, at about waist level. Reverse. These exercises will improve circulation, especially in your legs, and prevent the development of blood clots. (But be prepared for some of these to be quite painful, at least for the first 24 hours or so.)

To Get Up Between 8 and 24 Hours After Surgery.

With the help of the midwife, you'll sit up first, supported by the raised head of the bed. Then, using your hands for support, you will slide your legs over the side of the bed and dangle them for a few minutes. Then, slowly, you'll be helped to step down on the floor, your hands still on the bed. If you feel dizzy (which is normal), sit right back down. Steady yourself for a few more minutes before taking a couple of steps. Those steps may be extremely painful. Stand as straight as you can, though the temptation to hunch over to ease the discomfort may be great. (This difficulty in getting around is temporary; in fact, you may soon find yourself more mobile than the vaginal deliveree next door – and you will certainly have the edge in sitting.)

To Wear Elastic Stockings.

These improve circulation and help prevent blood clots in the legs.

Abdominal Discomfort.

As your digestive tract (temporarily put out of business by surgery) begins to function again, trapped gas can cause considerable pain, especially when it presses against your incision line. The discomfort may be worse when you laugh, cough, or sneeze. Tell the midwife or doctor about your problem and they will suggest some remedies. Narcotics are not usually recommended because they can prolong the difficulties, which ordinarily last just a day or two. You may get a small enema or a suppository to release the gas. Or you may be advised to walk up and down the corridor. Lying on your left side or on your back, your knees drawn up, taking deep breaths while holding your incision, may help. If the pain remains severe, a tube may be inserted in your rectum to help the gas escape.

Time with Your Baby.

You can't lift the baby yet, but you can cuddle and feed him or her. (If you're nursing, place the baby on a pillow over your incision.) Depending on how you feel, and on hospital regulations, you may be able to have modified rooming-in. Some hospitals even allow full rooming-in.

Sponge Baths.

Until the stitches are removed (or absorbed), you probably won't be allowed a real bath or shower.

Removal of Stitches.

If your stitches aren't self-absorbing, they will be removed about five or six days after delivery. And although the procedure isn't very painful, you may find it uncomfortable. When the dressing is off, look at the incision with the midwife or doctor; ask how soon you can expect the area to heal, which changes will be normal, which might require medical care.

You can expect to go home about eight to ten days postpartum.

WHAT IT'S IMPORTANT TO KNOW: GETTING STARTED BREASTFEEDING

Ever since Eve put Cain to suckle for the first time, breastfeeding has been coming naturally to mothers and newborns. Right?

Well, not always – at least not immediately. Though nursing does come naturally, it comes naturally a little later for some mothers and babies than for others. Sometimes there are physical factors which foil those first few attempts; at other times it's just a simple lack of experience on the part of both participants. But whatever might be keeping your baby and your breasts apart, it won't be long before they're in perfect synch – as long as you don't give up first. Some of the most mutually satisfying breast-baby relationships begin with several days of fumbling, of bungled efforts, and of tears on both sides.

Knowing just what to expect and how to deal with setbacks can help ease the mutual adjustment:

☆ Start as soon as possible after birth. Right in the delivery room is best, when that's feasible. (See Breastfeeding Basics, page 300.) But sometimes mother's not in any condition to nurse, sometimes baby isn't – neither of which means they won't be able to start success-

fully later. (That's not to say that if you feel well and the baby does, too, this first nursing experience will necessarily go smoothly. You both have a lot to learn.)

☆ Don't let hospital bureaucracy break your tentative connection with insensitivity, ignorance, and unnecessary rules. Enlist the support of your midwife or doctor in advance to be sure that you will be allowed to nurse in the delivery room if all goes normally. Also, arrange for full or partial rooming-in, or for a demand-feeding schedule (having the nursery bring the baby when he or she is hungry) if the staff will oblige. If the baby is with you all day, this may mean limiting visiting privileges to just your partner, which is probably for the best anyway since it allows the three of you to get to know each other, while maintaining the relaxed atmosphere needed for breastfeeding.

☆ Don't let sleeping babies lie, if it means that they'll sleep through a feeding. If you have rooming-in, you're not likely to have a problem with this. You'll be able to demand-feed the baby when he or she is hungry and let the baby sleep when he or she's sleepy. If you're dependent on the nursery staff to bring the baby – on their schedule, not the baby's – you may find that the allotted feeding period will be up before the baby wakes, and that someone will come to collect him or her unfed. Don't let this happen. If the baby isn't awake on arrival at your room, wake him or her. This sounds crueller than it actually is. Gently set the baby on the bed in a sitting position, one hand holding up the chin, the other supporting the back. Next, bend · the baby forward at the waist. The moment he or she stirs, quickly adopt the nursing position. If your baby is swaddled, loosen the blanket so he or she can be close to you.

☆ Be patient if your baby is still recovering from your labour. If you received anaesthesia or had a prolonged, difficult labour, you can expect your baby to be drowsy and sluggish at the breast for a few days. This is no reflection on you, your breastfeeding ability, or your baby. There's no danger the baby will starve in the meantime, since newborns have little need for nourishment during the first days of life. What they do need, though, is nurturing. Cuddling at the breast is just as important as suckling.

☆ Make sure your baby's appetite and sucking instinct aren't sabotaged between feedings. It's routine in some hospital nurseries to quiet a crying baby between mother's feedings with a bottle of sugar water. This can have a twofold detrimental effect. Firstly, it satisfies the baby's still-delicate appetite for hours. Later, when brought to you for feeding, your baby won't want to nurse, and your breasts won't be stimulated to produce milk – a vicious cycle is begun. Second, because the rubber nipple requires less effort, the baby's sucking reflex becomes lazy. Faced with the greater challenge of tackling the breast, he or she may just give up. Don't let anyone talk to you into the sugar water. Give strict orders through your paediatrician that supplementary feedings are not to be given to your baby in the nursery unless medically necessary.[2]

☆ Don't try to feed a screaming baby. It's hard enough for an inexperienced suckler to find the nipple when calm. When you baby is overexcited, it may be impossible. Rock and soothe him or her before you start nursing.

☆ If you're having trouble establishing breastfeeding, ask for assistance from hospital personnel or from your doctor. If you are lucky, a midwife or nursery nurse will join you at your first baby feeding to provide hands-on instruction, helpful hints and, perhaps, literature. If this is not a policy in your hospital (or you are somehow bypassed), you can find empathy

---

2. You may also want to discuss with your paediatrician the pros and cons of a pacifier being given to your baby in the nursery. On the one hand, it could get him or her hooked on a rubber nipple; on the other, it may be comforting when there's no one to cuddle with in the middle of the night.

Breastfeeding Basics

1. Get into a comfortable position.

2. Use your thumb and index finger to pull the nipple erect.

3. Tilt the nipple slightly upward, toward the roof of he baby's mouth.

4. Bring the nipple toward the baby's cheek so that it brushes the corner of his or her mouth. This will stimulate the rooting reflex (or you can use a spare finger to do this) which makes the baby turn its mouth toward the touch.

5. Repeat steps 3 and 4 several times; the baby should eventually take the nipple in his or her mouth. (Let the baby take the initiative; don't stuff the nipple into an unwilling mouth.)

6. Be sure the areola and the nipple, and not just the nipple, are in the baby's mouth. Sucking on just the nipple won't compress the milk glands and can cause soreness and cracking. Also be sure that it is the nipple that the baby is busily milking. Some infants are eager to suck (even if no milk is forthcoming) and can give you a painful bruise by gumming sensitive breast tissue.

7. Use your finger to press the breast away from the baby's nose to prevent interference with breathing.

8. You can assure yourself that your baby is suckling if there is a strong steady rhythmic motion in his or her cheek.

9. If your baby has finished suckling but is still holding on to the breast, pulling it out abruptly can cause injury to the nipple. Instead, break the suction first by depressing the breast or by putting your finger into the corner of the baby's mouth to admit some air.

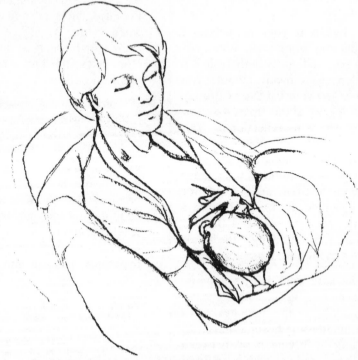

Whatever is comfortable for you and the baby is a good position; prop with pillows as necessary. And be sure not to block the baby's tiny nose with your breast.

and advice by calling your local La Lèche League chapter or NCT branch (page 342).

☆ No matter how frustrating nursing becomes, try to stay calm. Start out as relaxed as you can. Clear out the visitors 15 minutes before feeding time. Then remain cool throughout the feeding period, no matter how badly it's going. Tension not only hampers your ability to give milk, it can cause anxiety in your baby. An infant is extremely sensitive to your moods, and reacts accordingly.

When the Milk Comes in

Just when you and your baby seem to be getting the hang of it, your milk comes in. Up until now, your baby has been getting tiny amounts of colostrum (premilk), and your breasts have been quite comfortable. Then, within a few hours, your breasts become swollen, hard, and painful. Nursing is difficult for the baby and agonising for you.[3] Fortunately, this period of engorgement is brief. While it lasts there are a variety of ways of relieving it and the accompanying discomfort:

☆ Feed more often, for shorter periods – a four-hour schedule can lead to engorgement, and 20-minute feeding periods to sore nipples; both make feeding difficult in the long run for mother and baby. Start off with 5 minutes on each breast, gradually building up to 15 minutes each by the third or fourth day.

☆ Don't be tempted to skip or skimp on a feeding because of pain. The less your baby sucks, the more engorged you will become. Don't favour one breast because it is less sore or because the nipple isn't cracked; the only way to toughen up nipples is to use them. Use both breasts at every feeding, even if only for a few minutes – but nurse from the less sore one first, since the baby will suck more vigorously when hungry. If both nipples are equally sore (or not sore at all), start off the next feeding with the breast you used last.

☆ Use a breast pump on each breast before feeding to lessen the engorgement so that your baby can get a better hold on the nipple, and to get milk flow started. After feeding, empty the second breast if the baby hasn't already done so.

☆ Use ice packs to reduce engorgement. Or a hot shower or hot soaks, if you find them more soothing.

☆ Support is important in a nursing bra, but pressure against your sore and engorged breasts can be painful. Whenever leaking isn't a problem – and especially after feeding – leave the flaps of your nursing bra open.

---

3. A few lucky new mothers don't experience engorgement when their milk comes in, possibly because their babies were vigorous nursers from birth; there is also less engorgement with subsequent babies.

Sore Nipples

Tender nipples sometimes compound

Baby and Breast – A Perfect Feeding Team

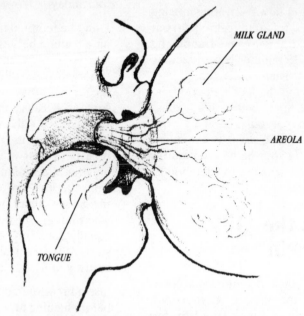

MILK GLAND

AREOLA

TONGUE

Just be sure that the feeding baby has the areola and not just the nipple in his or her mouth. This way the milk can be efficiently and, eventually, painlessly extracted.

the difficulties of early nursing. Most toughen up quickly. But in some women, particularly those who are fair skinned, the nipples become sore and cracked. To relieve the discomfort:

☆ Expose sore or cracked nipples to the air as much as possible.

☆ Let nature – and not the cosmetic companies – take care of your nipples. Nipples are naturally protected and lubricated by sweat glands and skin oils. A commercial preparation should be used only when nipple cracking is severe, and then should be as pure as possible. Unmedicated lanolin is effective; petroleum-based ointments are not. Wash only with water – never with soap, alcohol, tincture of benzoin, or premoistened towelettes – whether your nipples are sore or not: Your baby is already protected from your germs, and the milk itself is clean.

☆ Vary your nursing position so a different part of the nipple will be compressed at each feeding.

☆ Relax for 15 minutes or so before feeding, occasionally with a small glass of wine or beer. Relaxation will enhance the let-down of milk, whereas tension will only hinder it.

Occasional Complications

Once breastfeeding is established, it generally continues uneventfully until weaning. But once in a while, complications occur, among them:

Clogged Milk Ducts. Sometimes a milk duct clogs, causing milk to back up. Since this condition (characterised by a small, red, and tender lump on the breast) can lead to infection, it's important to try to remedy it quickly. The best way to do this is to offer the affected breast first at each feeding, and let your baby empty it as completely as possible. If he or she doesn't do the job, any remaining milk should be expressed by hand or with a breast pump. Keep pressure off the duct by being sure your bra is not too tight, and by varying your nursing positions to put pressure on different ducts. Also, check to see if dried milk is blocking the nipple after nursing. If so, clean it off with sterile cotton dipped in boiled and cooled water. Do not use this time to wean the baby; discontinuing breastfeeding now will only compound your problem.

Breast Infection. A more serious complication of breastfeeding is mastitis, or breast infection, which usually occurs in one or both breasts between the 10th and 28th postpartum day, in about 1% of mothers – usually first-timers. A crack or fissure in the skin of the nipple occurs and allows the passage of germs into the milk ducts.

Symptoms of mastitis are severe soreness, hardness, redness, heat, and swelling of the breast, with generalized chills and a fever of about 101 to 102 degrees. If you develop some of these symptoms, contact your doctor. Prompt medical treatment is necessary, and may include bed rest, antibiotics, pain relievers, and ice or heat applications. During treatment you should continue to breastfeed. Since germs from the baby probably gave you the infection, it won't harm him or her. And emptying the breast will help to prevent clogged milk ducts. Feed first on the infected breast and empty it with a pump if the baby doesn't.

Delay in treating mastitis could lead to the development of a breast abscess, the symptoms of which include: excruciating, throbbing pain; localised swelling, tenderness, and heat in the area of the abscess; and temperature swings between 100 and 103 degrees. Treatment includes antibiotics and, generally, surgical drainage under anaesthesia. Breastfeeding with the affected breast must be halted, and a breast pump should be used regularly to empty it until healing is complete and breastfeeding can be resumed. In the meantime, feeding can continue on the unaffected breast.

Don't let breast and feeding problems with your first baby discourage you from nursing future babies. Engorgement and nipples soreness are far less common with subsequent births.

Breastfeeding Twins

Breastfeeding, like just about every aspect of caring for newborn twins, seems impossible until you get into

Best-Odds Nursing Diet

The levels of protein, fat, and carbohydrates in your breast milk aren't usually affected by the levels of these nutrients in your diet; however, levels of some vitamins are (A and B$_{12}$, for example). But though the quality of your milk isn't always directly related to the quality of your diet, the quantity of milk usually is. Women whose diets are deficient in protein and/or calories, for example, will produce milk of good composition but in smaller amounts. To make good breast milk, and plenty of it, continue taking your pregnancy (or pregnancy/lactation) vitamin-mineral supplement, and adhere closely to the Best-Odds Diet on page 82, with the following modifications:

☆ Increase your caloric intake to about 500 calories per day over your pre-pregnancy requirements. This is flexible, and as during pregnancy, you can let your scale be your guide. If you have a lot of fat stored from pregnancy (or before), you can take fewer calories, as the fat will be burned to produce milk (and you will lose weight). If you are underweight, you will probably need more than 500 additional calories daily (the recommended daily allowance assumes some use of fat stores, which you don't have). No matter what your weight, you may find that you need more calories as the baby grows and demands more milk. Again, you will be able to determine this by checking your scale. If your weight starts dipping below the ideal, increase your daily intake.

☆ Increase your calcium requirement by one serving per day.

☆ Reduce your protein intake by one serving per day.

☆ Drink at least eight glasses of fluids (milk, water, broths or soups, and juices); take more if it's very hot, and if you've been losing a lot through perspiration. (Through it's all right to drink moderate amounts of tea, coffee, and alcoholic beverages, you can't count them in your fluid allowance, since they have a dehydrating effect.) Excess is not best, however; flooding yourself with too much fluid (more than 12 glasses per day) can paradoxically *slow* milk production. Thirst and urinary output can help gauge your needs.

☆ Splurge occasionally. You've served your nine-month sentence of abstinence; you're entitled to your just desserts, at least once in a while. The key is moderation. Small amounts of sugar won't interfere with milk production, but a steady diet of sweets will, by cutting down on your appetite for necessary nutrients. Ditto for other nutritionally superfluous foods, such as potato chips, french fries, white bread; eat them only *after* you've fulfilled your nutritional obligations.

the rhythm of it. Once you have a routine, it is not only possible, but very rewarding. To successfully breastfeed twins, you should:

☆ Fulfill all the dietary recommendations for lactating mothers (see the Best-Odds Nursing Diet), with these additions: take 400 to 500 calories above your prepregnancy needs for *each* baby you are nursing (you may need to increase your caloric intake as the babies grow bigger and hungrier, or decrease it if you supplement nursing with formula and/or solids, or if you have considerable fat reserves you would like to burn);

an additional serving of protein (four total) and an additional serving of calcium (six total) or a calcium supplement.

☆ Drink 8 to 12 cups of fluid a day, but not more, because too much may suppress milk production.

☆ Get as much help as you can with housework, meal preparation, and infant care, to conserve your energy.

☆ Explore the various feeding options: nurse one baby, bottle feed the other; alternate feedings of bottle and breast with each baby; or nurse each separately (which can take 10 hours or more a day just for feeding), or both together. Combining individual and group feedings, and giving each infant one private feeding a day, is a good compromise which encourages mother-baby closeness. Father might give a bottle to the other baby at these feedings. Such relief bottles, given by the father or another helper, can be formula or expressed milk.

☆ Recognise that the twins have different needs, personalities, and nursing patterns, and don't try to treat them identically. Keep records to be sure both are fed at each feeding.

Breastfeeding Advice

There are a number of organisations that can give you support and advice about feeding your baby. Your local community midwife and health visitor are both experienced sources of information on this subject, so do talk to them if you have any queries.

Two national organisations that can help are: The La Lèche League of Great Britain, BM 3424, London WC1V 6XX (01-769 8530). And The National Childbirth Trust, 9 Queensborough Terrace, London W2 (01-221 3833). If you do not have details of your local contact for either of these organisations, call the national office.

16
Postpartum: The First Six Weeks

After your baby is born, you and the baby will either be cared for by the staff on the postnatal ward of your hospital or maternity home, or at home by your community midwife and GP. If you have been in hospital, your local community midwife will visit you at least until the 10th postnatal day, and will care for you in conjunction with your GP.

A health visitor, who will probably have visited you during your pregnancy, will also visit some time in the second week after your baby is born. She or he will keep in touch with you until your child is 5 years old.

WHAT YOU CAN EXPECT AT YOUR SIX-WEEK CHECKUP

All doctors or midwives will schedule the mother for a six- or eight-week postpartum visit.[1] During that visit, you can expect the following to be checked, though the exact content of the visit will vary depending upon your particular needs and your doctor or midwife's style of practice.

☆ Blood pressure

☆ Weight, which should be down by 17 to 20 pounds or more

☆ Shape, size, and location of uterus, to see if it has returned to prepregnant condition and location

1. If you had a caesarean, your physician may also check your incision at about three weeks postpartum.

☆ Condition of cervix, which will be on its way back to its prepregnant state, but will still be somewhat engorged, and the surface possibly eroded

☆ Condition of vagina, which will have contracted and regained much of its muscle tone

☆ The episiotomy or laceration repair site, if any; or, if you had a caesarean delivery, the site of your incision

☆ Your breasts, for any abnormalities

☆ Haemorrhoids or varicose veins, if they developed during pregnancy

☆ Questions or problems you want to discuss – have a list ready

At this visit, the doctor will also discuss with you the method of birth control that you will be using. (See page 318.) If you plan on using a diaphragm and your cervix has recovered sufficiently, you will be fitted for one; if not, you may have to use condoms until you can be fitted. If you're not breastfeeding and plan to take birth control pills, they may be prescribed now.

WHAT YOU MAY BE FEELING

Physically

☆ Continued vaginal discharge (lochia), turned brownish, then yellowish-white

☆ Fatigue

☆ Some pain, discomfort, and numbness in the perineum, if you had a vaginal delivery (especially if you had stitches)

☆ Diminishing incisional pain; continuing numbness, if you had a caesarean delivery (especially if it was your first)

☆ Continued constipation (although this should be easing up)

☆ Gradual flattening of your abdomen as your uterus recedes into the pelvis (but only exercise will bring you back to pre-pregnancy shape)

☆ Gradual loss of weight

☆ Breast discomfort and nipple soreness until breastfeeding is well established

☆ Achiness in arms and neck (from carrying the baby)

☆ Hair loss

Emotionally:

☆ Elation, depression, or swings between the two

☆ A sense of being overwhelmed, a growing feeling of confidence, or swings between the two

☆ Lowered libido, or, occasionally, increased sexual desire

WHAT YOU MAY BE CONCERNED ABOUT

Fever

'I've just returned home from the hospital and I'm running a fever of about 101 degrees. Could it be related to childbirth?'

Thanks to Dr Ignaz Semmelweiss, the chances of a new mother developing childbirth (or puerperal) fever today are extremely slight. It was in 1847 that this young Viennese physician discovered that if birth attendants washed their hands before delivering babies, the risk of childbirth-related infection could be greatly reduced (though at the time, his theory was considered so outlandish that he was driven from his post, ostracized, and later died a broken man). And thanks to Sir Alexander Fleming, the British scientist who developed the first infection-fighting antibiotics, the occasional case that does occur is easily cured.

The most severe cases of infection usually begin within 24 hours of delivery. A fever on the third or fourth day, when you are already at home, could possibly be a sign of postpartum infection – but it could also be caused by a virus or other minor problem. A low-grade fever (of about 100 degrees) can occasionally accompany engorgement when your milk first comes in, or even result from the excitement of coming home with your baby.

In postpartum infection, the symptoms will vary according to the site of origin. A slight fever, vague lower abdominal pain, and perhaps a foul-smelling vaginal discharge characterize endometritis, an infection of the endometrium (the lining of the uterus), vulnerable because of detachment of the placenta. Infection is even more likely to occur here if a fragment of the placenta has been retained. With infection of a laceration to the cervix, vagina, or vulva, there will usually be pain and tenderness in the area; sometimes a foul-smelling, thick discharge; abdominal or flank pain; or difficult urination. In certain types of infection, the fever spikes as high as 105 degrees, and there are chills, headache, malaise. On occasion, there are no obvious symptoms but fever.

Treatment with antibiotics is very effective, but it should begin quickly. Report any fever during the first three postpartum weeks to the doctor – even if it's accompanied by obvious cold or flu symptoms – so that its cause can be diagnosed and any necessary treatment started.

Depression

'I have everything I have always wanted: a wonderful partner, a beautiful new baby – why do I feel so blue?'

Why should roughly one half of all new mothers be so miserable during one of the happiest times of their lives? That's the paradox of postpartum depression, for which experts have yet to provide any definitive explanations or solutions.

Hormones, so often the culprit fingered in the case of a woman's mood swings, may offer some rationale. Levels of oestrogen and progesterone drop precipitously after childbirth and may trigger depression, just as hormonal fluctuations prior to menstruation may do. The fact that sensitivity to hormonal fluctuations varies from woman to woman is believed to explain at least partially why, though all women experience the same shift in hormone levels after delivery, only about 50% suffer from postpartum depression.

But there are a host of other factors that probably contribute to the postpartum blues – which are most common around the third day after delivery, but which can strike at anytime during the first year, and which afflict second-time mothers more often than first-timers.

The Shift from Centre Stage to Backstage.
Your baby is now the star of the show. Visitors would rather run to the nursery than sit at your bedside inquiring after your health. This change in status will accompany you home; the pregnant princess is now the postpartum Cinderella.

Hospitalization.
When you're eager to get home and begin mothering, you may be frustrated by the lack of control you have over your life and your baby's in the hospital.

Going Home.
It's not unusual to feel overwhelmed and overworked by the responsibilities that greet you (particularly if you have other children and no help).

Exhaustion.
Fatigue from a strenuous labour and from too little sleep in the hospital is compounded by the rigours of caring for a newborn, and often leads to the feeling that you aren't equal to the demands of motherhood.

A Sense of Disappointment in the Baby.
He or she's so small, so red, so puffy, so unresponsive – not quite the all-smiles Ivory Snow baby you'd pictured. Resultant guilt adds to depression.

A Sense of Disappointment in the Birth and/or in Yourself.
If unrealistic expectations of an idealized childbirth experience weren't realized, you may feel (unnecessarily) that you're a failure.

A Feeling of Anticlimax.
Childbirth – the big event you'd schooled for and looked forward to – is over.

Feelings of Inadequacy.
A novice mother may wonder, 'Why did I have a baby if I can't take care of it?'

A Sense of Mourning for the Old You.
Your carefree, possibly career-oriented self, has died (at least temporarily) with your baby's birth.

Unhappiness over Your Looks.
Before you were fat and pregnant, now you're just fat. You can't stand wearing maternity clothes, but nothing else fits.

Probably the only good thing that can be said about postpartum depression is that it doesn't last very long – about 48 hours for most women. And though there's no cure other than the passage of time, there are ways of fading those baby blues:

☆ If the blues arrive at the hospital, try to have your partner bring in dinner for the two of you; limit visitors if their chattering grates on your nerves, have more of them if they cheer you up. If it's the hospital that's getting you down, inquire about early discharge. (See Going Home, page 294.)

☆ Fight fatigue by accepting help from others, by being less compulsive about doing things that can wait, by trying to squeeze in a nap or rest period when your baby is sleeping. Use feeding times as rest periods, nursing or bottle-feeding in bed or in a comfortable chair with your feet up.

☆ Follow the Best-Odds Nursing Diet (see page 304) to keep your strength up (minus 500 calories and three calcium servings if you're not breastfeeding). Avoid sugar (especially combined with chocolate), which can act as a depressant.

☆ Unwind with your partner over a cocktail during the baby's evening feeding, but be careful not to overdo – too much can lead to morning-after depression.

☆ Treat yourself to dinner out, if possible. If not, make believe. Order dinner in (or let your partner cook), dress up, create a restaurant ambience with candlelight and soft music, open a bottle of wine. And keep your sense of humour handy, in case the baby decides to interrupt your romantic interlude.

☆ Look good so you'll feel good. Walking around in a robe all day with unkempt hair would depress anyone. Shower before your partner leaves in the morning (or you may not have a chance again); comb your hair; put on makeup if you ordinarily wear it.

☆ Get out of the house. Go for a walk with the baby or, if someone volunteers to stay with him or her, without the baby. Exercise helps chase away the baby blues and will help you get rid of any postpartum flab that might be adding to your depression.

☆ If you think your misery might like some company, get together with any new mothers you know, and share your feelings with them. If you don't have any newly delivered friends, make some. Ask your midwife, health visitor or doctor for names of new mothers in your neighbourhood, or contact women who were in your childbirth class, possibly organizing a weekly afterbirth reunion. Or join a postpartum exercise class. The National Childbirth Trust organizes local coffee mornings or meetings in many areas. Contact your branch through the local telephone directory or the national organisation (see page 342). Mother and toddler groups usually advertise in the child care clinics, and your health visitor will also have a list of these in your area.

☆ If yours is the kind of misery that would rather be by itself, indulge in some solitude. Though depression usually feeds on itself, some experts believe that this is not true of the postpartum variety. If going out with cheerful people, or having cheerful people visit, makes you feel worse – don't do it. Don't, however, leave your partner out in the cold. Communication in the immediate postpartum period is vital for you both. (Partners, too, are susceptible to postpartum depression, and yours may need you as much as you need him.)

Severe postpartum depression, which requires professional therapy, is extremely rare – less than 1 in 1,000. If your depression persists for more than two weeks and is accompanied by sleeplessness, lack of appetite, a feeling of hopelessness and helplessness – even suicidal urges – seek counselling promptly. The Postnatal Illness Association, 7 Gowan Avenue, London SE6, provides information about depression, and offers telephone counselling and support for those who feel that it would help them. There are a number of local self-help groups also being set up, so do ask your health visitor whether there is one in your area. Many National Childbirth Trust branches offer the support of their members and the opportunity for you to meet and talk to someone else who has suffered from postnatal depression.

'I feel terrific, and have since the moment I delivered three weeks ago. Is all this good feeling building up to one terrific case of letdown?'

It's an unfortunate fact that feeling good doesn't get the kind of attention that feeling bad does. There's no shortage of articles in magazines and newspapers, or chapters in books, about the 50% of newly delivered women who suffer from postpartum depression; but there's little or nothing written about the other 50% who feel terrific after giving birth.

Baby blues are common, but they're by no means an absolute requirement of the postpartum period. And there's no reason to believe that you're in for an emotional crash because you've been feeling buoyant. Since the majority of baby blues cases occur within the first postpartum week, it's pretty safe to assume you've escaped them. If you'd like to play it even safer (or if you'd like to prevent a case next pregnancy around), see the tips for fading those baby blues, in the previous section.

Returning to Prepregnancy Weight and Shape

'I knew I wouldn't be ready for a bikini right after delivery, but I still look six months pregnant a week later.'

Though childbearing produces more rapid weight loss than the Scarsdale, Stillman, and Mayo Clinic diets combined (an average of 12 pounds at delivery), most women don't find it quite rapid enough. Particularly after they catch a glimpse of their postpartum silhouettes in the mirror – which can still look distressingly pregnant. But happily, most will be able to pack away their pregnancy jeans within the month.

Of course, how quickly you return to your prepregnant shape and weight will depend on how many pounds and inches you put on during pregnancy. Women who gained 25 pounds or less should be able, without dieting, to shed the weight by the end of the second month. Others will find that delivery won't make thighs and hips thickened by over-indulgence during pregnancy magically disappear. But sticking to the Best-Odds Nursing Diet (see page 304) if they are breastfeeding (or to the Diet minus the 500 extra nursing calories and three of the calcium servings[2] if they are not) should start them on the way to slow, steady weight loss. Non-nursers can, after the first six weeks, go on a good, well-balanced reducing diet, such as Weight Watchers. Nursing mothers with considerable amounts of excess body fat can cut their caloric intake somewhat without cutting into milk production and also lose weight. They will usually take off any remaining excess poundage when they wean their babies.

Unlike weight loss, getting back into shape is a problem even for those women who didn't gain excess weight. No one comes out of the delivery room looking much slimmer than when they went in. Part of the reason for that protruding postpartum abdomen is the still-enlarged uterus, which will be reduced to prepregnancy size by the end of six weeks, reducing your abdomen in the process. (You can follow the progress of your uterus by asking your doctor or midwife to show you how to palpate it in your abdomen. When you can no longer feel it, it has slipped back into the pelvis.) Another reason for your bloated belly is leftover fluids, 5 pounds or so of which will flush out within a few days. But the rest of the problem is stretched out abdominal muscles and skin, which will sag for a lifetime unless a concerted exercise effort is made. (See Getting Back into Shape, page 321.)

Breast Milk

'Does everything I eat, drink, or take get into my breast milk? Could any of it harm my baby?'

Feeding your baby outside the womb doesn't demand quite as Spartan an existence as feeding him or her inside did. But as long as you're breastfeeding, a certain amount of restraint in what goes into you will ensure that everything that goes into your baby is safe.

The basic fat-protein-carbohydrate composition of human milk isn't dependent on what a mother eats. If a mother doesn't eat enough calories and protein to produce milk, her body's stores will be tapped and the baby will be fed – until the stores run out. Some vitamin deficiencies in the mother's diet will, however, affect the vitamin content of her breast milk. So will excesses of some vitamins. A wide variety of substances, from medications to seasonings, can also show up in milk, with varying results.

To keep breast milk safe and healthful:

---

2. Though you won't need the calories and other nutrients of milk after pregnancy and/or lactation, it is now recommended that *all* women take a calcium supplement to bring their daily intake to 1,200 mg.

☆ Follow the Best-Odds Nursing Diet (page 304).

☆ Avoid foods to which your baby seems sensitive. Garlic, onion, cabbage, and chocolate are common offenders, causing bothersome gas in some, though by no means all, babies. Infants with discriminating palates may also be displeased by the taste a strong seasoning may impart.

☆ Take a vitamin supplement especially formulated for pregnant and/or lactating mothers. Do not take any other vitamins without the advice of your physician.

☆ Do not smoke. Many of the toxic substances in tobacco enter the bloodstream, and eventually your milk. (Besides, smoking near the baby can cause respiratory problems for him or her and may even be associated with sudden infant death syndrome, or cot death.)

☆ Do not take any medications or recreational drugs (other than moderate quantities of alcohol) without consulting your physician. Most drugs pass into the breast milk, and even in small doses can be harmful to a tiny infant. (Particularly dangerous are: antithyroid, antihypertensive, anticancer drugs; penicillin;[3] narcotic drugs, including heroin, methadone, and prescription painkillers, marijuana and cocaine; tranquillizers, barbiturates and sedatives; lithium; hormones, such as birth control pills; radioactive iodine; bromides.) Often, safe substitutes can be found for a medication you must take; or perhaps a particular medication can be discontinued for the duration of nursing. It's a matter of weighing risks and benefits. (Do make sure that any doctor who prescribes a medication for you is aware that you are breastfeeding.)

☆ Drink alcoholic beverages only in moderation. More than two drinks can make your baby drowsy and depress his or her nervous system.

☆ Restrict your intake of caffeine. One cup of coffee or tea a day probably won't affect your baby. Six cups could make him or her jittery.

☆ Don't take laxatives (Some of them will have a laxative effect on your baby); increase your fibre intake instead.

☆ Take aspirin or aspirin substitutes only with your practitioner's approval, but don't take more than the recommended dose, and don't take the drugs frequently.

☆ Avoid excessive amounts of chemicals in the foods you eat. An occasional diet soda won't hurt, but frequent use of saccharine or aspartame isn't a good idea. Read labels to steer clear of foods composed largely of synthetic chemicals – the possible effect of which are unknown.

☆ Minimize the incidental pesticides in your diet. A certain amount of pesticide residue in your diet (from produce, for example), and thus in

3. Exposure to penicillin at this early age could lead to a baby developing a sensitivity or allergy, to the drug.

your milk, is inevitable – and not proven to be harmful to a nursing infant. But though hysteria about breast milk contamination is unwarranted, it's prudent to keep your baby's exposure to pesticides from affected foods as low as you can without giving up eating. Scrub vegetable and fruit skins with detergent and water; eat low-fat milk products, lean meats, whitemeat poultry with the skin removed, and limited amounts of organ meats. (The pesticides ingested by animals are stored in fat and skin.)

☆ Avoid eating freshwater fish, which might be contaminated. (The same rules for safe fish and seafood consumption that apply to pregnant women apply to lactating women; see pages 122–123.)

Long-Term Caesarean

'I am just now going home, a week after a caesarean. What can I expect?'

A Need for Plenty of Help. Paid help is best for the first week, but if that's not possible, ask your husband, mother, or another relative to lend a hand. It's best not to do any lifting (including the baby), or any housework, at least for the first week. If you must lift the baby, lift from waist level, so you use your arms, not your abdomen. Bend at the knees, not at the waist.

Little or No Pain. But if you do hurt, a mild pain reliever will help.

Don't take medication, however, if you are breastfeeding, unless approved by your doctor.

Progressive Improvement. The scar will be sore and sensitive for a few weeks, but will improve steadily. A light dressing may protect it from irritation. Wearing loose clothing will be more comfortable. Occasional pulling, twitching, and other brief pains in the region of the scar are a normal part of healing and will eventually subside. Itchiness may follow. The numbness of the abdomen around the scar will last longer, possibly several months. Lumpiness in the scar tissue will probably diminish (unless you tend to get that kind of scar), and the scar may turn pink or purple before it finally fades.

If pain becomes persistent, if the area around the incision turns an angry red, or if a brown, grey, green, or yellow discharge oozes from the wound, call your doctor. The incision may have become infected. (A small amount of clear fluid discharge may be normal, but report it to your physician anyway.)

To Wait at Least Four Weeks Before Resuming Sexual Intercourse. Depending on how your incision is healing and when your cervix returns to normal, your doctor may recommend that you wait anywhere from four to six weeks for actual intercourse (though other kinds of lovemaking are certainly permissible). See page 317 for tips on making postpartum intercourse more successful. Also see Postpartum Contraception, page 318. You are, incidentally, much more likely to find early postpartum intercourse comfortable than are women who delivered vaginally.

To Be Able to Start Exercising Once You Are Free of Pain. Since the muscle tone of your perineum probably hasn't been compromised, you may not need to do Kegel exercises. Concentrate instead on those that tighten the abdominal muscles. (See Getting Back into Shape, page 321.) Make 'slow and steady' your motto, get into the programme gradually and continue it daily. Expect it to take several months before you're back to your old self.

Resuming Sexual Relations

'My doctor says I have to wait six weeks before having sex. Friends say that isn't necessary.'

It's fairly safe to assume that your doctor is more familiar with your medical condition than your friends are. And his or her restriction is probably based on what's best for you, taking into consideration the kind of labour and delivery you had, whether or not you had an episiotomy or laceration, and the speed of healing and recovery. Some doctors, of course, apply the six-week rule routinely to all their postpartum patients, regardless of condition. If you think that's the case with your doctor, and you're feeling up to making love, ask if he or she will consider bending the rule for you. This will be possible only if your cervix has healed and the lochia has stopped. And, for your own comfort,

you probably will also want to wait until intercourse no longer causes pain in your perineal area.

Should your plea be denied, however, it's wise to follow your doctor's orders. Waiting the full six weeks can't hurt (at least not physically), while not waiting might.

Lack of Interest in Making Love

'Ever since the baby was born I just don't feel very interested in sex.'

Sex takes energy, concentration, and time – all of which are in particularly short supply in the lives of new parents. Your libido – and your husband's – must regularly compete with sleepless nights, exhausting days, dirty nappies, and an endlessly demanding baby. Your body is still recuperating from the trauma of childbearing; your hormones are readjusting. Fears (of pain, of doing some damage internally, of not being the same, of becoming pregnant again too soon) may plague you. If you are breastfeeding, you may unconsciously be letting it satisfy your sexual needs. Or making love may stimulate uncomfortable leakage of milk. All in all, it's not surprising – and perfectly normal – if your sexual appetite, no matter how voracious it once was, is temporarily suppressed. (On the other hand, some women have strong sexual drives now, particularly in the immediate postpartum period, when there is engorgement of the genital region).

If your problem is lack of interest, there are many ways to make making love good again. Which ones will work for you will depend on you, your husband, and on your problems.

Make Time Your Ally. It takes at least six weeks for your body to heal, and sometimes much longer – especially if you had a difficult delivery or a caesarean. Your hormonal balance won't be back to normal until you start menstruating, which, if you are breastfeeding, may not be for many months. Don't feel obligated to make love because the doctor's given you the go-ahead, if it doesn't feel good, emotionally or physically. And when you do, start slowly, possibly with cuddling and petting but no penetration.

Don't Be Discouraged by Pain. Many women are surprised and disheartened to find that postpartum intercourse can really hurt. If you've had an episiotomy or a laceration, there may be discomfort (ranging from slight to severe) for weeks, even months, after the stitches have healed. You may also have pain with intercourse, although possibly less, if you delivered with the perineum intact – and even if you've had a caesarean. Until the pain disappears, you can minimize it in the ways described in Easing Back into Sex, page 317.

Find Alternative Means of Gratification. If intercourse isn't pleasurable yet, seek sexual satisfaction through mutual masturbation. Or, if you're both too pooped to pop, find pleasure in just being together. There's absolutely nothing wrong (and everything right) about lying in bed together, cuddling, kissing, and swapping baby stories.

Keep Your Expectations Realistic. Don't insist on simultaneous orgasms the first time you make love after delivery. Some usually orgasmic women don't have orgasms at all for several weeks, or even longer. With love and patience, sex will eventually be as satisfying as ever – or more so.

Readjust Your Sex Life to Dovetail with Your Life with the Baby. When your companionable two becomes a crowded three, you can no longer make love when and where you want to. Instead you'll have to either grab it when you can (if the baby is napping at 3 o'clock on Saturday afternoon, drop everything) or make a point of planning ahead. Don't feel that unspontaneous sex can't be fun. Instead, think of the advance planning as giving you the opportunity to look forward to making love (the baby will be asleep at 8 – can't wait!). Accept interruptions with a sense of humour, and try to start again where you left off as soon as possible. And, should sex turn out to be less frequent than before, strive for quality, not quantity.

Don't Be a Perfectionist. A lot of postpartum exhaustion is natural; learning to become parents is certainly taxing. But some of it is unnecessary, often due to trying to do too much too soon. Pack away your white gloves and forgo the dusting sometimes. Use frozen vegetables instead of fresh. Cut some dispensable corners, so that you occasionally have energy left for loving.

Communicate. A really good sexual relationship must be built on trust, understanding, and communication.

Easing Back into Sex

Lubricate. Lowered hormone levels during the postpartum period (which may not rise in the nursing mother until her baby is either partially or totally weaned) can make the vagina uncomfortably dry. Use a lubricating cream, like K-Y Jelly, until your own natural secretions return.

Medicate, If Necessary. Your practitioner may prescribe an oestrogen cream to lessen pain and tenderness.

Inebriate. Don't get drunk, of course (since too much alcohol can interfere with sexual enjoyment and performance), but do enjoy a glass of wine with your husband before making love, to help both of you relax physically and emotionally. It will also numb some of your pain, lessen the fear of it in you, and the fear of causing it in him.

Vary Positions. Side-to-side or woman-on-top positions allow more control of penetration and less pressure on the episiotomy site. Experiment to find what works best for you.

If, for instance, you're too wrapped up in motherhood one night to feel sexy, don't beg off with a headache. Be honest. A husband who's been included in parenting since conception is most likely to understand. If intercourse is painful, don't be a martyr. Explain to your spouse what hurts, what feels good, what you'd rather put off until another time.

Don't Worry. Despite what you may be feeling now, you will live to love again, with as much passion and pleasure as ever. (And because shared parenthood can often bring couples closer together, you may find the flame not only rekindled, but burning brighter than before.) Worry now can only put an unnecessary damper on your sexual relationship.

Becoming Pregnant Again

'I thought that breastfeeding was a form of birth control. Now I hear you can get pregnant while nursing, even before you start menstruating again.'

How completely you can rely on nursing as a means of birth control depends on how completely devastated you would be if you became pregnant again now. If you're like most brand-new patients, tummy-to-tummy pregnancies just months apart are not your idea of perfect family planning. And if that is indeed the case, breastfeeding by itself shouldn't be relied on for contraception.

It's true that women who nurse, on the average, resume normal menstrual cycles later than those who don't. Menstruation usually begins in non-lactating mothers somewhere between four and eight weeks after delivery, whereas in lactating women the average is somewhere between three and four months. As usual, however, averages are deceptive. Nursing women have been known to begin menstruating as early as 6 weeks and as late as 18 months postpartum. The problem is, there's no sure way to predict when you will again begin menstruating, though several variables influence the timing. For example, frequency of feeding (more than three times a day seems to suppress ovulation better), duration of breastfeeding (the longer you feed, the greater the delay in ovulation), and whether or not feedings are being supplemented (your baby's taking bottles, solids, even water, can interfere with the ovulation-suppressing effect of breastfeeding).

Why worry about birth control before that first menstrual period? Because the point at which you ovulate for the first time after delivery is as unpredictable as when you menstruate. Some women have a sterile first period; that is, they don't ovulate during that cycle. Others ovulate before the period, and therefore can go from pregnancy to pregnancy without ever having had a menstrual period. Since you don't know which will come first, the period or the egg, caution in the form of contraception is highly advisable.

Postpartum Contraception

Oral Contraceptives. The Pill is the most effective, and most popular, form of birth control – but it also presents many health risks, particularly for women over 35. Though it causes unpleasant side effects in some women, it is convenient (if one remembers to take it as prescribed) and doesn't interfere with intercourse. It is not usually prescribed during the first six weeks of lactation, because it can interfere with the production of milk. But because the effects of the hormones on a suckling infant aren't known, it is probably unwise to take birth control pills at all while breastfeeding. The Pill is also contraindicated if you have a history of coronary artery, gall bladder, or liver disease; diabetes; high blood pressure; thrombosis; epilepsy; menstrual irregularity; diagnosed or suspected cancer of the reproductive organs; or if you smoke. If you are interested in using oral contraceptives, discuss their possible side effects and risks with your doctor, and weigh them against the benefits before having it prescribed. Also ask that the type of oral contraceptive prescribed be the one that is most appropriate for your individual needs.

Diaphragm. The diaphragm, a dome-shaped rubber cap that fits over the cervix, is an effective birth control method when used properly with a spermicidal gel. It is also safe and without any side effects, and in no way affects lactation. But it must be prescribed and fitted by a medical professional. *It is very important to be refitted after childbirth*, as the size and shape of the cervix may have changed. The diaphragm has the disadvantages of having to be inserted before each intercourse and of having to be left in for six to eight hours afterward.

The IUD. This intrauterine device (it is not strictly speaking a contraceptive, since it interferes with implantation rather than conception) has lost some favour in recent years because of the associated risks of infection and ectopic pregnancy. Since these conditions could cause infertility, many women who want to have more children prefer not to use the IUD. Its use is not recommended for women who are exposed to multiple partners or for those with a history of PID (pelvic inflammatory disease or infection), those with known or suspected uterine or cervical malignancy or premalignancy, with menstrual or other bleeding irregularities, or with a susceptibility to infection. The main advantage of the IUD is that after your doctor inserts it, you can forget about it for at least a year (often more, depending on the type of device), except to check periodically for the string attached to it. The IUD also has no effect on lactation, nor does it affect the feeding infant.

Rhythm Method. This approach, which depends on knowing exactly when you ovulate and avoiding intercourse at that time, is impossible to use during lactation. It is the least effective of the various popular methods, though when based on a combination of steadfast timing, temperature taking, and vaginal mucus samples, it has only about a 24% failure rate.[4] It is completely harmless, except for the risk of pregnancy, and has the additional advantage for some religious groups of being morally acceptable.

The Sponge. The most recent addition to the birth control arsenal, the sponge, like the diaphragm, is a barrier method of contraception, one that blocks the entrance to the cervix. It appears to be less effective that the diaphragm or condom (studies have been done on relatively small numbers of women so far) and its safety is still under question because it contains chemicals that can cause cancer in animals, and because it's been linked tentatively to cases of toxic shock syndrome. The sponge is relatively easy to use (you insert it yourself, like a diaphragm), allows for greater spontaneity (it provides protection for 24 hours after insertion and allows for unlimited sexual activity during that time), is available without a prescription, and is not believed to have any effect on the nursing infant. The contraceptive sponge should not be used in the postpartum period (or directly after a miscarriage or abortion), however, without a physician's approval.

Condom. Very effective if used conscientiously (but somewhat less foolproof than the Pill), the condom (or rubber) is totally harmless. Its effectiveness is enhanced if it is used with a spermicidal foam or jelly. It has the advantages of not requiring a doctor's prescription, of being easily available and easy to carry. It in no way interferes with breastfeeding. Some find, however, that because it must be put on before intercourse (and not until erection), it interferes with spontaneity. Others claim it reduces sensation. Care should be taken when sheathing the penis to leave a small reservoir at the tip of the condom to hold the semen. The penis should be withdrawn before the erection is totally lost and while the condom is held on. The use of lubricated condoms or of a separate lubricating cream will help make insertion more comfortable when the vagina is dry after pregnancy.

---

4. This rate is for the typical user. The theoretical rate is much lower, possibly 5%.

Surgical Sterilization. Tubal ligation for women and vasectomy for men must be considered permanent, though occasionally it is possible to reverse them. They are also increasingly safe and virtually foolproof, though you do hear an occasional story of failure.[5] Sterilization is the frequent choice of couples who feel their family units are complete. Sterilization in women is often performed immediately after delivery.

Of course, accidents can happen. Medical science has yet to develop a method of contraception (with the possible exception of sterilization) that is 100% effective. So even if you've been using contraception – and especially if you haven't been – pregnancy is still a possibility. Unfortunately, the first symptom of pregnancy you would ordinarily look for (absence of menstruation) will not be apparent if you've been breastfeeding and not menstruating. But because of hormonal changes (there are different sets of hormones in operation during pregnancy and lactation), your milk supply will diminish noticeably soon after the new pregnancy is established. You might, in addition, experience any or all of the other symptoms of pregnancy. (See Signs of Pregnancy, page 24.) Of course, if you do have any suspicion that you might be pregnant, the best thing to do is to visit your practitioner as soon as possible. Because it is virtually impossible to do a good job of nourishing both a breastfed infant and a

developing foetus at the same time, it is highly inadvisable to continue nursing during a new pregnancy.

Hair Loss
'My hair seems to be falling out suddenly.'

Don't order a hairpiece. Hair fall is normal, and will stop well in advance of baldness. Ordinarily, the average head sheds 100 hairs a day, which are being continually replaced. During pregnancy (as when you're taking oral contraceptives), the change in hormone levels keeps those hairs from falling out. But the reprieve is only temporary. Those hairs are destined to go, and they will – within three to six months of delivery (or after you stop taking the pill).

Taking Baths
'I seem to be getting a lot of contradictory advice about whether or not baths are all right in the postpartum period. Are they?'

At one time, new mothers weren't permitted to set a foot in a bath until at least one month after delivery, because of fear of infection from the bath water. Today, because it's known that still bath water does not enter the vagina, infection from bathing is no longer considered a threat. Some doctors, in fact, recommend baths in the hospital (when a bath is available) because they believe bathing removes lochia from the perineum – and from between the folds of the labia – more efficiently than showering. In addition, the warm

---

5. This isn't generally a failure of the method, but due to a slip-up in the surgery, or carelessness on the part of a man who fails to use other birth control methods until all viable sperm have been ejaculated.

water is comforting to the episiotomy site, relieves soreness and oedema in the area, and soothes haemorrhoids.

Still, your doctor may prefer you to hold off on bathing until you are home, or even later. If you're anxious to bathe (especially if you have no shower at home), discuss the issue with him or her. You may be able to get a dispensation.

If you do bathe during the first week or two following delivery, be sure the bath is scrubbed meticulously before it's filled. (But be sure you're not the one who does the scrubbing.) And get help getting into and out of the bath during the first few postpartum days, when you're still likely to be shaky.

Exhaustion

'It's nearly two months since I had the baby, but I feel more tired than ever. Could I be ill?'

Many a new mother has dragged herself into her doctor's surgery and complained of overwhelming chronic fatigue – convinced that she's fallen victim to some fatal malady. The nearly invariable diagnosis? A classic case of motherhood.

Rare is the mother who escapes this maternal fatigue syndrome, characterized by tiredness that never seems to ease up and an almost total lack of energy. And it's not surprising. There's no other job as emotionally and physically taxing as that of being a mother. The strain and pressures are not, as in most other jobs, limited to eight hours a day or five days a week. (And mothers don't get lunch hours or coffee breaks, either.) Motherhood for first-timers also adds the stress inherent in any new job: there's always something new to learn, mistakes to be made, problems to solve. If all this isn't enough to produce symptoms, add the energy that goes into breastfeeding, the strength sapped by toting around a rapidly growing infant and accompanying paraphernalia, and night after night of broken sleep.

Check with your doctor to be sure there is no physical cause for your exhaustion. If you get a clean bill of health, be assured that time, experience, and your baby sleeping through the night will gradually help relieve much of your fatigue. And once your body adjusts to the new demands, your energy level should pick up a bit, too. In the meantime, try the tips for relieving postpartum depression (page 308), which is closely tied to fatigue.

WHAT IT'S IMPORTANT TO KNOW: GETTING BACK INTO SHAPE

It's one thing to look six months pregnant when you *are* six months pregnant, and quite another to look it when you've already delivered. Yet most women can expect to be wheeled out of the delivery room not much trimmer than when they were wheeled in – with a little bundle in their arms and several still around their middles. As for the pencil-thin skirts optimistically packed for the going-home trip, they're likely to stay packed, with maternity jeans the depressing substitute.

How soon after you become a new mother will you stop looking like a mother-to-be? With active exercise, that old prepregnancy figure (or a newly slender one) is only a couple of months away.

'Who needs exercise?' you may wonder. 'I've been in perpetual motion since I got home from the hospital. Doesn't that count?'

Unfortunately, not much. Exhausting as it is, that kind of general activity won't tighten up the perineal and abdominal muscles that have been left saggy by pregnancy. Only an exercise programme will.

You can start a postpartum exercise programme as early as 24 hours after delivery. But be careful not to overdo it. The following is geared for women who've had uncomplicated vaginal deliveries. If you've had a surgical or a traumatic one, check with your doctor before beginning.

Ground Rules

☆ Always start each session with the least strenuous exercise, as a warm-up.

☆ Keep your exercise sessions brief and frequent, rather than doing one long session a day (this tones muscles better).

☆ If you have the time and really enjoy exercise, take a class for new mothers or buy a postpartum exercise book and develop an extensive programme. If that prospect is unappealing, doing just a few simple routines regularly can also get you back into shape, especially if you gear them directly to problem areas, such as abdomen, thighs, buttocks, and so on.

☆ Do exercises slowly, and don't do a rapid series of repetitions with inadequate recovery time between each.

☆ Rest briefly between exercises (the muscle buildup occurs then, not while you are in motion).

☆ Don't do more than recommended, even if you feel you can.

☆ Quit before you feel tired: If you overdo it, you usually won't feel it until the next day – by which time you may be unable to exercise at all.

☆ Don't let mothering stop you from mothering yourself – your baby will love lying on your chest as you exercise.

☆ Do not do knee-chest exercises, full sit-ups, or double leg lifts during the six-week postpartum period.

All the following exercises are done in the basic position, though Kegels can be done in any comfortable position. The early exercises can be done in bed; the others are best done on a harder surface, such as the floor. (An exercise mat is a good investment because the baby can try his or her first tentative crawls on it later.)

Phase One: 24 Hours After Delivery

Kegel Exercises. You can begin these immediately after delivery, though you won't be able to feel yourself doing them at first. (See page 167 for directions.) This exercise can also be performed in bed. Or while you're urinating – contract to stop, then relax to release the flow of urine. Repeat several times. As the muscles regain tone, you will be able to allow just a few drops of urine to pass between repetitions.

Deep Diaphragmatic Breathing. In the basic position, place your hands on your abdomen so you can feel it rise as you inhale slowly through your nose; tighten the abdominal muscles as you exhale slowly through your mouth. Start with just two or three deep breaths at a time to prevent hyperventilating. (Signs that you've overdone it are dizziness or faintness, tingling, or blurred vision. See page 266 for dealing with hyperventilation.)

Phase Two: Three Days After Delivery

Three days after you deliver, you can begin doing more serious exercises. But only if you are sure that the pair of vertical muscles of your abdominal wall (called the recti abdominis) have not separated during pregnancy. Fairly common, especially in women who have had several children, this separation (or diastasis) will get worse if you do anything even mildly strenuous before it heals. Ask your midwife or doctor about the condition of these muscles, or examine them yourself this way: As you lie in the basic position, raise your head slightly with your arms extended; then feel for a soft lump below your navel. Such a lump indicates a separation.

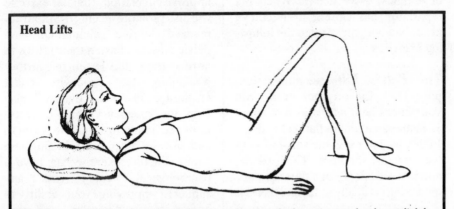

Head Lifts

Assume the basic position (see page 167). Take a deep breath, then raise your head very slightly, exhaling as you do. Lower your head slowly, and inhale. Raise your head a little more each day, gradually working up to lifting your shoulders slightly off the floor. Don't try full sit-ups for at least three or four weeks – and then only if you have always had very good abdominal muscle tone.

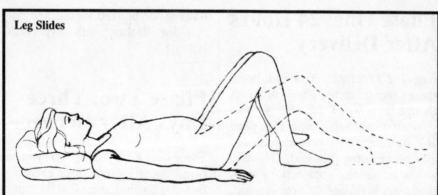

Leg Slides

Assume the basic position (see page 167). Slowly extend both legs until they are flat on the floor. Slide your right foot, sole flat on the floor, back toward your buttocks. Keep the small of your back against the floor. Slide your leg back down. Repeat with your left foot. Start with three or four slides per side, and increase gradually until you can do a dozen or more comfortably. After three weeks, move to a modified leg lift (lifting one leg at a time slightly off the floor and lowering it again very slowly), if it is comfortable.

You can help correct a diastasis, if you have one, with this exercise: Assume the basic position, inhale. Now cross your hands over your abdomen, using your fingers to draw the sides of your abdominal muscles together as you breathe out while raising your head slowly. Inhale as you lower your head slowly. Repeat 3 or 4 times, twice a day. When the separation has closed, or if you've never had one, move on to the following exercises.

The Pelvic Tilt (see illustration, page 168). Lie on your back, with your knees bent and your feet about 12 inches apart, soles flat on the floor. Inhale as you press the small of your back against the floor. Then exhale, and relax. Repeat 3 or 4 times to start; increasing gradually to 12, and then 24.

A postpartum exercise programme will do more than flatten your tummy and tighten your perineum. The perineal exercises will help you avoid stress incontinence (difficulty holding urine), a dropping (prolapse) of pelvic organs, and sexual difficulties. Abdominal exercises will reduce the risk of backache, varicose veins, leg cramps, oedema, and the formation of clots in veins (thrombi), as well as improve circulation. Regular exercise will also promote healing of your traumatized uterine, abdominal, and pelvic muscles, hasten their return to normal tone, and lessen the further weakening that inactivity could encourage. Planned activity will also help the pregnancy- and delivery-loosened joints to return to normal, and prevent further weakening and strain. Finally, exercise can have a psychological benefit (ask any runner), improving your ability to handle stress and to relax – and minimizing the chance of postpartum blues.

17
Fathers Are Expectant, Too

Mothers- and fathers-to-be today share not only the joys of pregnancy, childbirth, and childbearing, but the worries as well; and the chances are good that there is considerable overlap in what concerns each member of your expectant (or newly delivered) team. Yet fathers are entitled to a few worries of their own – and to some very special reassurance, not only during the pregnancy and the birth, but in the postpartum period as well.

And so this chapter – dedicated to the equal, but often neglected, partner-in-reproduction. But it isn't intended for fathers' eyes only – any more than the rest of the book is intended only for mothers'. An expectant mother can gain some valuable insights into what her husband is feeling, fearing, and hoping by reading this chapter; an expectant father can gain a better understanding of the physical and emotional changes his wife will undergo during pregnancy, and after, by reading the rest of the book (while also better preparing himself for his own role in the unfolding drama).

WHAT YOU MAY BE CONCERNED ABOUT

Feeling Left Out

'So much attention has been focused on my partner since she became pregnant that I hardly feel I have anything to do with it.'

In generations past, the father's involvement in the reproductive process ended once his sperm had fertilized his partner's ovum. Fathers watched pregnancy from afar, and childbirth not at all.

Great strides have undeniably been made in the past decade for father's rights. But social re-education hasn't changed the fact that pregnancy takes place within a woman's body. Or the fact that some fathers are lost in what is still largely a woman's shuffle. Or that they end up feeling forgotten, left out – even jealous of their partners.

Sometimes the woman is unwittingly responsible, sometimes the man is. Either way, it's vital that the father's feelings are resolved before resentment grows and is allowed to spoil what should be one of the most wonderful experiences of *both* parents' lives. The best way to accomplish this is for you to get involved in as many aspects of your partner's pregnancy as you can:

See an Obstetrician (or Midwife). Your partner's – as often as she does, if possible. Most doctors or midwives will allow the husband to attend the monthly appointment, and many will encourage him to do so. If your schedule won't permit a monthly visit, perhaps you can arrange to attend the landmark appointments – when the heartbeat will first be heard, for instance. Also try to schedule antenatal tests when you'll be able to be there.

Act Pregnant. You don't have to show up for work in maternity clothes or start drinking a quart of milk a day. But you can do your partner's pregnancy exercise routine with her; give up junk food for nine months; quit smoking, if you're a smoker. And when someone offers you a drink, tell them, 'No thanks, we're pregnant.'

Get an Education. Even Oxford Ph.D.s have a lot to learn when it comes to pregnancy and childbirth.

Read as many books and articles as you can. Attend childbirth classes with your partner. Talk to friends who've been through it recently.

Shop for a Layette. And a crib, and a pram. Help your partner decorate the nursery. In general, become active in picking out, planning, and preparing for the baby's arrival.

Talk It Out. Your partner may be leaving you out unintentionally – she may not even be aware that you'd like to be more involved. It's very likely that she'd be as happy to make you a part of her pregnancy as you would to be a part of it.

Fear of Sex

'Even though the doctor has assured us that sex is safe throughout pregnancy, I often have trouble following through for fear of hurting my partner or the baby.'

Never is sex more a mind-over-matter situation – for both partners – than during pregnancy. This is true particularly as gestation advances and the mind (and libido) must confront a very sizable matter: the expanding pregnant belly and its precious contents.

Fortunately, you can put your mind to rest and enjoy the matter. As vulnerable as mother and baby may seem to an anxious father contemplating intercourse, in a normally progressing low-risk pregnancy, neither one is. (There are a few caveats, particularly in the last two months, detailed in Making Love During Pregnancy, page 145.)

Not only can making love to your partner not do her any harm (assuming the caveats are observed), but because pregnancy is a time for emotional and physical closeness, it can do her a world of good. And as for your baby, though basically oblivious to the whole event, he or she may be pacified by the gentle rocking motion of intercoure and of contracting uterus during orgasm.

Impatience With Your Wife's Mood Swings

'I know it's my partner's hormonal changes that are making her so weepy and volatile. But I don't know how much longer I can be patient.'

If patience is a virtue, you're going to have to be very virtuous for the rest of your partner's pregnancy. Although the stabilization of hormone levels by the fourth month eases the pronounced premenstrual-like weepiness and moodiness of early pregnancy, the stresses of being pregnant continue. And many women continue to be subject to sudden bursts of emotion and attacks of vulnerability right up to delivery. It doubtless won't be easy, and at times you may find it close to impossible. But there's also little doubt that your efforts will pay off. Touchiness met with understanding will dissipate faster than touchiness met with anger and frustration; shoulders offered to your partner for a 15-minute cry won't have to carry around the weight of her unvented anxiety for days at a time.

Try to keep in mind that pregnancy is *not* a permanent condition, and that the changes in your partner's emotional status are as transient as the changes in her figure.

Sympathy Symptoms

'If it's my partner who's pregnant, why am I having morning sickness?'

You may well be among the estimated 11% to 65% (depending on the study) of expectant fathers who suffer from the couvade syndrome during their partners' pregnancies. The symptoms of couvade (which comes from the French for 'to hatch') most often appear in the third month and again at delivery, and can mimic in a man virtually all the normal symptoms of pregnancy in a woman – including nausea and vomiting, abdominal pain, appetite changes, weight gain, food cravings, constipation, leg cramps, dizziness, fatigue, and mood swings.

Many theories have been suggested to explain couvade – all, some, or none of which may be appropriate to you: sympathy for and identification with the pregnant woman; jealously over being left out, and a resultant desire for attention; guilt over being responsible for putting the woman in such an uncomfortable situation; stress from living with a woman who's become irritable, moody, and possibly off-limits sexually; and anxiety over the impending addition to the family.

Of course your symptoms could also indicate illness, so it's a good idea to see a doctor. But should an examination show no physical cause, couvade is a likely diagnosis. The cause, if you can identify it, may be a clue to the cure. For instance, if the cause is jealousy, becoming more involved in your partner's pregnancy may relieve your morning sickness. Or if it's anxiety over handling a newborn for the first time, taking a course in infant care, reading a copy of Dr. Spock, or even spending some time with a friend's baby might prove helpful.

Even if you can't put your finger on any one cause for your symptoms, talking out all your feelings about pregnancy, childbirth, and parenthood with your partner may alleviate your sympathy pains. So might discussing them with other expectant parents in your childbirth class. Should none of this help, be assured that your reactions are normal, and that all symptoms which don't go away during pregnancy will disappear soon after delivery.

Equally normal, of course, is the father who doesn't have a sick day during his partner's pregnancy. Not suffering from morning sickness or not putting on weight doesn't mean an expectant father doesn't empathise and identify with his partner.

Anxiety Over Your Partner's Health

'I know pregnancy and childbirth are safe today, yet I still can't stop worrying that something will happen to my partner.'

There's something undeniably vulnerable about a pregnant woman – and something very natural about your desire, as a loving partner, to want to protect your partner from any possible harm. But you can relax. Your partner is in virtually no danger. Women very, very rarely die as a result of pregnancy or childbirth anymore – and the vast majority of those who do are from crowded inner cities or remote rural areas and haven't had the benefits of prenatal care or adequate nourishment. (See page 82.)

But even though pregnancy doesn't pose a serious physical threat to your partner, you can still help make it an even safer and more comfortable experience for her; by making sure she gets the best medical care possible and that she eats the best possible diet; by letting her get extra rest while you do the laundry, make dinner, or clean the house; and by giving her the kind of emotional support she can't get from any other source (no matter how far obstetrical science advances, pregnant women will always be *emotionally* vulnerable).

Anxiety Over the Baby's Health

'I'm so afraid that something will be wrong with the baby, I can't even sleep at night.'

Mothers-to-be by no means hold a corner on the worry market. And like almost every expectant mother, virtually every expectant father worries about his unborn baby's healthy and well-being. Happily, nearly all worry is needless. The odds that your baby will be born both alive and completely normal are overwhelming – far better than in previous generations.

Of course, even the most reassuring statistics probably won't be able to banish all your worries; only the birth of a healthy baby will. But sharing your fears with your partner, and letting her share hers with you, may serve to unburden you both and will make the waiting – and sleeping – a little easier.

Your Partner's Looks

'As petty as this might seem, I'm afraid my partner's going to get fat and flabby with pregnancy, and stay that way afterward.'

If it were in your partner's obstetrical interest to gain 50 pounds with pregnancy, you (and the countless other expectant fathers who share your 'petty' concern) would have no option, of course, but to accept fat and flab as the price of a healthy baby. But though such calories-are-no-object weight gains are the current vogue, they just aren't medically justifiable – and can, in fact, lead to unnecessary complications during both pregnancy and delivery. A moderate, steady, carefully monitored weight increase of between 20 and 30 pounds, gained through a diet of highly nutritious food and no junk food, gives your baby the best odds for healthy development and safe delivery – and your partner the speediest return to slenderness after childbirth. (See the Best-Odds Diet. page 82; Weight Gain, page 128).

Sticking to a rigid diet even for two weeks isn't easy. Sticking to one for nine months can be close to impossible, unless the dieter has the support, understanding, and assistance of those close to her. In the case of your partner that's you. Not only do many partners fail to provide their partner, with that help, they may unwittingly sabotage their efforts. Men have probably done more to undermine their partners diets than all the chocolate manufacturers put together – either by bringing temptation into the house, ordering it in restaurants, or even offering it directly to their partners 'Come on – one bite won't hurt!').

With the following tips, you'll be able to become your partner's best ally in her campaign to gain weight moderately and eat sensibly during pregnancy – while protecting your own selfish interests (a thin partner):

Lead Your Partner Not into Temptation. If you must indulge in dietary indiscretion, do so out of your home and away from your partner. You can't expect her to live happily on broiled meats, steamed vegetables, and fresh fruit while you gorge on burgers, fries, and ice cream beside her.

Practice What You Preach to Her. What's good for the goose and the gosling is good for the gander, too. Your staying close to the Best-Odds Diet (recognising that you don't need all that protein or calcium) will not only support your wife, but will improve your health as well.

Don't Be Too Preachy. If she slips, nagging will only help her to fall faster and farther. Remind, don't remonstrate. Prod her conscience, don't try to become it. Signal her quietly when in public, rather than making a pointed announcement to all within earshot about her ordering her chicken breaded and fried. Most important, do it with a sense of humour and a lot of love.

Accentuate the Positive. Nothing will undermine her willpower like a faltering ego. So make a point of building her up, admiring her new pregnant shape, commenting often on how pregnancy becomes her.

Exercise with Her. It's much more fun for two to tango – or to follow a pregnancy exercise programme. Proper exercise during pregnancy is important not only for keeping your partner (and you) trim, but also for getting her in good shape for labour and delivery.

Falling Apart During Labour

'I'm afraid I'll faint or become ill during the delivery.'

Few fathers enter the delivery room without fear. Even obstetricians who've assisted at births of thousands of other people's babies can experience a sudden loss of self-confidence when confronted with their own baby's delivery.

Yet very few of these fears – of freezing, falling apart, fainting, or becoming sick to the stomach while watching the delivery – are ever realised. And though being prepared for the birth (by taking childbirth education classes, for instance) generally makes the experience more satisfying, even most unprepared fathers come through labour and delivery better than they'd thought they would. One study of fathers who attended their babies' births with no previous preparation found that though 70% expected that the delivery would be a frightening, unpleasant, and negative experience, all described it afterwards in highly positive terms.

But like anything new and unfamiliar, childbirth becomes less frightening and intimidating if you know what to expect. So become an expert on the subject. Read the entire chapter on labour and delivery, beginning on page 243. Attend childbirth education classes, watching the labour and delivery films with your eyes open. Visit the hospital ahead of time so that you'll be acquainted with the technology that's used in labour and delivery rooms. Talk to friends who have recently gone through the experience. You will probably find they had the same anxieties beforehand but came through feeling terrific.

Though it's important to get an education, it's also important to remember that childbirth isn't the final exam in your childbirth education course. Don't feel that you must perform perfectly (as some women feel obligated to) at the delivery. Nurses and doctors won't be evaluating your every move or comparing you to the man next door. More important, neither will your partner. She won't care if you forget every coaching technique you learned in class. Your being beside her, holding her hand, urging her on, giving her the comfort of a familiar face and touch, will do her more good than having Drs. Lamaze, Bradley and Dick-Reade themselves at her bedside.

'I would really rather not be at the birth, but I feel pressured to be there.'

Just because it's currently de rigueur in the birthing business for fathers to attend births doesn't mean it's mandatory. Studies have shown that fathers who attend births don't have more meaningful relationships with their offspring than fathers who don't attend; just as fathers who bond with their babies immediately after birth don't seem automatically to become better, more loving fathers. What's important is that you do what's right for you and your partner. If it doesn't feel right for you to attend the delivery, for whatever reason, you would probably do more harm than good to all concerned by being there. Ignore those who try to pressure you into a decision that would be wrong for you. Remember, more generations of fathers *haven't* seen their babies born than *have* with no ill effects.

However, that's not to say that attending the birth of your child is not a worthwhile experience, or one you should abandon without careful consideration. Though it's important that you not let anyone else make up your mind for you, it's equally important that you not make up – and close – your mind until the last minute. Go through all the preparations: accompany your partner on her prenatal visits, take childbirth classes, do

extensive reading. Many once-hesitant fathers find that familiarity with labour and delivery breeds a new perspective, which allows them to feel comfortable enough with childbirth to attend and participate fully.

Others, however, still end up deciding that being at the birth would be counterproductive for themselves and their spouses. Still others decide to give labour a try but find, sometime before or during delivery, that they'd rather step outside. All should feel free to follow their instincts, with the reassurance that doing so won't reflect in any way on their capacity for fathering.

'My partner is having a planned caesarean. Hospital regulations won't allow me to be there, and I'm afraid that our new family won't get off to the best start.'

If you made the decision to be at the birth only to discover that the decision wasn't yours to make (as in the case of a caesarean, in a hospital that doesn't permit partners to attend), don't give up without a civilized fight. Discuss your feelings with the obstetrician and ask him or her for the reasons you are to be excluded. As with all aspects of preparing for childbirth, it is important to be flexible. (It may help to remind them that a majority of hospitals now allow fathers to be present at non-emergency surgical deliveries.) If your campaign is unsuccessful (or if a hasty delivery precludes your presence), you have every right to be disappointed. But you have no right to let that disappointment taint the joy that should surround the birth of your child. Your not being at the birth can threaten your relationship with your baby only if you let it, by harbouring feelings of guilt, resentment, or frustration.

Bonding

'Because my baby was delivered by emergency caesarean and I wasn't allowed to be with her, I didn't hold the baby for 24 hours and I'm afraid I didn't bond with him.'

Until this decade, few fathers ever witnessed the birth of their children, and since the word 'bonding' originated only in the 1970s, none were ever even aware of the possibility of bonding with their offspring. But such a lack of enlightenment didn't stop generations of loving father-son and father-daughter relationships from developing. Conversely, every father who attends his child's birth and is allowed to bond with him or her isn't automatically guaranteed a lifetime of closeness with his offspring.

Being with your partner during delivery is ideal, and being deprived of that opportunity is reason for disappointment – particularly if you spent months training together for childbirth. But it's no reason for a less than fulfilling relationship with your baby. What really bonds you with your baby is daily loving contact – changing nappies giving baths, feeding, cuddling, lullabying. He or she will never know that you didn't share in the moment of birth, but your child will know if you aren't there when he or she needs you from then on.

Exclusion During Breastfeeding

'My partner is breastfeeding our baby. There's a closeness between them that I can't seem to share, and I feel left out.'

There are certain immutable biological aspects of parenting that exclude the father: he can't be pregnant, he can't labour and deliver, and he can't breastfeed. But, as millions of new fathers discover each year, a man's natural physical limitations don't have to relegate him to spectator status. You can share in nearly all the joys, expectations, trials, and tribulations of your partner's pregnancy, labour, and delivery – from the first kick to the last push – as an active, supportive participant. And though you'll never be able to put your baby to the breast (at least not with the kind of results the baby's looking for), you *can* share in the feeding process:

Be Your Baby's Supplementary Feeder. There's more than one way to feed a baby. And though you can't breastfeed, you can be the one to give any supplementary bottles. Not only will it give your partner a break (whether in the middle of the night or in the middle of dinner), it will give you opportunities for closeness with your baby. Don't waste the opportunity by propping the bottle up to the baby's mouth. Strike a nursing position, with the bottle where your partner's breast would be and your baby snuggled close to you.

Don't Sleep Through the Night Until Your Baby Does. Sharing in the joys of feeding also means sharing in the sleepless nights. Even if you're not giving supplementary bottles, you can become a part of night-time feeding rituals. You can be the one to take the baby out of the crib, do any necessary nappy changing, and put him or her back to bed once he or she has fallen asleep again.

Watch in Wonder, and Appreciate. There can be enormous satisfaction in simply watching the miracle of breastfeeding – as there is in watching the miracle of birth. Instead of feeling left out, feel privileged to be a witness to the love that passes between your partner and your baby as they nurse.

Participate in All Other Daily Rituals. Nursing is the *only* daily chore limited to mothers. And chances are that if you make at least one other chore your responsibility (and as many as possible), you'll be too busy to be jealous.

Feeling Unsexy After Delivery

'The delivery was absolutely miraculous to watch. But seeing our baby come out of my partner's vagina seems to have turned me off sexually.'

Human sexual response, compared to that of other animals, is extremely delicate. It's at the mercy not only of the body but of the mind as well. And the mind can, at times, play merciless havoc with it. One of those times, as you probably already know, is during pregnancy. Another, as you seem to

be discovering, is during the postpartum period.

It's very possible that the cause of your sudden sexual ambivalence has nothing to do with having seen your baby delivered. Most brand new fathers find both the spirit and the flesh somewhat less willing after delivery (although there's nothing abnormal about those who don't), for many very understandable reasons: fatigue, especially if the baby still isn't sleeping through the night; uneasiness about having a third person in your home; fear that he or she will awake crying at the first caress (particularly if the baby is sharing your room); concern that you may hurt your partner by having intercourse before her body is thoroughly healed; and finally, a general physical and mental preoccupation with your newborn, which sensibly concentrates your energies where they are most needed at this stage of your lives.

In other words, it's probably just as well that you aren't feeling sexually motivated, particularly if your partner (like many women in the immediate postpartum period) isn't feeling emotionally or physically up to it either. Just how long it will take for your interest, and hers, to return is impossible to predict. As with all matters sexual, there is a wide range of what is 'normal.' For some couples, the urge will precede even the doctor's go-ahead at six weeks. For others, six months can pass before l'amour and le bébé begin to coexist harmoniously in the same home. (Some women find desire lacking until they stop breastfeeding.)

Some fathers, even if they've been prepared for the childbirth experience, do come out of it feeling that their 'territory' has been 'violated,' that the special place that had been meant for loving has suddenly taken on a practical purpose. But as the days pass, that feeling usually does too. The father begins to realise that the vagina has two functions, equally important and miraculous. Neither excludes the other, and in fact they are very much interconnected. He also comes to recognise that the vagina is a vehicle for childbirth only briefly, while it is a source of pleasure for himself and his wife for a lifetime.

If the sexual urge doesn't return and its absence begins to cause tension, professional counselling is probably needed.

'Before the baby, my partner's breasts were a centre of sexual pleasure – for both of us. Now that she's breastfeeding, they seem too functional to be sexy.'

Like the vagina, breasts were designed to serve both a practical and a sexual purpose (which, from a stric-tly procreative standpoint, is also practical). And though these purposes aren't mutually exclusive in the long run, they can conflict tempora-rily during lactation.

Some couples find breastfeeding a sexual turn-on. Others, for aesthetic reasons (leaking milk, for instance) or because they feel uncomfortable about using the baby's source of nour-ishment for their sexual pleasure, find it a very definite turn-off.

Whatever turns you on – or off – is what is normal for you. If you feel that your partner's breasts are too func-tional to be sexy now, don't try to force yourself to feel otherwise. Leave them out of sexual foreplay for now, with the reassurance that you will feel differently once the baby has been weaned. Be sure, however, to be open and honest with your wife; taking a sudden unexplained hands-off approach to her breasts could leave her feeling unappealing. Be careful, also, not to harbour any resentment against the baby for using 'your' breasts; try to think of nursing as a temporary 'loan' instead.

18
Preparing for the Next Baby

In the best of all possible worlds, we would be able to plan life to our precise specifications. In the real world, where most of us live, the best-laid plans often often give way to the unexpected twists and turns of fate, over which we have precious little control – leaving us to accept, and to make the best of, what comes our way.

In the best of all possible pregnancies, we would know in advance when we would conceive and could make all the changes and adjustments in our lifestyle to help ensure our baby the best of all possible odds of being born alive and well. Such advance planning is a rare luxury, which many women (because of menstrual irregularity and/or the frailities of contraception) may never indulge in. And as has been stressed throughout this book, what a woman does before she realises she's pregnant (a few drinks, a few dietary indiscretions, a dental x-ray) does little to affect her baby's odds. Few women act pregnant from

the moment of conception, and yet the vast majority give birth to normal, healthy babies.

But it would be remiss not to outline a plan for the best of all possible pregnancies – simply because the possibility does, for many women, exist. The plan is appropriate whether you're already in the process of trying to conceive or if you're thinking ahead. Although it's never too late to start taking care of your body, it's also never too early. And, in fact, your good prepregnancy care will benefit not only your own children but your children's children. Act now, and:

Get a Thorough Physical. Both you and your partner should see your family doctor. An exam will pick up any potential problems that need to be corrected beforehand, or that will need to be monitored during pregnancy. Update your immunisations; especially be sure you're immune to rubella. Also take care of allergy shots, minor elective surgery, and anything else medical – major or minor – that you've been putting off. (If you start allergy desensitisation now, you will probably be able to continue once you conceive.)

See Your Dentist. Make an appointment for a thorough examination and cleaning. Have any necessary work, including x-rays, fillings, dental or periodontal surgery completed now.

Consider Your Choices in Childbirth and Have a Prepregnancy Consultation. Consider what choices are available (see page 28), and ask about the alternatives on offer in your locality. It is easier to make these decisions before you are pregnant.

Make an appointment to see your GP, and have a discussion about your planned pregnancy. She or he will give you advice about nutrition and any tests or consultations that may be relevant to your situation.

You could also contact Foresight (see page 342), and have a look at their literature. If they have a clinic in your area, you could make an appointment for a consultation on preconceptual care for both of you.

Have Genetic Screening. If either of you has any genetic problem in your personal or family history, see a genetic counsellor.

Evaluate Your Birth Control Method. If you are using a method of birth control that might prsent some risk (however slight) to a future pregnancy, change it before you start trying to conceive. Birth control pills

should be discontinued several months before conception if possible, to allow your reproductive system to go through at least two normal cycles before you start making babies. The IUD should be removed before you begin trying. Since the risks of spermicides are as yet unclear, playing it extra safe means discontinuing their use (alone or with a diaphragm) one month to six weeks before you want to become pregnant. The birth control method to switch to for the interim: the condom (used with care, as described on page 319).

Improve Your Diet. Start eliminating junk food and refined sugars from your diet, and increase whole grains and fibre. Since it's best to embark on your pregnancy as close to normal weight as possible, try to get there before conceiving. Add or cut calories as necessary. (Use the Best-Odds Diet, page 82, for a good basic food plan; but you will only need 2 calcium and 2 protein servings daily until you conceive.) Don't go on a crash diet.

Improve Your Partner's Diet. The better your partner's nutrition, the healthier his sperm. His diet should mirror your prepregnancy diet, with caloric intake adjusted to accommodate his weight and activity.

Take a Vitamin-Mineral Supplement Formulated for Pregnancy. Studies show that certain birth defects may be avoided by taking a supplement prior to conception. In addition, the supplement will ensure that you will be getting necessary vitamins, particularly folic acid, and minerals, particularly iron, when you conceive.

Shape Up. An exercise programme will tone and strengthen your muscles in preparation for the challenging tasks of carrying and delivering your baby-to-be. It will also help you take off excess weight.

Avoid Unnecessary X-Rays and Chemical Exposure. Some (though far from all) kinds of exposure can be harmful to your husband's sperm or your ova before conception, and later to a developing embryo or foetus. Avoid potentially hazardous exposure on the job. If you're trying to conceive you may have already succeeded. Inform doctors who are treating you, or x-ray technicians taking x-rays, that you might be pregnant, and do not permit unneeded x-rays (see page 69). Don't inhale directly fumes from such materials as paints, insecticides, and cleaning products (see pages 73–75).

Cut Back on Caffeine. Moderating (and gradually cutting out, if possible) your intake of coffee, tea, and colas now will spare you the symptoms of withdrawal once you're pregnant. That means no more than two cups a day total of coffee, strong tea, or soft drinks containing caffeine before you conceive, and preferably none afterwards (see page 67).

Cut Down on Alcohol Consumption. Even a daily cocktail or glass of wine will not be harmful in your pregnancy-preparation phase, but

avoid heavy drinking. Once you start trying to conceive, stop drinking altogether (see page 62).

Give Up Smoking. Not only you: Recent studies indicate it would also be a good idea for your partner to give up, if he's a smoker. (See page 66 for tips on how to quit.)

Avoid Marijuana and Other 'Recreational' Drugs. These can interfere with conception, and their effects on the foetus range from unknown to serious (see page 65).

Limit Prescription and Over-the-Counter Drugs. Discuss your plans with a doctor to see if any medication you are taking regularly may present a problem should you conceive. Are there alternatives? Can the dose be reduced? Avoid taking any non-prescription drugs without medical advice once you start trying to conceive.

Check for Immunity to Toxoplasmosis (if you have a cat or eat raw meat regularly). If you are immune, you needn't worry about this problem during pregnancy; if you're not, check your cat for the disease (have him treated if he has it), and stop eating raw or rare meats. (See page 69.)

Relax. This is perhaps the most important of all. Getting tense and uptight about conception could prevent you from conceiving at all.

Appendix

COMMON TESTS DURING PREGNANCY[1]

TEST AND WHEN PERFORMED	PROCEDURE	REASON
Blood type; first visit, unless already known from previous pregnancy or test for Rh antibodies if indicated	Examination of blood drawn from your arm.	To determine blood and Rh type in case blood transfusion is needed at some point, and to be prepared for the possibility of Rh incompatibility (see page 46).
URINALYSIS 1. Sugar (glucose) in the urine; at each visit	A specially treated stick, dipped in a specimen of your urine, shows presence of sugar.	While an occasional increase in sugar is normal in pregnancy (see page 138), persistent high levels could indicate hyperglycaemia; further tests will determine if gestational diabetes is present, requiring special diet and care.
2. Albumin (protein) in the urine; at each visit	A special strip, dipped in a urine specimen, shows presence of albumin.	High albumin levels could be related to toxaemia; if routine test shows increase, a 24-hour test may be ordered.
3. bacteria in urine; first visit	Urine specimen is examined in lab.	Bacteria in urine could indicate susceptibility to infection; treatment may be initiated.

1. Your doctor may omit some of these tests or add others, depending upon your condition and his or her professional opinion.

Blood pressure; at each visit	Blood pressure is measured with cuff and stethoscope, or with an electronic device.	A sudden rise in your normal blood pressure of more than 30 points in the upper (systolic) range, or 15 in the lower (diastolic) range, could be warning of complication such as pre-eclampsia (see pages 136, 181).
Haematocrit or haemoglobin; first visit and often fourth month (repeated if values are low or anaemia diagnosed)	Blood drawn from arm or from pricked finger is examined.	Values are slightly reduced in pregnancy, but abnormally low levels require further examination and treatment.
Rubella titre; first visit	Blood drawn from your arm is tested for levels of antibodies to rubella.	High levels of rubella (German measles) antibodies in your blood indicate you are immune to the disease; if you aren't immune, it is important to avoid exposure to the disease – particularly in your first trimester – and to be immunized before another pregnancy.
VDRL; first visit, sometimes again in seventh or eighth month	Blood drawn from your arm is tested.	To test for syphilis infection; if present, prompt treatment will prevent harm to foetus.
Cervical smear; first visit	Cervical secretions are collected on a swab and examined under a microscope for abnormal cells.	Abnormal cells could, on further study, turn out to be malignant, requiring treatment.

NON-DRUG TREATMENTS DURING PREGNANCY

SYMPTOMS	TREATMENT	PROCEDURE
Colds, flu, diarrhoea	Additional fluids	Drink water, juices, soups – 8 ounces every hour. (With diarrhoea, use only diluted juices, avoid prune.) Take milk as recommended by your doctor.

Itchy abdomen	Baking soda and ammonia paste	Mix ½ cup of baking soda with household ammonia to make a paste (avoid breathing the fumes); apply to itchy skin. Check persistent skin problems with your doctor/midwife.
Swelling or bruises	Cold compresses	Dip a soft cloth in a basin of ice cubes and cold water, wring it out, and place over affected site. Re-chill when cold dissipates.
Sinusitis	Alternating hot and cold compresses	Dip a cloth in hot water, wring it out, and apply to the painful area until the heat dissipates; then apply a cold compress until the cold dissipates. Continue alternating heat and cold for 10 minutes 4 times daily.
Sore or scratchy throat	Gargle	Dissolve 1 teaspoon of salt in 8 ounces of hot water (the temperature of tea) and gargle for 5 minutes; repeat as needed, or every 2 hours.
Itchy eye discharge	Warm soaks	Use a cloth dipped in warm, not hot, water (test it for comfort on your inner forearm), and apply to your eye for 5 or 10 minutes every 3 hours.
Colds, coughs	Inhalation	Use a standard humidifier or vapourizer or a steaming kettle; prepare a tent by draping a sheet over an open umbrella which is resting on a chair back; place humidifier on chair. Spend 15 minutes 3 or 4 times a day under tent; extend the time to 30 minutes, if you aren't too uncomfortable. (Don't stay under tent if you become uncomfortably warm.) Keep the humidifier near your bedside when you are sleeping or resting.

Tight muscles, tension, bruises and sprains	Hot soaks	Twenty-four hours after injury, wet a towel thoroughly in warm water, then wring it out and place it over the affected site, covering all completely with a plastic bag. Place a heating pad over the plastic at a medium setting, being careful that it does not touch the wet towel. Apply for 1 hour twice daily.
Bruises, sprains, burns, on the hands, wrists, and feet	Cold soaks	Place a tray or two of ice cubes in a basin (a styrofoam bucket or cooler is best) of cold water and immerse the injured part for 30 minutes; repeat 30 minutes later if necessary.
Haemorrhoids	Sitz bath	Sit in enough hot water (hotter than your usual bath) to cover the affected area for 20 to 30 minutes. 2 or 3 times daily.
Fever	Sponge bath	Using a plastic sheet to catch drips, apply cold towels soaked in 2 quarts of water, 1 pint of rubbing alcohol, and 1 quart of ice cubes to the skin. Stop if shivering begins.
	Cooling bath	Use a tub of tepid water and gradually cool it by adding ice cubes – stopping immediately if shivering begins.

Useful Addresses

AA (Alcoholics Anonymous),
11 Redcliffe Gardens,
London SW10 9BG

AIMS (Association for Improvement
in Maternity Services),
Elizabeth Key,
Goose Green Barn, Much Hoole,
Preston, Lancashire

ARM (Association of Radical Midwives),
c/o 8A The Drive,
Wimbledon, London SW20

The Birth Centre,
c/o Roz Clacton,
16 Simpson Street, London SW11

Compassionate Friends,
5 Lower Clifton Hill,
Clifton, Bristol BS8 1BT

Foresight,
The Old Vicarage, Church Lane,
Witley, Godalming,
Surrey GU8 5PM

Foundation for the Study of Infant
Deaths,
5th Floor, 4/5 Grosvenor Place,
London SW1X 7HD

La Lèche League of Great Britain,
BM 3424, London WC1V 6XX

Maternity Alliance,
309 Kentish Town Road,
London NW5 2TJ

Miscarriage Association,
2 West Vale, Thornhill Road,
Dewsbury, West Yorkshire

National Childbirth Trust,
9 Queensborough Terrace,
London W2

National Society for Non Smokers,
Latimer House, 40/48 Hanson Street,
London W1P 7DE

The Post Natal Illness Association,
7 Gowan Avenue, London SE6

Release,
1 Elgin Avenue, London W9 3PR

Stillbirth and Perinatal Death
Association,
37 Christchurch Hill, London NW3
1JY

Society to Support Home Confinements,
c/o Margaret Whyte,
17 Laburnam Avenue, Durham

Templegarth Trust,
82 Tinkle Street, Grimoldy,
Louth, Lincolnshire LN11 8TF

Toxaemia Society,
88 Plumberow Lee, Chapel North,
Basildon, Essex

Turning Point
9–12 Long Lane, London EC1

The Women's Health Information
Centre,
52 Featherstone Street, London EC1

Index